CONVERSATIONS IN MEDICINE

The Story of Twentieth-Century
American Medicine
in the Words of Those Who Created It

ALLEN B. WEISSE, M.D.

D0914872

New York University Press
New York *and* London
1984

Library of Congress Cataloging in Publication Data

Weisse, Allen B.
Conversations in medicine.

Includes index.
1. Medicine—United States—History—20th century—
Addresses, essays, lectures. 2. Medical scientists—
United States—Interviews. I. Title. [DNLM: 1. History
of Medicine, 20th century—United States—Personal narra-
tives. 2. Physicians—United States—Personal narratives.
WZ70 AA1 W43c]
R152.W45 1984   610'.973   83-27228
ISBN 0-8147-9200-6 (alk. paper)

*Clothbound editions of New York University Press books are Smyth-sewn and
printed on permanent and durable acid-free paper.*

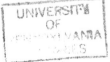

Conversations in Medicine

To the memories of
my father,
who instilled a love of words,
and of my mother,
who brightened so many lives with them.

CONTENTS

INTRODUCTION

How did this book come to be written—and why?

In the spring of 1978 I was invited to give several lectures concerning heart disease research at the University of Utah College of Medicine in Salt Lake City. It was to be a sort of homecoming for me inasmuch as I had trained there in cardio-vascular disease as a fellow under Dr. Hans H. Hecht between 1961 and 1963.

As I began to make preparations for my trip I became increasingly conscious of another opportunity this might afford me: to meet with certain distinguished members of the faculty whom I had long admired but known only slightly back in the early 1960s. As a postdoctoral fellow I had had little opportunity to meet with Dr. Max Wintrobe. Even though he headed the Department of Medicine of which I was nominally a member, his area of expertise was hematology. As a cardiology trainee, I was in another division of the department and therefore once removed from his direct tutelage and—some hematology fellows half-jokingly confided to me—his occasionally withering critiques of one's performance. Whatever the pros and cons of my former status, I was now a "visiting fireman" and under this guise would attempt to meet personally with Dr. Wintrobe and in some small way compensate for the lack of contact in the past.

While in Utah, I had been even further removed from another figure of international repute, Dr. Louis S. Goodman, who then headed the Department of Pharmacology. He too was still on the scene in 1978, and I hoped to meet with him as well. After all, wherever I went following that two-year stint in Salt Lake City people would ask me, "So you really were at Utah with Wintrobe and Goodman! What were they like?" Unfortunately, I hardly knew.

No sooner did I resolve to request meetings with these two eminent senior scientists than the thought occurred to me that, undoubtedly, many others, physicians and laymen alike, might be interested in knowing just how such great contributors to American medicine felt about themselves and their profession in the twilight of their careers.

I decided to record these conversations in medicine, and thus was the idea for this book born.

In the United States during the twentieth century perhaps in no field of endeavor have more profound changes taken place than in medicine. What I have attempted to do in this book is to interview a number of outstanding physicians and, through their own words, reveal to the reader not only what they did but how and why.

As a physician-researcher, myself, I had a considerable head start on this project. I had already been somewhat personally acquainted with several potential contributors; others I knew by reputation to be primary candidates for inclusion. I therefore had a fairly good idea of which group of people might provide through their own experiences an adequate spectrum to reflect the medical story of our country during the last fifty years or more. Through their insight I also hoped to gain some idea of what the future course of medicine will be in this country and perhaps the world.

The selection of any such group of medical scientists by a single individual must, to some extent, be biased, but I have tried to be guided by what are generally acknowledged to be among the major medical advances of the twentieth century:

- the understanding of the formation of the blood elements (hematology)
- the growth of pharmacology: antibiotics for infectious dis-

ease and useful drugs for the treatment of heart disease and high blood pressure
- the development of open-heart surgery
- the expansion of our knowledge in immunology
- the introduction of organ transplantation and artificial organs
- the discovery of the chemical configuration of DNA and the beginnings of molecular biology

The contributors to this book have all played essential roles in one or more of these areas. No doubt other scientists or medical historians might add to the list; I do not pretend that it is in any way complete. The discovery of insulin along with advances in neurochemistry and endocrinology might also be cited as milestones of progress, for example, but many of those one would have liked to meet with concerning these are dead or inaccessible. Nonetheless I believe that, despite such omissions, the men and women who did participate in this book will reveal patterns of behavior and experience that transcend their specific scientific areas of interest.

Beyond the purely research aspects of medicine there are others we must also acknowledge as integral parts of the whole picture. Until the beginning of the twentieth century the status of medicine in this country, especially when compared with that in Europe, was low indeed. It was not until the occurrence of two events—the founding of the Johns Hopkins School of Medicine in 1893 and the famous Flexner Report in 1910—that we began to emerge from mediocrity or often worse. The result of the Flexner Report and the efforts of those who supported it was that responsible medical schools began to introduce basic science studies into the training curricula for our future doctors and the diploma mills and schools of quackery that had previously infested the nation began to go out of existence.

Finally, no story of medicine in the United States would be complete without some mention of the relationship between the medical establishment and such groups as women, blacks, and Jews. The stories here speak for themselves.

A few words about the mechanics of this undertaking might be of interest. After deciding upon a particular contributor and gaining his or her acquiescence, I would receive a copy of the individual's curriculum vitae and bibliography. This I would use to fill in the gaps of my own knowledge regarding background material. Depending upon the party in question, I would spend various amounts of time in the library reading previous papers and reviews; in some instances, I would also contact others more familiar with the subject that I in order to determine the best lines of inquiry. Therefore, a considerable amount of preparation preceded each meeting, which varied from a few hours (in most cases) to a day's visit or two. The rough transcript prepared from the recorded conversations served as the basis for reorganizing the material in its final form before submission to the contributor for approval prior to publication.

These were indeed "conversations" with all the give and take that the word implies, but in their final form I have arranged the material in such a way as to provide a continuous and meaningful narrative. I have kept my own remarks to a minimum and inserted them only where necessary to propel a line of thought, introduce a new one, or reveal some bit of meaningful information of my own that might shed further light on the subject under discussion. Of special interest to me was the way the lives of so many of these people interdigitated (quite naturally) and the comments they had to make to me about one another. Where other prominent medical figures are mentioned in passing, for those readers who would like to identify them more precisely, I have included a Biographical Notes section at the back of the book. Such individuals are identified by a "b" following their names in the text.

Some important aspects of twentieth-century American medicine may have been slighted: the growth of federally supported research; the rise of prepaid health care; the potential, and potential problems, of national health insurance. These are covered only obliquely with some of those interviewed and perhaps more specifically with Sir George Pickering and Francis Moore, who have been rather finely tuned in to such considerations here and in Great Britain over the years.

But this is primarily a book about people, about a group of extraordinary people. Through their words we learn about them; about those upon whose professional shoulders they felt they stood; and, finally, about those whom they themselves uplifted. The author gratefully counts himself among the latter and hopes that no one reading the stories of these great men and women will fail to find himself similarly inspired by them.

Conversations in Medicine

CHAPTER 1

At the Turn of the Century

THE MEN AND WOMEN in this book generally began their work in the second decade of the twentieth century and have continued in varying degrees up to the present. What was the medical scene like when they first appeared upon it, and how has it been changing through their lifetimes?

Foremost among the nineteenth century's contributions to medical knowledge were the discoveries of such outstanding microbiologists as Louis Pasteur and Robert Koch proving that bacterial infection lay at the root of so many diseases that then plagued us. Thus, at the beginning of the twentieth century we knew a good deal about the cause of many naturally occurring diseases but were still without very effective means of combating them. The use of sulfonamide drugs would not be introduced until the 1930s; penicillin, the first of the antibiotics, would not be in adequate supply until after World War II.

In surgery, complicating infection was a major problem and frequent cause of postoperative death. Surgeons devised their own methods of preventing or combating infection. In Great Britain, Joseph Lister, beginning in 1865, emphasized "antisepsis," the introduction of certain chemicals in wounds to cleanse them. Before him, in Vienna and Budapest, obstetrician Ignaz Scmmclwcis during the 1840s had insisted on "asepsis," the disinfection of the hands and clothing of physicians and midwives who were about to assist women in the birth of their children. These women were often at risk of developing puerperal or childbed fever, a lethal postpartum infection.

Immunology would also play a role in the control of infections until the arrival of the antibiotic era. This was nothing new: Edward Jenner had used vaccination to prevent smallpox in 1796, and much of Pasteur's work, especially with rabies, had involved vaccination. Attempts to control bacterial diseases such as diphtheria, tuberculosis, and tetanus would continue along these lines during the first half of this century. Interestingly enough, because of their small size viruses could not actually be seen until the invention of the electron microscope in 1940. This and other scientific developments continued the interest in the applications of immunology, since viruses are rarely sensitive to antibiotics, and many of the problems of transplantation and even cancer are amenable to the immunologic approach.

The greatest boon to surgeons of the nineteenth century was the development of general anesthesia, and this discovery enabled their successors to attempt more complicated and time-consuming operations than were allowed their predecessors. Abdominal and thoracic explorations became common, and the days when surgeons required assistants to restrain conscious patients while attempts to perform limb amputations or remove bladder stones in record time were gone forever.

As the century progressed, improved standards of living and better sanitation changed the nature of our major health problems. Infectious disease came under better control, and nutritional deficiencies such as those resulting in pellagra or scurvy virtually disappeared. Today the complications of atherosclerosis (coronary artery and cerebrovascular disease) and cancer have come to the fore as the major killers of our aging population.

Coronary heart disease was long recognized as an occasional cause of sudden death in time past, but it was not until the development of the electrocardiograph in 1903 by Willem Einthoven of Leiden that heart specialists like James Herrick and George Dock could prove that many of those attacks of "indigestion" suffered by middle-aged men were in reality non-fatal myocardial infarctions (heart attacks). Heart surgery was still in the future, however, and no routine heart surgery would be performed until after the 1940s. After this time, it grew exponentially in the treatment of congenital as well as in a variety of acquired heart diseases.

While we can point to major advances in the diagnosis and treatment of heart disease, the progress in cancer has been less impressive. We began the century in the "heroic" stage of massive surgical excisions for various neoplasms; but neither that approach nor the use of radiation, chemotherapy, or endocrine therapy have markedly reduced the toll from such major killers as lung and breast cancer. The quality of surviving life has been improved for many of these patients, however, and miraculously some of the most rapidly growing tumors have proved the most amenable to the newer forms of nonsurgical treatment.

In 1900 endocrinology was in its infancy. The term "hormone" was not even coined until 1905. An extract of thyroid gland was used to treat myxedema (hypothyroidism) in the 1890s, but insulin for diabetes had to await Banting's and Best's discovery in 1921. Cortisone, that ubiquitous agent now used in so many current diseases, was not introduced until 1949 when Philip Hench and his colleagues made their report from the Mayo Clinic.

X rays were not discovered until 1895, and for this work Wilhelm Conrad Roentgen received the first Nobel Prize in physics. Use of X rays in medical diagnosis spread rapidly and played an increasing role in the professional lives of our protagonists. Today other applications involving radiation have contributed greatly to diagnosis (angiography, radioisotopes in nuclear medicine) and therapy (radiation treatment for cancer).

Human genetics and molecular biology were essentially nonexistent at the beginning of this era, but in the last twenty years over a half-dozen Nobel awards have been made in recognition of accomplishments in this field. The use of artificial organs, transplants, and even dialysis for renal failure are also relatively new developments in medicine.

Such is the panoramic view of medicine as it was during the period with which we are concerned; individual facets will be elaborated upon as we take up the lives of each of the contributors to this volume.

A recounting of medical discoveries is, however, but an enumeration of results. It may be more important to recognize that behind each new discovery lies a superstructure in the scientific community that enabled it to be brought to fruition. Without proper encouragement and support, our most brilliant medical pioneers might not have been able to fulfill their promise.

At the beginning of this century there was little in the way of a scientific "superstructure" to enable the advance of medicine. The Civil War had demonstrated to the world the remarkable potential of the United States for technological development, but in the ensuing years as a nation we were unwilling to bend our efforts toward the growth of knowledge unless it was in the cause of war or immediate commercial gain. In 1893 Dr. Theobald Smith demonstrated conclusively that the cattle tick was responsible for the transmission of Texas cattle fever. This was a landmark discovery in bacteriology and preventive medicine, but it might not have been undertaken if the losses of our cattlemen had not been so severe. In 1900 the Walter Reed Commission demonstrated the role of the mosquito in the transmission of yellow fever, another discovery of worldwide historical consequence. But the commission would never have been established had we not had so many of our soldiers afflicted with it during the Spanish-American War in Cuba.

In general, as this period began our medical standards were poor and our medical schools disorganized, inept, and ill-supported. In 1891 among the three major professions—theology, law, and medicine—the last ranged below the other two in institutional support. The total endowment for theological schools amounted to $18 million as against $500,000 for medical education. We languished behind Europe with its long tradition of relating medical education to the high standards of universities and the creation of well-funded and effectively organized research institutes for the purpose of studying disease. American physicians wishing to obtain any appreciation of the scientific basis of medicine were forced to make a pilgrimage to Europe, especially to the German-speaking countries, to experience it.

But we were about to emerge from our backwater status and attain the preeminent position in medicine that we occupy today. The reasons for this awakening can be stated largely in terms of one university (Johns Hopkins); two brothers (Abraham and Simon Flexner); three millionaires (Andrew Carnegie, John D. Rockefeller, and Mary E. Garrett); and four physicians (Hopkins's Osler, Halsted, Kelly, and Welch).

The Johns Hopkins Hospital opened in Baltimore in 1889, but the trustees lacked an additional $500,000 necessary for the opening of its medical school. A committee of women that included Mary E. Garrett raised only $200,000 for the school in a national campaign for funds. Miss Garrett offered to provide the additional $300,000 from her own personal funds provided that women be accepted to the medical school on an equal basis as men and that the academic requirements for admission of *all* candidates be upgraded considerably. The trustees reluctantly accepted these conditions, and the medical school was able to open in 1893. Thus, Miss Garrett was able to strike a double blow with her gift: one for women's rights and another for general excellence in medical education.

The Johns Hopkins Hospital was planned by John Shaw Billings, a U.S. Army surgeon; its first director was Daniel Coit Gilman, who moved into that position from the presidency of the university. Both were conversant with the generally high caliber of European medicine and the low state of our own. They were determined to alter the balance. Gilman decided to organize the hospital like a department store, with the appropriate physician-surgeon in charge of each division and with all the divisions responsible to him. This was a momentous decision, since eventually all other hospitals and medical schools were to adopt the departmental system.

Outstanding individuals were recruited for each of the departments, but four have come down in history as the most remarkable of all. These were William H. Welch in pathology; Howard A. Kelly in obstetrics; William Osler in medicine; and William S. Halsted in surgery. All were well versed in the European traditions of scholarship and science and set the pace for future generations of American physicians.

Of the four, perhaps Osler has become the best known and most venerated. If George Washington could be called the father of our country, then Osler might well be looked upon as the George Washington, John Adams, and Thomas Jefferson of American medicine. His skill as a physician, his effectiveness as a bedside teacher, and his textbook of medicine would, in themselves, have guaranteed him a place in the medical pantheon. But he was also a classical scholar; a distinguished public speaker; and, once intended for the ministry, an essayist with a strong philosophical bent. Although he was born in Canada and spent his early medical years there, the bulk of his career was spent at Hopkins before he left for England to accept the Regius Chair in Medicine at Oxford.

There were millionaires other than those in Baltimore who influenced the future course of American medicine. Andrew

Carnegie, the poor Scottish immigrant boy who later founded Carnegie Steel, was originally concerned with the plight of many college professors whom, he found, had no pension plans and often spent their declining years in poverty. To study this problem he set up the Carnegie Foundation for the Advancement of Teaching, which did, indeed, lead to the establishment of retirement plans for college faculty that persist as the major ones in existence today. Carnegie selected as the first president of his foundation an astronomer, Henry S. Pritchett. Pritchett's initial assessment of the status of American college faculty made it apparent to him that medical teaching here was of an extremely poor quality.

To study the problem Pritchett sought a man of perception but with no preconceptions or former ties to the American medical community. He selected Abraham Flexner, whose background had been in psychology and education. The Flexner Report, published in 1910 as the now famous Carnegie Foundation *Bulletin* No. 4, caused an uproar. Flexner had visited 155 medical schools in the United States and Canada and, in almost all of them, found the requirements for admission, the curriculum, and the library facilities woefully inadequate. The publication of this report, along with the parallel efforts of the American Medical Association's Council on Medical Education to improve medical instruction, soon led to the closing or merging of many schools and the reorganization of others, using Johns Hopkins as a model for reform.

In 1901 the Rockefeller Institute was founded in New York City. This was the first major private philanthropic effort to promote medical research in the United States and was influenced in its organization by such European centers as the Pasteur Institute in Paris and the Koch Laboratory in Berlin. William Welch, the Hopkins pathologist, was to be its first major scientific advisor as president of the board of directors, but the major moving force in its history would be a protégé of Welch, Abraham Flexner's brother. Simon Flexner was a su-

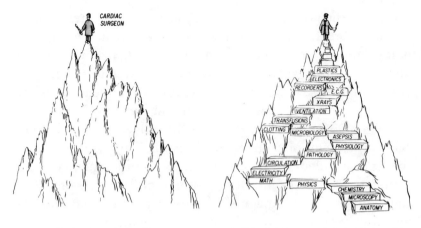

One giant leap to the pinnacle?   *Or did he climb the steps up the back of the mountain?*

Figure 1. Two ways of looking at the "ascendancy" of the cardiac surgeon.
(Reprinted by permission of the American Heart Association.)

perb pathologist-microbiologist and served as director of the Rockefeller Institute from 1902 until 1935. The institute (now university) would become the world's foremost center of medical research over the next fifty years.

There would be other schools and other cities and other sources for research funds during the course of the century, but these were the beginnings, and without them American medicine would never have achieved its current stature.

The growth in scientific achievement spurred by these early developments eventually was enhanced greatly by the participation of the federal government after World War II, mainly through the National Institutes of Health (NIH). There are two graphic examples I should like to present to illustrate the importance of all aspects of biological science to medicine and their growth in recent years. The first is an illustration from an article entitled "Ben Franklin and Open Heart Surgery" by Julius H. Comroe and Robert D. Dripps (Figure 1). This shows how the apparent sudden appearance of the cardiac surgeon at the peak of medical science was really

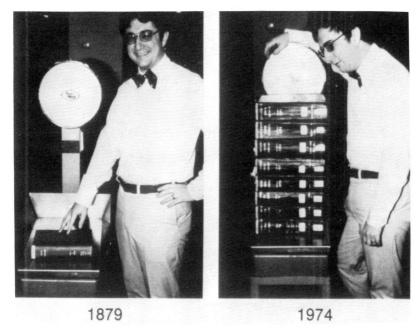

1879   1974

Figure 2. The growth of medical research as reflected in the *Index Medicus* of 1879 compared with that of 1974. (Reprinted by permission of the *New England Journal of Medicine*.) 298:775 (1978).

the culmination of accomplishments in a wide variety of scientific disciplines. The other (Figure 2), from a partially tongue-in-cheek article from the *New England Journal of Medicine* a few years ago and entitled "The Weight of Medical Knowledge," shows simply by the weight of the *Index Medicus* (a listing annually of all medical publications) the explosion of knowledge that has occurred since the beginning of the century.

With this as a background, let us now explore the lives and careers of some of the major figures of this exciting period in our history.

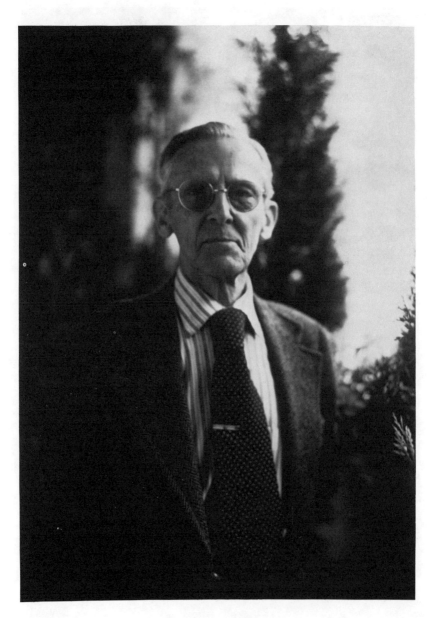

William Dock, M.D.

CHAPTER 2

William Dock, M.D.
(1889–   )

IT WAS A HOT, muggy Saturday morning in July 1960 as I boarded the IRT subway in midtown Manhattan, as I had so many times in the past, and headed out to Kings County Hospital in Brooklyn.

Having only one more year to go in my medical residency, I was at one of those crossroads of my career and was in much need of some solid advice as to where I should go and what I should do next. At the time I was on vacation from my position as a resident in San Francisco, and had just finished scouring Boston and New York for possible positions. Time was running out; I was due back on the job in the emergency room of the San Francisco General Hospital the following Monday morning. In desperation I had telephoned the Department of Medicine at the State University Medical Center in Brooklyn the previous afternoon to inquire if any of the senior faculty at my alma mater might be expected in the following morning.

"Dr. Dock is usually in the hospital Saturday mornings" was the reply, and an appointment for an interview was made.

Each floor of the main Kings County Hospital was divided into wings containing a large number of beds. At the extreme end of some of these were sun porches that, owing to an overall lack of space for administrative functions, had been converted to "offices" for the faculty. It was at one of these that I found Dr. Dock. He did not remember me, nor should he have.

I had not been a very special student. Nonetheless, he freely gave of his time and advice. The latter took the form of his own life story, some of it retold here, over a period of more than two hours, perhaps the most fascinating and rewarding two hours I can remember.

No one could be more suitable than William Dock to begin this story about twentieth-century American medicine. Effective medical and surgical treatment did not really arrive until the beginning of this century. During the preceding decades the great clinicians and pathologists of the nineteenth century laid the groundwork for such therapeutic advances by providing us with a knowledge of the natural history and morbid anatomy of the diseases we would ultimately be equipped to treat. Dr. Dock, an eminent cardiologist, is one of the few great living clinicians who was also well grounded in pathology.

Through his father, a protégé of Osler, he continued this line of distinguished physicians, and, as will become apparent, he knew just about every great American physician of his time and many of those in Europe as well. His illustrious background was for him neither a crutch nor a heavy burden; it was simply part of the package.

Unlike many of the others who contributed to this book, he did not occupy a high administrative position, such as departmental chairman, for many years of his life, nor did he wish to do so. He will be remembered best as the possessor of a very unique mind and as an inspiring teacher. An example of his style might best serve to give one an idea of the man in person.

There is a long-standing controversy in medicine about the genesis of the first heart sound. It is not a matter of earth-shaking consequence; the first heart sound is, after all, just one of countless details concerning us, about which biologists feel a little happier if they can explain precisely. The details of the dispute are unimportant here. Suffice it to say that Dock is a major proponent of the view that the sound is produced by sudden tensing of the valve substance and that others disagree. I vividly recall his small, almost natty figure pacing animatedly before the blackboard and him suddenly pulling a white handkerchief from his breast pocket. He grasps two opposite sides, lets it go limp in the center, and then suddenly pulls the cloth tense to produce a sound and make his point.

I think the secret of his success with students was related to his enthusiasm and to the fact that he did not "talk down" to them. If some idea seemed perfectly reasonable to him, he assumed that it should be just as easily grasped by his students. This attitude was very effective, and we worshiped him.

His contemporaries often did not fare as well. He was a superb debator, and although I never saw him in the midst of a public dispute, it was said that his argumentative skill was such that, even when the weight of all the facts was not on his side, he could usually gain the advantage of any adversary. In some quarters this made him feared, and some thought him intolerant and arrogant; perhaps, at times, he was. Perhaps this is why he never sustained himself for a great many years in a position of departmental leadership where political savvy as well as scientific acumen is an important ingredient of success.

The unsettling aspects of his presence could, however, be turned to advantage; and it was this, undoubtedly, that led Alan Gregg, medical director of the Rockefeller Institute, at one time to suggest that he leave the staid and prestigious Cornell and venture into the medical backwater of Brooklyn to "shake things up" a bit.

Because of the shifting of his locale during the course of his career, the following list may help in maintaining the orientation of the reader as we follow him:

1926–36 Stanford (Medicine)
1936–41 Stanford (Pathology)
1941–44 Cornell (Pathology)
1944–56 Long Island College of Medicine/SUNY Downstate (Medicine)

1956–57   Palo Alto Clinic (Cardiology)
1957–66   SUNY Downstate (Medicine)

Following his time at Downstate, Dr. Dock served at the Brooklyn Veterans Administration Hospital as chief of the Medical Service until 1969 and, for a short period, worked at the Lutheran Medical Center in Brooklyn before retiring to Paris, where he now resides.

He has removed the "M.D." after his name in the apartment house directory in Paris, and he pointedly referred to this when I visited him there. But Dr. Dock, even in his eighties, cannot escape the urgings of his restless and inquiring mind. He was fascinated by the story of the discovery of radioactivity, which he was in the process of putting into book form. He also had heard that someone was teaching that the sounds you hear when you take someone's blood pressure were due to a mechanism that he felt was completely wrong. He was in the process of devising a set of experiments to prove it.

■ You came from a medical family: George Dock was your father.

My father was the first full-time professor of medicine in the United States, at the University of Michigan in Ann Arbor. When Washington University [St. Louis] started with a full-time faculty in 1910, he became head of the Department of Medicine there. He was an extremely good department head, and he was an extremely good clinician—and he was a clinician who kept up to date. When ECGs were invented he didn't say "What nonsense!" or, like Henry Christian,[b]* "Well, Sam[b] (Levine), what are the wild waves sayin'?" or, "What the hell is your gadget for?" My father was a believer in using polygraphs to record motions of arteries and veins and the precordium; he fiddled with this. He was very good with a microscope, and so he was a good parasitologist when more people had more parasites. He studied hookworm disease and wrote a good book on it. He also studied pellagra. He was a good hematologist because of his skill with the microscope, but he never made any original observations with it. He had a lot of Negro patients and must have seen dozens of smears of sickle-cell anemia, but it was Jimmy Herrick[b] in Chicago who hardly saw any Negro patients who described the disease.

■ You were a very peripatetic family.

Well, my father liked to travel. I was born and raised in Ann Arbor, Michigan. I spent a year in New Orleans when my

*See Biographical Notes.

father was at Tulane. Then my family was in St. Louis from 1910 to 1922.

■ There's a well-known story concerning appendicitis and your father walking around with it and this great diagnostician not even recognizing it in himself. Is this true?

No, it was my brother that walked around with it for three days when we were in New Orleans. His appendix ruptured, and Rudolph Matas,[b] one of the best surgeons in America at that time, heard from my *mother* who let him know that *he* better see my brother. Matas put him in the hospital and took the appendix out. It was ruptured, so he had a drain in for six weeks. The next year, my father was in California fortunately, and so when I came down with appendicitis mine came out before it ruptured.

■ So I had the story right but the characters wrong. It *was* your father who did not recognize it in your *brother!*

He didn't even think about it! But, of course, it was the women in our family who were the brightest. My father's sister, Aunt Lavinia, spent a lifetime in nursing and had a tremendous influence on the profession. She graduated from Bellevue and, after being night supervisor there, wrote a materia medica for nurses which became a standard text. She later went down to Hopkins for a few years and wrote a classic multivolume history of nursing with Adelaide Nutting.[b] Although she did most of the work, she preferred to have the authors listed as "Nutting and Dock" because the words seemed to flow better that way. Incidentally, she didn't think much of doctors even though she knew Osler.[b] She hardly ever needed doctors either. Aunt Vinnie lived to ninety-nine and had not seen a doctor for her own care from the age of nine. It was a broken hip she had, but it was not the hip that she died from—it was from indignation!

■ Was growing up the son of such a famous physician a help or a hindrance to you?

Oh, it was a great help, because in those days doctors were really rich. In 1910 at Washington University in St. Louis a full-time chief was felt to be on miserable pay. He only got ten thousand dollars. But in 1910, before the introduction of the income tax and with the buying power of the dollar then, ten thousand dollars was the equivalent of eighty-five thousand dollars a year after taxes in more current times. I discussed this in a talk I gave in Atlantic City some years ago entitled "Hours Rescued from Oblivion."

■ You went to war before you went into medicine.

Yes. My brother, who was four years older than I, went over in 1915 and finally joined up with a French flying squadron, not the American Lafayette Escadrille. I went over in 1917 as a volunteer ambulance driver for the French army. I had gotten to be pretty good at fixing things, and this came in handy on the job. A few years before that, when I was seventeen, I worked on a ranch, later Camp Vandenberg, in California. The ranches then depended on windmills to keep the cows in water, and I became the best boy on the ranch in repairing windmills. I've been good at gadgets ever since. While I was in France during the war there was a pretty difficult ambulance run from Montzeville to Esnes, and the ambulance drivers always hated getting stuck along the way and perhaps getting hit by a stray shell. I became pretty good at fixing Fords and getting them going again once they got stuck. I offered to be there to help out, go back and forth until the last trip. The other drivers were very appreciative of this. One day when our commanding officer informed us that headquarters intended to pass out a few medals to some of our group on the following day, they selected me to get one. My citation said I was a devoted and conscientious driver, et cetera: bravery was not mentioned. I changed tires fast and unclogged carburetors fast! [He received the Croix de Guerre.]

■ What about your early medical training?

I took my first two years of medical school at Washington University in St. Louis. My brother was in France at this time, and my mother wasn't feeling very well and I thought I had better stay home. Then my brother came back safely from the wars, and I realized I couldn't take my clinical years in St. Louis because my father was head of the Department of Medicine. So I shopped around and found that the best place for me was Rush Medical School in Chicago. In this I made no mistake. Rush was a marvelous place; they thought you were an adult, and you could do what you wanted to do in those two years as long as you wrote the examinations at the end of it. I spent almost all my time there doing autopsies with a marvelous pathologist, E. R. LeCount.[b] Although I never took clinical microscopy and was never a clinical clerk, you still could not get better clinical training than they offered there. People like Frank Billings[b] and James Herrick, who put coronary disease on the map, were active then.

After Chicago I was a house officer at the Brigham* between 1922 and 1924. Murphy [William Parry] was the best internist at the Brigham. He was a resident when I was an intern. Hermann Blumgart[b] was also a fine assistant resident at the time. Bill Murphy, Blumgart, and Samuel B. Grant were the three best residents and internists at the Brigham along with Sam Levine. "Uncle Henry" Christian was a superb executive but was not in the same class as a diagnostician. His rounds were called "shifting dullness."

From Boston I knew I wanted to go into practice in San Francisco and had already made some preliminary arrangements, but first I was going to take a *Wanderjahr* on my own. My father, however, insisted that I go work with his old friend K. F. Wenckebach,[b] the head of the First Medical Clinic in Vienna. Wenckebach, who was Dutch, was the first man to do clinical electrocardiography. People in Amsterdam wouldn't have anything to do with it when he started. This "silly toy" the physiologists had made! It wasn't movable, you know; you

*Peter Bent Brigham Hospital

had to bring the patient to it. But "Wencke" persisted. He described atrial fibrillation; he described atrial flutter; he described atrial and ventricular tachycardia. One day one of his patients came in with an attack of atrial fibrillation and told Wenckebach, "Oh, that's nothing. I'll be back tomorrow and it will be all over."

Wenckebach asked, "What do you do for it?"

"I take quinine." [The patient had had malaria]

Wencke found that quinine was good but quinidine was better. So he introduced the first good antiarrhythmic drug. He was a pioneer in this, and my father was a good friend of his from the time when they were doing carotid and jugular tracings together—which got them both interested in cardiac arrhythmias.

So my father as usual was right in sending me abroad, although at first I was indignant at spending such a long time in Vienna. As it turned out, I had a wonderful time there. I also went there on a honeymoon. I took my wife with me and she came back highly pregnant.

■ What was Wenckebach like?

He was a charming person. He was small and thin and quick. He spoke French, German, English, and, of course, Dutch quite fluently. He was a very poor teacher in clinic, however. He would come in and do his cerebration in public; he would think about the patient and about the disease and about the history of it. Well, the students didn't take kindly to this rambling. They used to recite:

In der Klinik Wenckebach
Nur die erste Bäncke wacht.

(In Wenckebach's clinic only the first row can stay awake.)

But I wouldn't have made a penny when I got back to San Francisco if I hadn't been given the key to some gold nuggets.

The mercurial treatment for diuresis was discovered while I was there. And, of course, it was discovered by the nurses. They used to give mercurials intravenously for the treatment of syphilis, and frequently the syphilitic patients had congestive heart failure resulting from syphilitic aortic insufficiency. They kept jugs at the end of the beds to measure the urine output, and the nurses kept pointing out to the doctors that whenever they gave mercurials to one of these patients in heart failure he'd have one hell of a diuresis. Eventually Saxl, who really was not one of the brightest men there, thought he better look into this, and they were off to the races and so was I.

When I went into practice I was the only man in San Francisco who could treat pulmonary edema properly. You gave 'em intravenous mercury, and they told all their friends that you were a miracle worker.

■ How did you switch from private practice to academic medicine?

I originally never intended to go into academic medicine. I thought my father had carried the family as far as they could go in that direction. After being in Boston, I decided that I wanted to do in San Francisco what Sam Levine did: have a connection with a good hospital and good medical school but to practice in town or a major suburb. I started in San Francisco as the "boy" of Drs. René Bine and Alfred Reed down in Union Square. I did their odds and ends in the afternoons and evenings: lumbar punctures, chest taps, transfusions, and whatnot, also seeing some patients. In the mornings I went to the outpatient clinic at Stanford, and some evenings I could also do a little work there, using it as a sort of laboratory.

In the year prior to my arrival Dr. Bloomfield[b] had come out as chief of medicine from Hopkins, and he had anticipated bringing Chester Keefer[b] with him as his first instructor. Chester was at the University of Chicago as a resident. Toward the end of the year Bloomfield asked me to come see him, and when I got there he said, "Bill, I'm in a fix. Chester Keefer has written me and wants to be released from his contract so that he can go to Peking Union Medical School* as an assistant professor of medicine and stay there for a few years. Of course, I released him. Now, I've got to have somebody, and you'll have to come back here the first of September."

I had built up quite a practice with my friends in Union Square by that time, so I went home and asked my wife if she could afford to take the cut in income. She said yes, and with one year's exception I spent the rest of my professional life in academia.

■ You carried on the "peripatetic tradition" of your family in more ways than one. You shifted back and forth between the two coasts as well as between medicine and pathology. You stayed in medicine at Stanford from 1926 to 1936 and then suddenly shifted to pathology. Why?

Well, I got into pathology the same way I did academic medicine—by accident. Our dean and professor of pathology at Stanford had been Dr. William Ophüls, the man who discovered coccidioidal granuloma. He was a wonderful dean but, like all good deans, spent far more time teaching and in the laboratory than in the dean's office. Well, he died and they got von Glahn, a Hopkins graduate, to come out from Columbia to look at the job. Dr. von Glahn proceeded to write an insulting but perfectly accurate description of the state of pathology at Stanford as compared with eastern pathology. Then they got William Boyd[b] to come down from Saskatchewan, and he accepted but was snapped up by Toronto as soon as they read the announcement in *Science*.

Finally, President Wilbur of Stanford sent for me and told me, "Dock, you'll have to take over the Department of Pathology the first of September." At the time I was perfectly happy in medicine but again went home and asked my wife if she

---

*At that time a center for the study of infectious diseases and a highly desirable and exciting place for those in the field to work.

would be willing to take another pay cut in going from medicine to pathology. She agreed and I went into pathology.

Wilbur had promised a great many things to me upon my acceptance of the pathology job, but during the five years I remained there he did not make any change in the income of the department, which was inadequate for our staff. Each year the promised increase never came. I finally indicated that if this was not straightened out I would resign. I was considering a professorship in pathology at Cornell. He knew I had been offered some deanships which I had turned down—I was no administrator—and believed that if I had turned down a deanship I certainly would not accept a professorship in pathology. He was wrong. When he did not increase the budget and the only way I could raise the salary of the other members of the department was to resign, I did.

■ Why Cornell?

One answer to this might be the one that the "darkie" American who had signed up with the French gave to Mrs. Vanderbilt when she visited him in the hospital in Paris during World War I. He had been a dock worker in Savannah. Mrs. Vanderbilt asked him, "Mr. Bullard, how did you happen to join the French army?" He said, "Ma'am, it was more through curiosity than intelligence."

But actually I had to leave. Wilbur gave me no other choice.

Once I got to Cornell it was perfectly obvious to me that what they needed was a different kind of man. I was interested in the seats and causes of disease, in doing autopsies, in training young surgeons (at Stanford I always had a prospective surgical resident assigned to me).

At Cornell the surgeons were scared to death of pathologists, and when I gave a talk to the sophomore students on the causes of thromboembolic disease and said that everybody should be out of bed as soon as possible after an operation, the surgeons thought I was crazy and couldn't get rid of me soon enough. What they wanted was someone of an entirely different sort: one who would spend all his time studying viruses or enzymes or something like that rather than bothering the surgeons and obstetricians.

■ After three years (1941–44) at Cornell in pathology you went back to medicine—in Brooklyn of all places.

Well, I was wasting my time at Cornell, and Alan Gregg,[b] the head man at the Rockefeller Foundation, got wind of this and sent for me. He said, "Dock, I think you should consider going to the Long Island College of Medicine. There is only one little school in the whole of Long Island. You are worth twenty times as much in Brooklyn as you would be in Boston and ten times as much as you are in Manhattan, and I think you should consider it. You may get thrown out of there in two or three years, but I know you'll land on your feet."

I knew that I was in no shape to take over a department of medicine after all those years in pathology, so I arranged through some friends of mine at the University of Southern California to work for six months at the Los Angeles County Hospital. I did not bring my family west for this period, and although officially a professor of medicine, I lived the life of a resident again. I was lodged at the Sante Fe Railroad Hospital and started ward rounds there every morning at seven-thirty. I left for the County Hospital at eight-thirty and spent most of the day there, returning about four in the afternoon to complete my work at Santa Fe. I took calls with the residents and gave all those wonderful new drugs that were coming along. I gave sulfadiazine intravenously and for the first time in my life saw bacterial meningitis cured. It was the best education in medicine one could get after being away from it for eight years. After the six months were up I returned east to head the Department of Medicine at the Long Island College Hospital on July 1, 1944. I had good friends there who were sympathetic, and Alan Gregg was right. I was the only one they could have sent there to shake things up a bit, and I had talked to a lot of people there before moving, people like Jean Oliver,[b] who was probably the world authority on renal anatomy and pathology.

When I arrived in Brooklyn, I recognized that the situation was nowhere near hopeless. But it was clear that this school could not survive as a WASP institution in a community that was predominantly Catholic and Jewish. The faculty were all WASPs, and they needed to recognize the large Jewish community with a lot of doctors—some terrible and some very good—and work with them. George Baehr, an internist at Mt. Sinai in New York and a chief advisor to the Federation of Jewish Charities, was helpful, and he had the kind of political clout to help us with Albany. I convinced Jean Oliver and others at the school that this was the way to go, so we affiliated with Maimonides in Brooklyn and finally got the school to become the Downstate Medical Center of the State University of New York.

■ I have suggested that you never stayed in one place very long, but actually, except between 1956 and 1957, when you went to Palo Alto, you were continuously at Long Island—Downstate, for a period of over twenty years.

After I settled in at Long Island I resigned the chairmanship of the department in order to get Perrin Long[b] to take it over— he was an administrator deluxe. It was political interference from Albany that led to my leaving for a year. They had arranged that in the Open Division at Kings County Hospital they would have the right to appoint their own professors and make their own promotions with no control by the Department of Medicine at the college. Political influence had been brought to bear on the dean, and someone had to do something about it. Once I resigned, I was able to talk freely to the chairman of the board of trustees and then spent my year at the Palo Alto Clinic in private practice. That's what every professor of medicine should do for a sabbatical. He shouldn't go to Oxford to study viruses; he should go to a good private clinic and learn how to take care of sick people.

After a year out there things got straightened out between Albany and the medical school in Brooklyn, and Perrin Long brought me back. And I stayed on there until Ludwig Eichna succeeded him. Eichna had a number of good qualities—he was good with students, a good committee worker, an executive—but he tried to disaffiliate with the other hospitals, so he antagonized the entire community in Brooklyn, and he made it clear to me and Bob Austrian[b] that we could not get off the faculty too soon to please him. So he got rid of us. But, unlike me, he didn't go away when he was sixty-five.

No one should stick around too long. My father retired at sixty-two; Harvey Cushing[b] resigned from Harvard at sixty-two; Osler left Hopkins at fifty-six. Fifty-six was the age that Hippocrates chose as the beginning of senility. Osler was a great Hippocrates and *Religio Medici* man, so that he had firm feelings about what doctors should do and one of them is: "Here's your coat. What's your hurry?"

■ Do you really believe, as someone who has worked all his life in biological science, that you can hang a certain age on somebody and say "All right, now that you're sixty-five or whatever, you're finished"? There are some people that are old when they are fifty and others who are still young mentally at seventy.

Yes, I'm only too painfully aware of this. The problem is that you are not fit to be the judge of which of these you are. Other people can tell right away whether you're fifty and acting seventy or just the reverse, but you, yourself, have no idea. The only solution is to do what my father and Harvey Cushing did and not stay too long.

■ Who are the people who most influenced you?

Dr. E. R. LeCount in Chicago; Dr. Philip Schaefer, biochemist at Washington University; Dr. Opie, who was professor of pathology at Washington University at St. Louis; and Frank Wilson.[b] Frank Wilson was the greatest man I ever met in medicine. I guess it was one of the Haldanes who said, "The cosmos is characterized by inexhaustible queerness." And studying the queerness is the fun of being here. Frank Wilson understood that better than all the rest of us. He's the man who introduced the twelve-lead electrocardiogram, but aside from his work in cardiology he was a splendid astronomer and had his own observatory. He was a splendid ornithologist: he knew all the warblers there were in the United States and could recognize their songs, and knew where they wintered and where they summered. He was a splendid botanist. I walked through the Arnold Arboretum in Boston with him, and he could identify every tree at a distance just by its shape. He was a superb mathematician and a very good clinician. You never met such a man. He really had—a mind! He spent all his life in Ann Arbor, except for a few years when he was with my father in St. Louis. I was lucky, because he was in charge of sophomore students for physical diagnosis and history taking when I was there. It was immediately obvious to me then that "Boy, this is a man!" and I almost went to Ann Arbor to work with him but got sidetracked in various directions.

■ What about your own research work?

You have to know what sort of talents you have. I'm not any good at all at biochemistry. I wouldn't be any good at all in bacteriology and virology. My "tricks" are not the ones that are good for you in those areas.

■ You are good at gadgets. What about the ballistocardiogram?

We have already talked a bit about my way of fixing things. Ballistocardiography is a sad story. Its potential was never realized. It is one of the best methods of studying patients; not just cardiac patients. It's a wonderful cheap toy*: I do it in

*In the 1940s when the then current instrument was selling for $3,200 on the market, Dr. Dock devised an equally good one at a cost of $20 to construct.

three planes because doing it in one plane is just like taking only one lead on the electrocardiogram. I left my three-plane gadget behind me with more regrets than anything else when I retired. No one else ever had the slightest interest in it.

■ There is a long-standing dispute between you and Luisada[b] about the genesis of the first heart sound.

I refuse to dispute with him. Never argue with a man with an obsession and who won't repeat any experiments that are in the literature. In the eighteen-thirties a good Frenchman, Rouanet, pointed out that two leaflets could come together but would not make noise unless you subjected them to tension. I quoted him in my first paper, and this is a hundred and forty years old now.

What I liked to do is get the answer to things. I've got some new experiments cooking here. I discovered to my horror that people were teaching that when you measure a patient's blood pressure the Korotkoff[b] sound in the artery is due to blood hitting the blood below the cuff. Well, anybody who has ever squirted a hose under the surface of a pool knows that's nonsense. You don't get that kind of noise that way. I'm working on this now.*

One particular bit of work, you'll be pleased to know, was performed in 1920 when I was a medical student working with another fellow on our own and not under a professor. We showed that the "bone" that forms in a kidney when you tie a renal artery is not due to calcification of the chalk that precipitates in the kidney but to the cells that lie right under the transitional epithelium in the pelvis of the kidney. Many years later, I think in 1963, Charlie Huggins[b] in Chicago gave me a flourishing introduction as the man who had made this discovery, and I was quite pleased.

*This work was published during Dock's eighty-second year in the *New England Journal of Medicine* (1980).

■   What kind of work makes you the happiest?

Well, I'm happiest with the things that are the least work.
There was that talk that caused all sorts of trouble for me at
Cornell, "The Abuse of Bed Rest." It all happened quite by
accident when I was asked by McKean Cattell, the professor of
pharmacology and therapeutics, to give a talk as part of a
regularly occurring symposium in 1944.

From my Stanford days as a pathologist I had known that
excessive bed rest gave rise to thromboembolic complications
and had lectured on this to students at Stanford since 1936.
The death rate from thromboembolism was always much less
at the County Hospital than it was at Stanford Hospital. At
the County on rounds all you needed to do was ask a patient,
supposedly on strict bed rest, "How many times did you get
up last night to go to the bathroom?" And he might say, "Well,
only *once*, Doc," because there weren't enough orderlies and
nurses around at the County to bring the urinals to the patients when they wanted them. This wasn't true at the private
hospitals. So the patients at the County, when they got up to
go to the bathroom, dislodged only tiny clots from their veins
and these did not harm them when they got to the lungs and
were dissolved, while the wealthier patients who remained in
bed and formed large clots in their legs and pelvises suffered
the major consequences of large pulmonary emboli.

I gave this same talk in New York and had no idea it was
being written down. It got into the *New York State Medical
Journal* and it got into *Time* magazine, and there was my
picture on the cover with me looking cuter than ever in 1944
because the picture they used has been taken by my fiancée
under a lovely azalea bush twenty years earlier.

Within six months all over the world surgeons were able to
get their patients out of bed earlier, and obstetricians were
getting their ladies out of bed. The cost of hospitalization
went way down. This was during the war, you know, and only

at that time when they couldn't build new hospitals and had a severe shortage of beds would the surgeons have accepted the idea. After all, they charged the patients for all those daily visits while they were at bed rest.

What I am most proud of is where I saved the most lives. No one ever saved as many lives in twenty minutes as I did with that talk. Incidentally, during the war they were having a rash of thromboembolic complications in a military hospital in young men after surgery, and I was asked to look into it. I found the same thing, but in this instance the medical corpsmen were giving them too much narcotics so that they would not be bothered by them. The patients just lay there for days forming thrombi.

■ What about the localization of tuberculosis to the right apex?

One morning on rounds at the Long Island College Hospital one of the students or house staff asked me to explain why it was that pulmonary tuberculosis was so often limited to the apex of the lung rather than the lower lobes. He forced me to think of an explanation. The pulmonary artery pressure had just been measured in man and found to be only one fifth of systemic pressure, and I looked at the chest X ray and the location of the main pulmonary artery and the height of the apex above it. I reasoned that the blood supply was less there than the rest of the lung and provided a more favorable culture medium for the tubercle bacillus. Then I was challenged by some of my colleagues on this. "Why the right apex rather than the left apex? They are both the same height above the pulmonary conus." Again I was forced to come up with an answer and reasoned that it was because of the branching of the main pulmonary artery with the branches to the right apex coming off at a much sharper angle and providing less favorable perfusion to the right apex when compared to the left.

The apical localization theory was turned down by a good

many TB men at first, but in 1960 Dollery, at Hampstead, England, got a cyclotron in his backyard producing radioactive carbon dioxide. He showed that, when you sit up, the blood flow to the right apex is less than that to the left. He wrote: "This exactly confirms Dock's hypothesis of 1946."

That makes you feel better because I never believe any of my own work until it's confirmed by other people with independent methods. Similarly, my work on the localization of coronary disease was confirmed by Minkowsky, who showed that in adults it occurred in the thickest parts, as I had shown in the newborn. So it's nice to have your work confirmed. I get the most satisfaction in knowing I wasn't wrong.

■ Were you ever wrong?

Yes, at Stanford I was wrong once. Some people in Italy had reported that by giving Congo Red you could get a remission in pernicious anemia. This was before Minot and Murphy, of course.* I tried this on some patients, and their serum bilirubins went down and their reticulocyte counts may have risen. But I've never repeated the Congo red experiments, and it certainly was not the solution to pernicious anemia!

■ While you were at Long Island, you and Janet Watson were interested in another kind of anemia—sickle cell—before Linus Pauling came up with the right explanation.

Harvey Itano did all the work. Itano was one of the people who worked with Pauling[b] at Cal Tech, and Pauling just handed this problem over to him: "See what happens with the hemoglobin from sickle-cell people as compared with normals when you study the electrophoretic pattern." And he immediately hit the jackpot. You see, Pauling knew from Castle[b]** that this was a disease of hemoglobin and *that* is what you study. The first year I was at Long Island, Janet Watson had

*See Murphy's interview (chap. 4).
**The whole sickle-cell story is covered in the Wintrobe interview (chap. 5).

a contract with the people at Brooklyn Polytech to study birefringence, solubility, and electrophoretic mobility of hemoglobin from normals and patients with sickle-cell disease, but unfortunately she gave them whole blood. They then found that the sedimentation rate was quite high and that there was a high gamma globulin, and they told her, "You don't know anything about this; the trouble here is the plasma, not the hemoglobin." They never wanted to study the hemoglobin after this. But I said, "Plasma doesn't explain why the cells sickle; you've got to study the hemoglobin." The people at Polytech had no way of studying this, so they sent samples to London, and a paper appeared in *Nature* saying: "We are grateful to the people in Brooklyn who sent us this blood." So I at least helped get the experiments under way to show why the cells sickle: hemoglobin crystallizes out and deforms the cells.

■ It's funny, sometimes, how discoveries get made.

Like good old Pasteur said, "Chance favors the prepared mind." It helps to recognize something when you stumble over it.

We've talked about Washington University, St. Louis, and Frank Wilson. There was also this fellow there named Dr. Alan Chesney.[b] He later went back to Hopkins and ended up as a dean. He was studying something that had to do with rabbits but, along the way, noted that his rabbits got goiters during certain times of the year when they were eating nothing but cabbage for greens. He looked into this and found that it was a thio- compound in the greens that gave them the goiter. And this is where all those antithyroid drugs—thiouracil, and so on—come from. He was the one that opened up that field. Chesney was very bright and observant. This was serendipity, but when he stumbled over something he knew that he had "bumped his shins."

Look at the discovery of the Roentgen ray. There were

Crookes tubes all over Europe and America, standard toys in every physics department, a cathode-ray tube. From time to time one laboratory or another would complain to their photographic supply house that "a lot of the plates you sent us were all fogged." Ilford, the main photographic supplier in England, got the most complaints because it was in England that there were the most physicists using Crookes tubes. Ilford got these complaints and always wrote back: "We're sorry, but many other people have lots of the same emulsion and they are having no trouble with it. You better look into the source that is fogging your plates." Not one of these physicists had the sense to put up a plate beside his Crookes tube and leave it there for half an hour and then develop it. Roentgen[b] put a good black cardboard cover over his Crookes tube and went in with a platinocyanide fluorescent screen and it glowed at three meters. He knew when "his shins had been bumped."

Some people have very insensitive shins. Look how long it took them to recognize nonfatal myocardial infarction. My father reported five cases of myocardial infarction, diagnosed during life, in 1896. He reported this to the Buffalo Medical Society because it was old stuff to him. Pathologists in Germany and France had been studying myocardial infarct for years but couldn't interest the clinicians. And you know why? Clinicians had believed that coronary occlusion was immediately fatal.* And if a doctor had called one of these attacks a coronary occlusion [or myocardial infarction] he would be making a damn fool out of himself, because in eight out of ten cases the patients would be back to work in a week, saying, "That doctor was crazy; he said I had a fatal form of heart disease." It was only after Pardee in 1920 published "An Elec-

---

*Probably influenced by the work of experimental pathologist Julius Cohneim (1839–84), who showed that in dogs coronary arteries were "end arteries": the animals died almost immediately after the coronaries were ligated.

trocardiographic Sign of Coronary Occlusion" that a doctor could make this diagnosis without losing his practice.

Before World War I, Frank Wilson recognized the ECG changes of infarction, as did Sam Levine, Fred Smith, and Herrick, of course.

■ Speaking of coronary disease, I've always emphasized to my patients that many have survived for long periods after a myocardial infarction: Eisenhower, Johnson; and Churchill fought a world war after having his fairly early during World War II. You, yourself, must be a record holder of sorts. When did you have yours?

In 1957. Sam Levine came down from Boston to verify it because I wasn't in a hospital. I would never go to a hospital for a coronary; the death rate is twice as high. Tinsley Harrison[b] didn't go to a hospital when he had his infarct. He's dead now but not from his coronaries. Frank Wilson didn't go into a hospital either, and while we may not all have lived "happily ever after" we survived and went back to work.

When they put you in an intensive care unit, the mental stress is far greater than at any time in your life, immobilized and with all those tubes running in and out. That's a terrible thing to do. If a patient begins to have showers of ventricular ectopic beats, I think it's a good idea to monitor him with a defibrillator handy but in a nice quiet single room. The danger period is that time between the time you suddenly realize "Help, boys, I've had an infarct" and the end of the week. If you live through the week you've probably got it made.

I am by no means a record holder in terms of survival. Dr. Osler used to treat coronary disease, and in 1896 he wrote this up. Tinsley Harrison's father was one of his patients and had severe angina at the age of thirty-eight. He went up to visit the great professor at Hopkins who took a very careful history, including how many children he had, what their ages were, whether Mrs. Harrison was as plump as he was, and how his weight compared then to what it was during the time he was a high school athlete. After getting all this down and doing a physical examination, Osler said, "Well, I think you'll get over your angina all right when you lose the fifty-five pounds you put on between the time of your marriage and the time this began." He told him to go for walks every Saturday and Sunday and as much as he could during the week but that he should lose weight steadily by just eating less of all the things he liked to eat. Dr. Harrison did this and lived to the age of ninety-one. John Hunter[b] lived twenty years after the onset of his angina. So long survival after the onset of angina is not unusual. In my case, I'm a confirmed and practicing coward, so that I promptly went down from 150 to 125 pounds in about six months. I weigh 110 now.

■ Your friend William Bean[b] once described your father when he gave the thirty-fourth annual George Dock Lecture a few years ago. In addition to his medical work he obviously had a rapier wit, and when Bean reported "He certainly did not suffer fools gladly. He didn't suffer them at all!" I could not help but be struck by the fact that the same might be applied to you. All of your students worshiped you, but you always seemed to have a knack of making your peers very uncomfortable.

Oh, no. People like Bill Castle, Art Bloomfield, Jean Oliver, Perrin Long were not in the least uncomfortable, and they were my peers. Some of these other people were simply not *quite* my peers. I never sought to make people uncomfortable but I knew I did; I recognized the cause and the result. It was like the father who came home one day and said, "Well now, children, your father has become a professor emeritus," and his young son looked up at him and said, "I know Latin: 'e' means you're out and 'meritus' means you goddam well deserved it!"

■ That's perhaps the best definition of "emeritus" I've ever heard. What is nonetheless amazing about your career is that you are so well known despite the fact that, unlike others like Wintrobe, for example, you never spent your life at one institution and created your own medical dynasty.

I never had a chance to do this. I was never invited to be

chief of medicine at a new medical school, as my father was at Washington or Tinsley Harrison at Birmingham or Bob Williams[b] at the University of Washington in Seattle or Wintrobe at Utah. I don't know why this was so. Perhaps I was never in the right place at the right time. And perhaps it's just as well. I am not a good administrator; I'm not in a class with people like Wintrobe. You see, when someone is good at organizing a textbook like Williams's *Endocrinology* or Wintrobe's *Hematology* or Tinsley Harrison's *Textbook of Medicine*, he is obviously a good organizer. I am completely disorganized and always have been. After heading the Department of Medicine at Long Island College for a short time, I was more than happy to have Perrin Long take it over.

■ We students never thought much of him, you know. We knew he had something to do with the introduction of sulfa drugs during the war, but we thought him something of a buffoon.

But he was an administrator deluxe and the kind of administrator who made ward rounds. And when he made mistakes on rounds and heard about it, he told everyone about it. He didn't pretend to be a brilliant clinician. He once diagnosed an Arthus reaction in a woman who had a swollen arm after receiving an injection. On rounds the next day Paul Spear, who was chief of medicine at the Brooklyn VA at the time, stuck in a needle and pulled out a load of pus! Perrin loved to tell that story. As for sulfa, it was invented in Germany but was very toxic, and then the French made it less toxic. Long brought this to the United States and persuaded three different drug firms to look into analogues. The first one was sulfinpyrazone, which he used at Hopkins to cure pneumonia, but it made the patients awfully sick. Then he got sulfadiazine and hit the jackpot, because this would cure pneumonia *and* meningitis without making you sick. No one made as much of a contribution to saving lives in the United States as Perrin Long did. This was before the war. When World War II broke out he instantly left Hopkins and served as a medical consultant in North Africa.

■ Do you have any particular regrets about the past?

Regrets? Oh, many of them. I played my cards badly. I don't lose any sleep over it, but I have the ordinary feeling that "I could have played that hand better."

■ Without meaning any disrespect, may I say something? Your friend Dr. Pickering spoke very highly of you and very fondly of you, but he did say, "The trouble with Bill Dock was that he never knew when to keep his mouth shut."

Yes, that's perfectly true. I had a disease that is very well described: it is better to keep your mouth shut and be thought a damn fool than to open it and leave no doubt about the question. I had to move around quite a lot in my life, but I didn't mind moving and I would have missed a great deal in California, New York, and Brooklyn. I learned a lot and I never worried about moving:

For to admire and for to see
And for to behold this world so wide
It never done no good for me
But I can't stop it if I tried.*

*Rudyard Kipling.

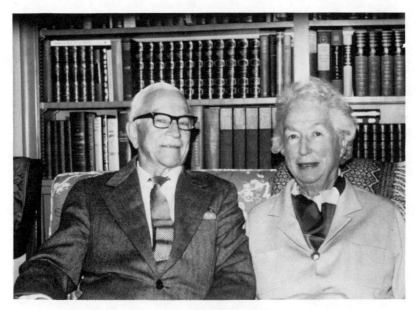
Owen H. Wangensteen, M.D., Ph.D., and Sarah D. Wangensteen

CHAPTER 3

Owen H. Wangensteen, M.D., Ph.D. (1898–1981)

D R. WANGENSTEEN was born and raised in Minnesota where he also spent his entire professional life at the University of Minnesota. His contributions to clinical surgery, the training of surgeons, and surgical research are almost too numerous to mention. He authored or coauthored almost nine hundred publications.

He became truly the Dean of American Surgery as a result of his efforts in Minneapolis and, as indicated in the interview, was responsible for the training of more outstanding American surgeons in his time than perhaps any of his contemporaries. He built up the Department of Surgery at the University of Minnesota until it was one of the best in the world and a leader in many areas of surgical research and progress.

Dr. Wangensteen's personal contributions to surgery were mainly in the field of gastrointestinal disease. No one who has ever been on a surgical service as a student or house officer can ever forget the use of the "Wangensteen tube" for decompression in acute bowel obstruction. This was perhaps his main scientific work, and his monograph on intestinal obstruction is a classic in its field. Although this particular area of his expertise is mentioned only briefly in our discussion, it should not be overlooked. Some of the other projects he worked on, discussed at greater length, do, however, give some idea of the breadth and intensity of his interest in a variety of surgical problems.

Perhaps the greatest contribution of Dr. Wangensteen to the progress of surgery was his early recognition that, while the surgeons of the nineteenth century had depended on the study of anatomy and pathology to make their advances, the surgeon of the twentieth century would have to know "how things work"—he would have to be a physiologist as well as a surgeon in order to succeed.

The marriage between Physiology and Surgery that he and Maurice Visscher consummated at the University of Minnesota enabled that institution to be first and foremost in the development of open-heart surgery. The progeny of that union reads like a "Who's Who" in the field: Clarence Dennis, Richard L. Varco, C. Walton Lillehei, Richard DeWall, Vincent Gott, Norman Shumway, Aldo Castaneda, F. John Lewis, and Christiaan Barnard, among many others.

Like Dr. William Dock, Dr. Wangensteen also had a firm grasp on medical history, and his final major gift to us was in the form of the book, *The Rise of Surgery, Emergence from Empiric Craft to Scientific Discipline,* which he wrote with his wife, Sarah D. Wangensteen.

Reflecting on my meeting with Dr. Wangensteen, I have mixed emotions. There is a great sense of joy and fulfillment in having had the opportunity to meet with this great man and hear him speak of his experiences and views. But sadness came with the news of his sudden and unexpected death from a heart attack less than three months after that meeting.

During the years following his retirement as chairman in 1967, he wryly referred to himself as "a superannuated professor," that is, obsolete. This was certainly not true through all the days and years preceding his death, and as long as we can read of his work and benefit from his teaching this will never be true.

■ You have frequently remarked that you entered medicine "through the portals of pigs and manure and a good spread of each." Could you elaborate on this?

I was born and raised on a farm in western Minnesota and had no ambition other than to be a farmer. I loved all the things that are growing, plants and animals—and took a keen interest in sick cows and horses as well as pigs. When I was thirteen years of age, my father had fifty Poland China sows that could not farrow their young, probably due to some nutritional deficiency, but we had no idea about this then. The veterinarian advised my father to send the sows to the South St. Paul meat market, but I asked my father if I might try my hand at it, and he granted my request, knowing of my interest.

I had seen in *The Breeders' Gazette* an advertisement for something that looked like a gopher snare and telephoned an outfit in Fargo to send one down. It didn't work nearly as well as my hands, though. I stayed out of school for about a month—multiple births, as every obstetrician knows, is a time-consuming task—and at the end of that time presented my father with three hundred piglets. From that time on my father would hear nothing but that I should be a doctor. I resisted until the summer of 1917 when all the available young men were in the army, and I had to do all this farm work alone, hauling hay, pitching manure, milking the cows every morning and night. . . .

One evening my father asked me, "Owen, what are you going to do when you go back to college in the fall?" By this time I had learned that I should have listened to my father much earlier, and I replied, "Father, I'll do anything you want me to do."

■ What about the rest of the family?

There were five children in the family, three boys and two girls, but I was the only one who went into medicine. My youngest son, as you may know, is a surgeon.

I was only seven when my mother died from tuberculosis, and I really missed her. When I entered primary school I had a teacher who knew my mother and she was marvelous, but during the second grade I fell victim to a real disciplinarian. I was a brash youngster, but my first teacher did not mind because I had a phenomenal memory then and could read a page and just regurgitate it word for word right back to her. But the second teacher beat me a few times when I spoke out of turn, and I lost interest in the learning process until the sixth grade when I met Lizzie Hansen. This new teacher encouraged me and altered my whole outlook on things. I suppose she was a surrogate mother in that sense.

■ Taking you very quickly through your undergraduate and medical school training at the University of Minnesota, you then became an instructor in surgery and spent a year in Europe during 1927–28.

Yes, I was encouraged to do this by the dean of our medical school, Dr. E. P. Lyon, and Dr. George Fahr, an internist I highly respected and who had himself been trained abroad by Einthoven[b] in Leiden among others. Dr. Will Mayo[b] also encouraged this and urged me to visit various clinics as an observer. He provided me with many letters of introduction. When you presented a letter from Will Mayo, the chief of the clinic would dash out and say, "Ah, Dr. Mayo!" It was the best recommendation one could possibly have at the time because the Mayo Clinic was appreciated in Germany and German-speaking countries far more than it was here.

Today more emphasis is placed on the performance of operations rather than on observing them, and I think it has been overdone. Will Mayo and other surgeons of his generation were keen observers, and they advocated visiting various clinics to do just this.

I went abroad to study with Professor Fritz de Quervain at the Bern Surgical Clinic in Switzerland, but after some months there I realized that an operating surgeon was not going to give me what I was looking for. I then went to see Professor Leon Asher at the Physiological Institute. Asher was a pupil of Hugo Kronecker[b] with whom Harvey Cushing[b] had worked. I wound up staying five months at the Physiological Institute.

Certain things impressed me when I was abroad. I saw that de Quervain was very much like many of the great surgical professors of the time. He would give his lecture in the morning, and then he would look in on an operation for a few moments and then dash off across the city to a private clinic. I thought that the private practice of surgery was not a useful service to the university when overdone and did not contribute to the intellectual status of the professor. I vowed then that if an opportunity came to me to supervise a surgical clinic I would attempt to set a good example for my colleagues and trainees by strictly adhering to the primary functions of a university professor.

During the ten to fourteen months I remained abroad I visited many clinics in Denmark, Switzerland, France, Italy, Germany, Austria, Holland, and Great Britain. I was appalled by the lack of interest in the experimental approach to surgery. Very few surgeons at that time had laboratories; and this was traditional. Billroth,[b] for insance, at a somewhat earlier period in time used pathology laboratories to which he would send his residents to work out the details of a new operation he contemplated attempting. When they had perfected the procedure as best they could, he would come himself to see how they did it, elaborate on it, and then perform it in patients. Laryngectomy, colectomy, gastric resection, and other procedures were all developed in this way.

In only two institutions were surgical laboratories for the training of surgeons in evidence: at the University of Heidelberg under Eugen Enderlen and at the University of Edinburgh supervised by David P. D. Wilkie.

Clinical teaching in German-speaking Europe during those days was not the best. Contact between students and professors was quite remote. The best clinical teaching to small groups of students was to be seen on the British surgical wards and outpatient departments where an experienced clinician would spend time with them. This was the forerunner of our own clinical teaching method introduced by Osler at Hopkins.

I became convinced of the importance of physiology training to the surgeon and that this would be the stepping-stone for the surgeon in the twentieth century as anatomy had been in the nineteenth century.

■ Shortly after your return to Minnesota you became, at the age of thirty-one, chairman of the Department of Surgery. You have indicated that you got the job because no one else wanted it.

That's essentially it. On my return in the fall of 1928 I was made associate professor and finally chairman in January 1930, but not before the search committee had sought in vain for another replacement for Dr. Arthur C. Strachauer, who had vacated the chair. He had served in this capacity only on a half-time basis, and a full-time man was being sought. Two promising candidates had been interviewed, Dr. Francis Newton from Harvard and a trainee of Halsted's,[b] Dr. Mont Reid, who was then at the University of Cincinnati. Both said to me, in substance: "There is nothing here and there never will be." But they didn't stay here long enough to catch the spirit of the atmosphere, which was friendly to learning.

Locally the prime candidate for the position was the Nestor of surgery in this area, a chap named Arnold Schwyzer. He was born and raised in Switzerland and trained in gynecology. One night Dr. Schwyzer was invited by the search committee for dinner at the home of our professor of medicine, Hilding Berglund. I was there as the youngest of the group. When Schwyzer was offered the full-time position as chairman of the Department of Surgery, he said he would think it over.

An interesting domestic episode occurred that night. At the end of the dinner an enormous frozen ice-cream pie was brought in for dessert. It was so hard that when Dr. Berglund attempted to carve it the whole thing slipped out from under his knife and onto the floor. Helen Berglund was in tears, and I, being the youngest there, ran to the kitchen to see if I could help. I asked Mrs. Berglund to get me some long knives and real hot water and, using the old cautery principle, we were able to cut the pie for all the professors. When Schwyzer finally decided he could not relinquish his practice for the full-time job and they selected me, I wondered if my coming to the rescue with the ice-cream pie had anything to do with it.

■ It was not all smooth sailing for you during those early years, was it?

That is correct. The departmental budget was thirty thousand dollars in January 1930 when I assumed direction of the department. By July 1931 it had decreased to twenty thousand dollars because of the severity of the financial depression, and most of it went to pay the clinical professors who also had their private practices. We had only one surgical resident at the time, and I asked Dean Lyon if I could not take this money and use at least part of it to hire six additional fellows. (They were only earning six hundred dollars a year in those days.) He reluctantly agreed. Despite the shift in funds, no opportunity to work was taken away from the part-time staff.

Three years later this decision came back to haunt me with the appointment of a new dean, Dr. Richard E. Scammon, who was probably one of the finest lecturers in the history of the medical school but who had no experience in administration or money matters. In May of 1933 he called me to his office and handed me a letter consisting of several typewritten pages single-spaced. He was asking for my resignation. I told him, "This is a lot of trivial drivel" and said that I would stand on my record.

The next day I sent the dean a letter saying I would step aside until the problem was resolved, sending a copy to the president of the university, Lotus D. Coffman. For three weeks of soulful cogitation while I awaited the outcome of all this I thought of future research problems and formulated a plan, if vindicated, to spend the rest of my professional career trying to build a strong Department of Surgery at the University of Minnesota.

As a result of the support of Dr. Strachauer, Dean Lyon, President Coffman, and Will Mayo, who was a regent of the University of Minnesota, I was completely vindicated. It was very unfortunate for Dr. Scammon because he was a wonderful man and a great teacher. Dean Scammon was later made the university's first Distinguished Service Professor in 1935, relieving him of all administrative responsibilities.

■ No one would doubt that you fulfilled that promise to yourself. I suppose you are most proud of the number of people you have trained who have distinguished themselves in surgery.

The surgical program did grow. At one time we had, including urology and orthopedics, over one hundred fellows training in surgery at the University of Minnesota. At one time thirty-three professors or heads of departments were former trainees of ours; there were also about thirty at the rank of full-time associate professor at American universities, and I suppose there were perhaps one hundred at lower ranks. Unfortunately, not all of these remained as chairmen; you have to have the Norwegian kind of persistence, I think, to stay under difficulties. Some have retired from their chairmanships but were willing to remain as professors.

■ You were chairman at Minnesota from 1930 to 1967. That's a long time for any one person to head a department. Do you think this is becoming a thing of the past?

Oh, yes. The trend is away from that regardless of the ability of the incumbent. You may know David State. He was at Yeshiva's Albert Einstein School of Medicine some years ago, and David was a marvelous fellow. I can't conceive of how anyone could have objected to him. Well, a new dean arrived on the scene and asked him, "How long have you been in this position as chairman of surgery?" David told him, "Oh, about a dozen years." The dean informed him, "Well, from now on no one is going to be a chairman of any department for more than five years," and demanded his resignation on the spot. Three months later they fired the dean!

■ Some deans used to get away with murder. At Seton Hall, before it became the New Jersey Medical School, we had a dean who fired two chairmen in the same day. For some reason or other he peremptorily removed the chairman of surgery. Then the chairman of psychiatry came in and said, "Here now, you just can't go about firing a chairman of a department like this." "I can't? Well, you're fired too." But the psychiatrist had some satisfaction in the end because he took the school to court and won considerable damages. You were instrumental in establishing a journal, the *Surgical Forum* of the American College of Surgeons. Could you tell me about this?

In the July 1940 issue of *Surgery* I wrote an editorial in which I pleaded the need for a surgical forum for the younger people in surgery. At that time only the oldsters presented at the programs of the American College of Surgeons and other meetings. I thought that the youngsters showed more promise and should have a chance to present their work (and have it published). Evarts Graham[b] read this and asked me to come to Chicago and plead the case for this before the regents of the college. Of those who then constituted the regents, only three of the sixteen were academicians: Al Blalock,[b] Alton Ochsner,[b] and Fred Coller[b] of Ann Arbor. They agreed with me, but we could not win over the other thirteen. They all contended that such a meeting would have no promise of winning a good surgical audience. Despite this initial failure, Graham, who was then chairman of the board of regents of the college, invited me to readdress the board at the fall meeting of the Clinical Congress. This time I urged *trial* rather than *argument:* we could try it for one year, and if it failed we would just give up on the idea. The last pre–World War II session was held in 1941 in Boston, and the forum was a great success. The annual forum presentations have continued to alert surgeons to new trends in surgery and helped make the American College of Surgeons the great organization it has come to be. They were also a means of drawing into the College of Surgeons many academicians who previously thought that the college had not been worthy of their attention: professors and scholars like Churchill[b] and Cutler[b] from Harvard and others.

■ You and Alton Ochsner also were coeditors of *Surgery* for a great many years.

That's true. Dr. Will Mayo proposed to C. B. Mosby, the publishers, that they establish a journal of surgery for the Midwest. He never thought of it as a journal that would acquire a national standing, but it did develop in this way.

■ What about your own areas of interest in surgical research?

Intestinal obstruction was my chief point of interest. I was amazed at the enormous mortality, about fifty percent, during my surgical residency period. No one in our clinic was interested in it in the nineteen-twenties, so the field became mine. I promptly introduced a much smaller catheter than the one that had been in favor for draining enterocolostomies and substantially reduced the incidence of fistulas which frequently followed removal of the larger-sized tubes. This reduced the mortality somewhat. With the introduction of gastroduodenal suction in 1932 the mortality continued to decline. There were further developments along these lines, and the mortality of acute bowel obstruction is now probably in the five to eight percent range at most.

The work on appendicitis with Clarence Dennis[b] was among the most interesting things we did. Rupture of the appendix with peritonitis was a frequent observation on the wards forty to fifty years ago and carried a high mortality. In fact, in 1930 appendicitis ranked among the fifteen most important causes of death in the United States, with some eighteen thousand patients dying annually from it. In 1927 I heard Ludwig Aschoff[b] of Freiburg say that appendicitis was a specific bacterial disease caused by the streptococcus B of Gundel (who was in his department and interested in microbiology). Well, being a surgeon, I was inclined to think the problem was mechanical and made notes to myself that this was one of the things I wished to involve myself with as soon as I could get to it.

We started with obstructing the appendix in the dog, but nothing came of that. The second animal we experimented with was the rabbit. We found that the minute we ligated its appendix at the cecal-appendicular juncture and cannulated the appendix, the intraluminal pressure began to rise and within ten hours rose above that of the diastolic blood pressure. Of the ten rabbits' appendices we obstructed in this manner seven ruptured within ten hours. We then tried to show this in other species. Clarence Dennis, bless his heart, operated upon twenty-six different species of animals, starting with chickens, ducks, and turkeys, and then went out to the St. Paul Como Park Zoo for more species of animals on which to attempt this. It was not until we got to the chimpanzee that we observed what we had in the rabbit: an increase in the pressure within the appendix following the ligation.

In the mid-nineteen-thirties exteriorization of malignancies of the large bowel prior to excision was a commonplace procedure: primary resection for colon cancer came only late in the nineteen-thirties. In fifteen patients who had the procedure and in whom the appendix appeared normal we were able to demonstrate following ligation of the cecal-appendicular junction a similar rise in pressure within the obstructed appendix.

These were elderly patients, two in their sixties or seventies. None came to any harm from the procedure, and all had final restitution of intestinal continuity.

The fecalith [a small hardened ball or mass of feces] is the usual obstructing agent, but the nature and origin of the appendiceal fecalith continues to be a mystery. You don't always find them at surgery. There is a lot of lymphoid tissue in the appendix, more than in the whole of the colon. It is also possible that the swelling of this might cause obstruction and perforation, but I really don't know.

■ Peptic ulcer disease was also one of your interests.

I suppose the thing I did with cooling the stomach, hypothermia, is probably the most significant thing I did there. I think if anyone ever gets enthusiastic about the method, as my colleagues and I were, the method could be improved, but we finally lost financial support for it.

■ What about the second-look program for cancer?

In about 1948 we initiated two things at the university: a screening program for cancer, and the second-look program.

I had a patient who had a large carcinoma of the cecum which had invaded the abdominal wall and involved many lymph nodes. I removed the cancer, the nodes involved, and a section of the abdominal wall; but when she left the hospital I told her, "Miss McKee, you should come back in six months for a second look." She said to me, "Why? What experience have you had with this?" "None," I said, "but I make this recommendation to you on the basis that in terms of recurrence there's a big disparity between the cancer patient with lymph nodes involved and the patient with none involved."

After months had passed I had almost forgotten about her, but she showed up for the second look. To make a long story short, I reoperated on her five times and she lived for twelve and one-half years, dying, not from cancer, but a "stroke." A complete autopsy showed no recurrence of the tumor. At the present time, with what we now know, we could have accomplished this with perhaps four second looks. The second-look program has been adopted in a number of surgical centers with a good deal of success, especially with cancer of the colon.

■ As a cardiologist I'm most impressed about how cardiac surgery progressed at Minnesota even though you personally are not known for this.

Well, I did some of the first *extra*cardiac operations in Minnesota. After Bob Gross[b] showed the way, I was the first in Minnesota to ligate a patent ductus arteriosus [a connection between the pulmonary artery and aorta abnormally persisting after birth]. I also was the first to operate on coarctation [narrowing] of the aorta and do a pericardiectomy for constrictive pericarditis here. But that was the limit of my cardiac surgery. After World War II, when all the men came back from the service, the department got going on intracardiac surgery, and having Maurice Visscher[b] at the university was crucial to the development of the program.

Maurice Visscher has one of the most analytical minds I have ever known. He had been a classmate of mine at the University of Minnesota, and we were good friends. During the time of my trouble with Dr. Scammon he offered to help get me a position in Illinois where he was then located. Fortunately, this was not necessary, but in 1936 I helped get him back here to the Department of Physiology.

When he returned to the University of Minnesota, I persuaded him to have a weekly surgical-physiological conference with our department at the University Hospital. The first windfall from that association was in anesthesia. We had a group of clinical anesthesiologists here who were giving simultaneously a number of different inhalation anesthetics to their patients without knowing the concentration of any of them, and I suspected that some of these patients were dying from the anesthesia. The anesthesiologists protested, saying that there was no such thing as an anesthetic death. Obviously, they didn't know much about their own discipline. So Maurice and I went to see Alfred Nier,[b] who was in the Department of Physics. He had developed a large spectrograph and said, "There is this apparatus I'm not using at the moment. I'll let you use it." We brought that over to the hospital, and within a few weeks the anesthesiologists were convinced that they *were* killing patients. Namely, they had known nothing of the concentration of the gases they were giving at the time. With the spectrograph they could now tell exactly within a few seconds the concentrations of each.

When it came to cardiac surgery, Visscher's help was invaluable. As you know, he was one of Ernest Starling's[b] last pupils and knew more than anyone else at the time about the physiology of the circulation. He consented to take some of my boys with an interest in intracardiac surgery into his laboratory to teach them the nature of the circulation, and this became an integral part of their training.

The first man in the world to do successful open-heart surgery was John Lewis.[b] He did it under hypothermia here on September 2, 1952. DeWall[b] developed the bubble oxygenator here, and that is still widely in use. And there were a number of excellent cardiac surgeons who came out of this program.

■   When it comes to recognition, people always associate the development of heart transplantation with Chris Barnard[b] and Groote Schuur in Cape Town, but he actually trained here.

When he first came here he worked with me a year and then with Walt Lillehei.[b] When he first arrived I told him it would take five years to get his Ph.D. in surgery, and it has been related that he left my office in tears, although I was never aware of this. However, his ability and industry were such that he got his Ph.D. in two years and nine months, and I don't think anyone had ever done that before.

■ Was he frustrated when he learned of the long training period because of the limited time he had to work? I have heard that he felt his arthritis would limit the span of his surgical operative career.*

Well, that's been said. At any rate, he did the first successful heart transplant in late 1967. And some interesting things were said about it in the *South African Medical Journal.* It said that, whereas the University of South Africa and the Groote Schuur Hospital had been the stimulant for this work, the real "fairy godmother" was the University of Minnesota.

When Barnard was leaving here in 1956, he came to see me and say goodbye. I asked him how well equipped he was to continue his cardiac work, and he said, "Well, I need a heart-lung machine." He actually needed several other things as well. I asked him if he had any money for his research, and he said he had none.

In those days a surgeon who had had some successes at research could be heard in Washington most of the time, so while Barnard was in my office I called up someone in Washington and said, "I've got Dr. Chris Barnard here and he's leaving for South Africa. He's had a good deal of success with his research and needs some support." I got him approved for ten thousand dollars over the telephone.

■ "Them days are gone forever."

It was a great period, of course, and Barnard did go on to be a national hero. When I visited Cape Town in 1964 we attended a banquet, and the equivalent of what we would call a governor in the American College of Surgeons asked me about the purpose of my visit to South Africa. I said, "Well, I am here to learn and I also am not above proselytizing for American surgery." And he said, "Doctor, if you so much as raise a finger to remove Chris Barnard from this area you'll never leave here alive!" So he did do great work in that area and was greatly

*Which it finally did when he reached the age of sixty in 1983.

appreciated even before the heart transplant. The real achiever
in transplantation, of course, is Norman Shumway,[b] who was
here at the same time with Barnard.

■   There is one chapter of the transplantation story with which you perhaps
are not familiar, and it was sort of sad for the man involved. Adrian Kantrowitz[b]
had had great success with transplants in puppies, where the rejection problem
did not seem to interfere. Barnard actually spent some weeks with him before
returning to South Africa. In the winter of 1967 Kantrowitz was trying to
interest me to come to work with him at Maimonides Hospital in Brooklyn. As
you know, for years there seemed to be a tremendous psychological barrier to
doing the first human transplant in this country, but he assured me that the
next time an anencephalic baby (one without a functional brain but normal
heart) was delivered at Maimonides he would use the heart to replace that in a
baby with a severe congenital heart defect. A few weeks later news came from
Cape Town that Barnard had successfully transplanted a heart into Louis Washkansky.*

One can become very concerned about priority and that sort
of thing. You know that at one time in Great Britain, Bayliss
and Starling were coworkers at the University College, and all
the papers, even those in which the principal work was done
by Starling, came out with Bayliss's name first because it was
traditional then to list the authors alphabetically.

■   I would like to get into your interest in medical history. I have just finished
reading your book on the rise of surgery, and I was astonished at the amount of
documentation. Twenty-five percent of the book consists of source material
that I am certain will be of great help to future medical historians.

I want to make a real acknowledgment of the debt I owe my
wife, Sally, not only in this work, but she has been an ideal
wife. I suppose wives often are the causes of some men leaving the academic arena, but I've had all the encouragement
any man could hope for from her. She was a great contributor to
the book, and I think that in her time she was probably one of
the best of medical editors. She was managing editor of *Mod-*

*Three days later Kantrowitz attempted his own operation in a newborn, but it failed.

ern Medicine for over ten years, and prior to that she worked for a university president and dean as their amanuensis.

We worked twenty years on the selection of data before we ever started to write the book, and then it took us four or five years to put it all together. It is now in its third printing. We've taken no royalties except for expenses because the University of Minnesota has been so good to me.

■ You knew or met personally with a number of great surgeons, and I would like to get your impressions. You seemed to have had a closer relationship with Will Mayo rather than with his brother, Charles.

Will Mayo said they lived out of the same pocketbook when that wasn't very easy to do. But Will had a paternalistic interest in his younger brother. Charles Horatio Mayo[b] died in April 1939, and Will died the following July. My relationship was much closer to Will; he was a regent of the University of Minnesota. Will Mayo remembered everybody; Charles Mayo remembered nobody. His wife once asked him whom he was having for dinner and he said, "My chief resident, but I don't recall his name." He was a great operating surgeon but not really innovative, and his judgment was not the same as Will's. I can remember seeing a case in consultation with Charles Mayo who said the patient should have an operation. The referring physician was dissatisfied with this recommendation and called in Dr. Will Mayo. Will listened carefully— which Charles would never do (he'd raise his hand and talk before letting a fellow finish)—and then Will told the doctor just to send the patient home.

Will was a good surgeon despite the fact that he always had a tremor; it didn't seem to interfere. But more importantly it was Will who had a great influence on the development of the Mayo Clinic and its relationship to the University of Minnesota. He was a great judge of men, and when he heard a man talk in Great Falls, Montana, or wherever, he would try to interest him in the Clinic, ask him a few searching questions, and presently the fellow might get an invitation to join the Clinic mainly on the adjudication of Will Mayo. He made many wise decisions of this nature. He also encouraged research.

As you undoubtedly know, the Clinic's association with the University came about under intense protest by the clinical faculty at the university. When Dean Vincent was here between 1911 and 1917, one of his objectives was to upgrade the students' training during the clinical years. He became well acquainted with Will Mayo and was very surprised to find that here was a clinical surgeon who was actually a medical educator. The affiliation which came about between 1915 and 1917 continued to be fought against by many of the university's faculty, some of whom resigned in protest. But the alliance gained approval of the legislature in 1917, and it has been in existence ever since. I think today everybody agrees that both the Mayo Clinic and the university were winners in the process.

■   Did you know the neurosurgeon Harvey Cushing[b] at all?

When I came back from Europe, one of the first things I did was to go and spend ten days in his clinic watching him operate. He was a perfectionist. He came out of Harvard and trained under Halsted at Hopkins, but he also spent a few semesters in physiologic research abroad with Kronecker in Bern and with Charles Sherrington[b] in Liverpool. It's interesting to note that he wrote of that period abroad: "I acquired more of real value for my surgical work than in my previous six years of service as a hospital intern."

I visited him in September 1928, and during that time there was only one observer there other than myself. But if either of us moved during surgery Cushing would look up disapprovingly. He was also one of those surgeons who insisted on complete silence during an operation. He felt that the speaking of surgeons, even through a mask, was hazardous in terms of infection, and I think that was a great contribution to asepsis.

Of course, technically he was a great surgeon. Most of his assistants feared him. He was very critical. But there was actually no great school of surgeons in Boston until Harvey Cushing came along and really established the discipline of neurosurgery. There was a strong line of "surgeons-Warren" even since the Revolutionary War, but you can't build a strong faculty based on nepotism even though they were all great performers.

■ What about George Crile?[b]

He was a great individualist and a very inventive fellow. He came through with what he called anociceptor association. That involved adding a local anesthetic to general anesthesia and finally proved that this did provide additional blockage of painful stimuli to the brain. He also performed "thyroidectomy by stealth" for Graves' disease [hyperthyroidism], and I observed him doing this in 1926. It was known that these patients did not tolerate adverse stimuli well, so he would anesthetize them in their own beds several times and tell them that these were trials to note reactions. When the real operation came, the patients thought they were still undergoing another trial in bed and therefore were not overly stimulated by the knowledge that they were about to have surgery.

However, I think he wandered too far around in the whole field of surgery. In order to make a contribution I think one has to concentrate on a more limited area. But he had a great mind.

■ You knew the great German surgeon Sauerbruch.[b] I understand he was quite a character. One of my former professors had been a student of his and told me that he would take a few students with him on trips between hospitals in his limousine and during the trip ask them questions. If a student missed an answer, he was unceremoniously dumped out in the street.

Sauerbruch was a wonderful surgeon; you could communicate with him, but as you indicated, he was unpredictable. One day he would be severe to his residents, and the next day he would be more normal in his reactions. I became acquainted with a chap by the name of Rudolph Nissen who worked with Sauerbruch at the time I visited his clinic and with whom I continue to correspond up until this day. He was a marvelous type of surgical technician, and once, after observing him operate, I made a favorable comment to the head nurse who replied, "Ah, er steckt die alle in die Tasche" (He puts them all—including Sauerbruch—in his pocket).

Sauerbruch died, as you know, a senile person. They tried very hard to get him to abandon surgery at the Charité Hospital, but when he left he began to operate in his own home, I understand. Finally he stopped because the surgery was so poor.

■ He was charged at one time with Nazi sympathies, was he not?

It is true that he was under suspicion, but that charge against him was finally dismissed. In a book called *The Dismissal* by Jürgen Thorwald this case is aired, and I think it is made quite clear that he wasn't pro-Nazi. After all, he stood up boldly and courageously in public for Nissen, who was Jewish and who finally had to leave the country.

■ What about the future of surgery, especially surgical research?

On the governmental level, there have been significant contractions in financial support for research. Although we have made progress in many fields, the public's perception is that there has been a poor return on this investment of money and resources. If we can see some new breakthrough, such as was the reduction of poliomyelitis or eradication of smallpox, I think we may once again restore public confidence and obtain the support we need to advance.

As for the younger people coming up today, there are major differences compared to the past. The celibacy requirement for surgeons in training is gone, and now many of them are married and money has become more important. And they can earn so much more in private practice than they can at a medical school or university. But the lexicographer Samuel Johnson said that you can live on six pounds a year or any multiple thereof. So this difference between *need* and *want* is great, and I encourage all my trainees to recognize it.

Interest is the most important thing.

When I got my first appointment to the University of Minnesota, Dean Lyon asked me how it was that I had been only 23rd in my undergraduate class but had graduated first in my medical school class. I told him it was the development of interest in what I was doing. Richard DeWall had been in private practice for a few years in a town about twenty miles from here, but he didn't care for that kind of work. He came to me and applied for a position in our surgical program. His school records showed he had been 113th in a class of 117, but it made no difference to me. I hired him because of his interest. Well, he went on and developed the bubble oxygenator. And whenever I later recommended a man to the dean and he objected because his academic standing was not too high, I would remind him: "Remember DeWall!" Of course, we would all like to have the top people in every class come to work for us, but intense interest is the most important thing.

I don't think that anything can compare to the opportunities one can have in the academic arena. If you can develop an atmosphere friendly to learning, establish a mood of dedication—anything can happen!

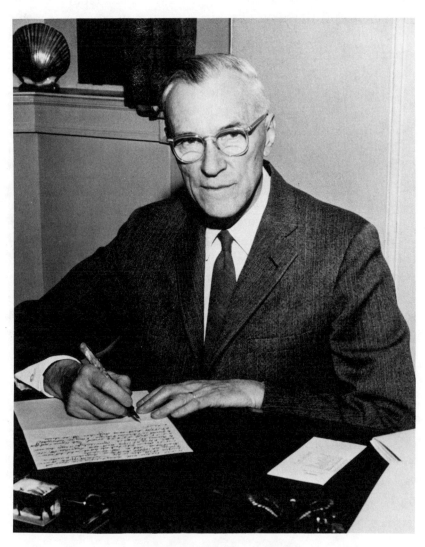

William Parry Murphy, M.D.

CHAPTER 4

William Parry Murphy, M.D.
(1892–   )

ALTHOUGH for hundreds of years there had been a clear separation between surgeons and physicians, the now well-recognized subspecialties within each group were not at all developed in the 1920s when Dr. Murphy entered practice. A medical man, for example, might have a special interest in heart disease or lung disorders or blood abnormalities, but he was still considered a general internist. Increasing knowledge about the pathogenesis, diagnosis, and treatment of a number of diseases is what permitted the establishment of various subspecialties within both of these major branches of medicine. Today even among pediatricians there are similarly recognized subspecialties in the medical and surgical areas.

In the field of hematology a major factor in its growth into an independent discipline was the ability to classify and treat a number of anemias that, in scientific terms, had previously been described in only the vaguest way. The discovery of an effective treatment for pernicious anemia by George R. Minot and William P. Murphy in 1926 can be considered the centerpiece of this development in hematology. The events leading up to, and proceeding from, this high point of achievement provide a paradigm of medical progress. For their work on pernicious anemia Minot and Murphy shared with George H. Whipple the Nobel Prize for medicine and physiology in 1934.

A brief explanation of the cause of pernicious anemia as we view it today will provide a clearer understanding of what went before. The normal production of red blood cells (erythropoiesis) depends on a number of factors, of which Vitamin B_{12} (cyanocobalamin) is but one. The steps involving this vitamin in blood production are, however, unique. The vitamin is not synthesized by the plants we eat and must be obtained from a variety of animal sources, of which liver, glandular tissue, and red meat are the most prominent. Two steps are required for B_{12} to be taken in by the body after its ingestion: (1) it must first be bound to a protein found in normal gastric juice, and (2) the gastric protein-B_{12} complex must then pass to a specific part of the small intestine (the terminal ileum) where specialized cells allow its absorption into the bloodstream.

Patients suffering from pernicious anemia have as their fundamental defect a severe atrophy of the stomach resulting in a loss or extreme deficiency of all gastric secretions, including the protein necessary for B_{12} absorption. The cause of the gastric atrophy in these patients is unknown. The clinical features of this anemia, to which Minot and Murphy turned their attention in the early 1920s, had been well described by Thomas Addison in 1855 and later came to be called "pernicious": although insidious in onset, the outcome was always fatal. Many of Minot's and Murphy's contemporaries, still understandably in awe of the accomplishments of those great nineteenth-century microbiologists, Pasteur and Koch, thought that the disease might be infectious in origin. The possibility of it being related to a nutritional deficit began to be entertained in the 1900s as evidence accumulated indicating that the absence of certain foodstuffs from the diet could cause specific diseases in man (e.g., beriberi) and be cured by their restitution. One hallmark of pernicious anemia recognized by all physicians was atrophy of the stomach and achlorhydria, the absence of the hydrochloric acid normally present in the gastric juice of man.

Popular belief had long attributed therapeutic benefits to various foods, but it was not until the pathologist George Whipple's studies at the University of Rochester that some quantitative effort was made to evaluate the direct effect of diet on blood formation. Whipple's experiments were done on dogs that had been made anemic by bleeding and that were fed on a salmon bread diet to maintain a stable low hemoglobin content of the blood to serve as a baseline for evaluating the efficacy of various foods in returning the blood toward normal. He found liver, kidney, and beef, in that order, to be the most effective foods. It was his success with liver that prompted Minot to try this treatment on his patients after a visit with Whipple in 1922–23.

Minot and Murphy acknowledged that diet had been used as part of the therapy of pernicious anemia in the past but pointed out that a certain food "had often been selected because it appeared to be easily digested or because it seemed particularly nutritious and strength giving. Rarely have diets been chosen for some assumed direct effect on the blood."

The selection of liver by Minot and Murphy provides, in retrospect, one of the odd quirks of medical research where error results in success all the same. Whipple had not really characterized the type of anemia that occurred in his bled dogs, one that we would now immediately know to be the iron deficiency type. If he had, Minot and Murphy might not have tried liver in their patients because they had already administered iron without success. It turns out that liver has high concentrations of both iron and vitamin B_{12}. Thus, high liver diets cured both the iron deficiency anemia in Whipple's dogs and the pernicious anemia in Minot's and Murphy's patients. What also helped these two investigators at the time was the introduction of new stains to recognize and count young red cells (reticulocytes). The rapid increase in these counts after effective therapy helped in documenting its value before the standard hemoglobin and red cell counts changed significantly.

Dr. William B. Castle, who at the time was working at the Thorndike Laboratory in Boston City Hospital as a junior staff member, carried the work one step further. "Why," he asked himself, "do normal people not need large amounts of liver to stave off pernicious anemia?" He turned his attention to the abnormal stomach. He fed patients beef patties both before and after having the patties exposed to normal gastric juice. He learned that it was not the absence of hydrochloric acid that caused the disease but another unknown factor in the gastric juices, a substance he called the "intrinsic factor" and that was later recognized to be a binding protein. The food substance needed in our diet in addition to this factor in the stomach he called the "extrinsic factor." These findings were published in 1929. Although there remain some unanswered questions about pernicious anemia, the final piece of the puzzle was more or less put in place when in 1948 Berk and his colleagues isolated vitamin B_{12} and identified it as the extrinsic factor.

Pernicious anemia is a disease that affects both the formation of the red blood cells and the spinal cord tracts. These patients have symptoms related to both the anemia and the nervous system. Before the introduction of liver therapy, medication with arsenic-containing compounds and even splenectomy were tried, obviously without success. Blood transfusions served only to prolong life a little. The impact of liver therapy was dramatic, the large amounts of B_{12} contained therein overcoming the patients' lack of the intrinsic factor. In 1926 almost 6,000 Americans were dying each year from the disease. By 1934 when Whipple, Minot, and Murphy received their Nobel Prize, the presenter estimated that since their discovery between 15,000 and 20,000 lives had been saved in the United States alone. The ingestion of such large amounts of liver (a half pound daily) was soon replaced by liver extract injections and eventually by B_{12} itself when it was finally isolated.

When I finally met Dr. Murphy, he was in his eighty-seventh year and suffering from the aftereffects of a "stroke." I was most impressed that this was, indeed, a gentle-man and reassured by the knowledge that one did not have to be ruthless, overbearing, or highly competitive in order to achieve one's aims in life. I recalled that Dr. Dock, a superlative bedside physician himself, had named Dr. Murphy as among the best of a number of historically astute physicians who worked at the Peter Bent Brigham Hospital in their time. I recognized also that there must have been a will of iron behind this gentle exterior, a will that enabled him to do the work he did with Minot in the face of all the skepticism that initially met them. In learning about his enterprising physician son, who has also been responsible for medical innovations, and about his daughter, who also pioneered in her own tragic way, it became apparent to me that these exceptional qualities had obviously been passed on to his children.

■ You were a grade-school teacher in mathematics and physics for two years before you even went into medicine.

Yes, I did some teaching to earn some money to go to medical school. I was born in Stoughton, Wisconsin, but moved with my parents to Oregon where I attended the University of Oregon. My father was a minister and ministers weren't paid much in those days, so I had to earn some money to go to medical school, which even then was fairly expensive. I took the first year of medicine at the University of Oregon but then was able to go to Harvard.

■ How did that happen?

Back in Wisconsin before we headed west I worked for a local weekly newspaper in a town called Trempealeau. I used to set type for the paper while I was a high school student. After we moved to Oregon the woman who ran the paper continued to send me copies. There were local items on the front page, but there was not enough local material to fill up the entire paper, so inside she would use clippings from various other newspapers to fill out the paper. It was in one of these that I read that a Dean Briggs from Harvard was going to give the baccalaureate address at Reed College, which was only about twenty miles from Portland.

I got up the courage to call him out at the college after he arrived and asked if it would be possible for me to see him at Reed College while he was there. He said, "Oh, sure. But you don't need to come out here. I'll drive into town to meet you anyplace you want." I said, "How about the YMCA?" and he replied that that would be fine. So I met him at ten o'clock in the morning at the YMCA in Portland and then he said, "Do you know who I am?" I told him, "No. I know nothing about you except that you are from Harvard, and I thought I might talk to you about getting a scholarship to Harvard Medical School."

He said, "Well, that's interesting. I happen to be the chairman of the scholarship committee." We talked a little longer and then he said, "You know, I'm going to recommend you for a scholarship to Harvard." I thanked him and told him that that would be very nice, and he said, "The committee has never turned down my recommendation."

■ That's remarkable. But what commended you to him—you, a perfect stranger who just "walked in off the street" asking for a scholarship to Harvard?

Well, you see, there was this fellow by the name of Murphy who had died in Boston and left some money for a scholarship to Harvard with the provision that each year it be given to someone with the name of Murphy.

■ Was this indicated in the newspaper item you saw? Did you know they were looking for someone like you?

No, no. I knew nothing about that. It wasn't in the newspaper. Dean Briggs just told me about the scholarship after we had spoken awhile at the YMCA, and he said, "You will be the first one to receive the William Stanislaus Murphy Fellowship at Harvard."

■ I guess that's what they call the luck of the Irish! Who were some of the prominent people active while you were a medical student there?

Dr. Cannon[b] was there, but I didn't have an opportunity to do any work with him directly. Later on, as a medical resident at the Brigham Hospital, I used to go to Dr. Joslin's[b] [diabetes] clinic a great deal. Then when Banting[b] and Best[b] discovered insulin they decided to designate eight clinics throughout the country to test it. Dr. Fitz[b] and I were interested in diabetes at the time, and so we were one of the eight.

■ **What was Dr. Joslin like? Did he really terrorize his patients to get them to follow his diets as they say?**

He was a nice old gentleman, but he was very adamant about the details of his treatment and very much against alcohol of any sort, just on general principles. While we were doing the pernicious anemia work I had occasion to send him a patient for evaluation for possible diabetes. This was an Irish lady, and she asked him, "Would it do any harm if I take a drink occasionally?" He told her, "It will probably do you less harm than anything else." Assuming that she had pernicious anemia, he estimated that she did not have more than a year to live anyway, since that was the expected survival in those days.

■ **Before you ever got into pernicious anemia you published a half-dozen papers concerning diabetes but also another paper with a very unusual title: "A Study of the Value of Osteopathic Adjustment of the Fourth and Fifth Thoracic Vertebrae in a Series of Twenty Cases of Asthmatic Bronchitis." I'm sorry that I haven't read it, but what was all this about?**

One of our visiting physicians was an osteopath, Dr. Channing Frothingham, and some osteopaths had approached him and asked him if someone might do this study for them at the hospital. He referred them to me, so I did some work with the osteopaths.

■ **Did it do any good?**

No. They finally agreed with me that it didn't do much good.

■ **How did you get involved with Dr. Minot[b] and the work on pernicious anemia?**

When I finished residency training at the Peter Bent Brigham Hospital in 1923, I was looking to go into practice. Dr.

Joslin asked me if I would like to join his group; Dr. Lahey[b] asked me if I would like to join his group; and Dr. Edwin Locke[b] asked me if I would like to go with him. He headed a new group of physicians, of which Dr. Minot was one. I was interested in hematology and knew that Dr. Minot was also interested in the blood, so I became the youngest member of this group. I became Dr. Minot's assistant, and we used to see his patients together. I would see the patients before he did and examine them and tell him what I thought each patient had. We would discuss the patient together, and then I usually followed them after he had seen them for the initial evaluation.

He was about seven years older than I, pleasant, but sometimes a little difficult to work with. He used to write notes to me on scratch paper, and I was supposed to read these notes before the patient came in. Because he wrote so badly it usually took me all day to decipher them, and often I did not quite have them deciphered when he was ready to see the patient. He was often upset about that, but then we all have our problems.

When we started our work on pernicious anemia it was a fatal disease. The patients became quite weak and didn't eat very well, and many of them couldn't walk because of the spinal cord changes. Many of them came to us in wheelchairs. They were usually in their fifties, although I had some patients in their thirties. They usually had blood transfusions, which kept them alive, but if they missed their transfusions they were likely to die. Very few of them lived more than a year or so.

The thing that interested us in the use of liver was Whipple's[b] work on dogs where this seemed to be of use in the experimental anemia he produced. We also were helped in evaluating patients because of the reticulocyte counts, because these would tell us very early, before the hemoglobin content went up appreciably, whether or not a specific therapy was helping a patient.

In 1925 we decided to hospitalize a group of pernicious anemia patients at the Brigham Hospital and systematically evaluate the liver treatment. I was at the Brigham at the time, and Dr. Minot was medical chief at the Collis B. Huntington Hospital next door where we evaluated the effects of the treatment in the hematology laboratory.

Dr. Henry Christian[b] was chief of medicine at the Brigham at the time and agreed to let us do the work there as long as we did not let the patients die. If the liver was not helping the patient, we had to give him a blood transfusion instead. When we brought in the first patient, Dr. Frothingham was in charge of the ward; he and Dr. Christian were both very skeptical about what liver would do. And, of course, the house officers wanted to give him transfusions because there weren't too many blood transfusions done in those days and they wanted the experience.*

We brought the first patient in and started feeding him liver. By midnight of the fourth day I found that the reticulocytes had gone up to four percent, and I thought he was probably going to be all right, so I insisted on withholding the transfusions. I went home and slept restlessly and got back to the hospital at seven the next morning. The residents used to eat breakfast at seven, and I wanted to be sure I got to see the patient before they did; but the thought also crossed my mind that I might find him dead. I went over to his bed, and he looked up at me and sat up and said, "Aren't we going to have any breakfast?" I knew then that he would be all right.

■ After your success with those forty-five patients at the Brigham, Dr. Peabody[b] over at the Thorndike (Memorial Laboratory, Boston City Hospital) wanted to verify your results, and apparently this spurred Dr. Castle[b] on to do his work on feeding beef patties to pernicious anemia patients after they had been incubated in normal gastric juice as opposed to their own atrophic stomachs. I always wondered: Did Castle use himself as the source for this gastric juice?

---

*Some things never change.

Yes, I think he did.*

■ I wonder if he was attempting this experiment today, what with all the "informed consent" business, he would ever be able to get patients to ingest, even through a nasogastric tube, food that had been partially digested in someone else's stomach juices. Knowing the precise details, many patients might not be all that cooperative, and we might still not know the real cause of pernicious anemia. Did you have any idea that this work would lead to a Nobel Prize? And how did it affect your life?

I never thought anything about the Nobel Prize while we were doing this work. Of course, after we received the prize it changed my life in that people wanted more consultations. I was also invited to speak before many groups, and I did quite a bit of traveling.

I still see a few patients whom I have treated for a great many years and who insist on continuing to see me. Of those first forty-five patients we reported in 1926 I still see two. In one family I have treated three generations with the disease.

In one of the patients whom I had treated for pernicious anemia for fifty years there developed a complete heart block, and they had to put a permanent cardiac pacemaker in her. I later found out that the pacemaker they put in her was one made by my son, William Parry Murphy, Jr. He is also a physician but went into this business of making pacemakers and artificial kidneys and so forth. He founded the Cordis Corporation and was its president until recently.

■ Well, that's certainly keeping the care of the patient within the same medical family. You also had a daughter, but if you don't wish to talk about her we don't have to. She was very young . . .

Yes, she was. She was nineteen and the youngest licensed pilot in the United States at the time. She had taken off from

*Dr. Castle wrote me: "For the first few observations when the result of employing normal human gastric juice and beef muscle was uncertain I was the source of the gastric juice. Thereafter, over the years, the source became a series of medical students who were paid for their services as 'gastric juicers'. . . . I was an expert at passing the tube on myself and . . . the patients."

Logan Airport and was practicing in the same area that Amelia Earhart was using. She ran into a snowstorm and crashed into a small mountain near Syracuse, New York.

■   Do you have any regrets at all about your life?

Just that I haven't been aggressive enough. I think I have been rather shy and not likely to speak up about problems in medicine that bothered me. Perhaps I should have.

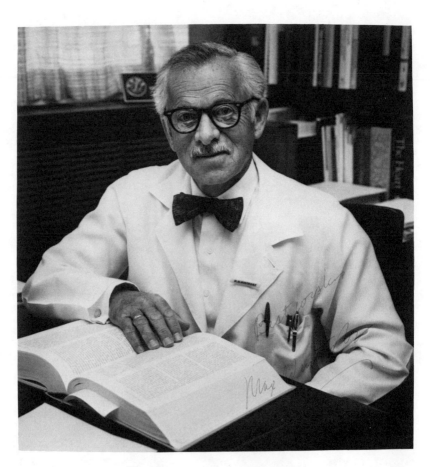

Maxwell M. Wintrobe, M.D., Ph.D.

CHAPTER 5

Maxwell M. Wintrobe, M.D., Ph.D.
(1901–   )

THE MEDICAL CAREER of Dr. Wintrobe, consciously or not, followed a course similar to that of his great idol and, more than any man, the father of American Medicine, William Osler. Osler, who helped found our first great medical school at Johns Hopkins and spent his best years there, was born in Canada and died Sir William Osler at Oxford, England. Dr. Wintrobe, another Canadian, also made a name for himself at Johns Hopkins, but then this young man went west—to Utah.

As with all aware young physicians of his generation, Dr. Wintrobe's imagination was sparked by the exciting discoveries of Whipple, Minot, and Murphy that had just been made known; indeed, his own initial work was in pernicious anemia, as we shall see. Equally if not more important at the beginning of his career was his appreciation of the incomplete and haphazard nature of our knowledge of the blood at that time.

He found, for example, that as late as in the 1920s the values accepted as normal for the red cell count of men and women had been based on the examination of two subjects, in 1852 and 1854, by inaccurate and obsolete methods. The classifications of anemia had no rational basis. It depended on the so-called color index: the percent hemoglobin divided by the erythrocyte (red blood cell) count and multiplied by two. All those with a color index greater than one were classified as having "primary" anemias, the rest, as having "secondary" anemias. The methods for determining hemoglobin and the red cell count were, themselves, subject to considerable error.

Early on Dr. Wintrobe introduced the use of a simple and reliable method of evaluating the blood, the hematocrit, where a sample was centrifuged and the column of red cells expressed as a percentage of the total column of cells and plasma. At about this time he also introduced a system for classifying anemias on the basis of size (normo-, micro-, macrocytic) and red cell hemoglobin content (normo-, hypochromic) and calculating indices on this basis. These innovations have persisted to the present and have formed a foundation upon which modern hematology could develop. His subsequent work in and of itself, together with its various offshoots in other branches of science, has contributed to many areas of medicine.

The arrival of Wintrobe in Utah had a profound effect, not only on that state and an area constituting almost a third of the continental United States of which Utah represented the geographical center, but on medicine in general. His presence enabled the medical school there to attract a number of other outstanding people in both the clinical and the basic sciences.

The affection and admiration that Dr. Wintrobe maintains for Johns Hopkins is evident even today. It was during the thirteen years he spent there, after his first brief tenure at Tulane, that he first spread his professional wings, and he brought the Hopkins standards of excellence with him to Utah to create his own medical citadel. With the publication of his monograph, *Clinical Hematology*, written solely by him until the seventh and latest edition, his reputation became international, and we who worked in Utah were witness to the constant flow of patients coming to visit Dr. Wintrobe from all over the globe.

Toward the end of each academic year in the sizable hospital amphitheater there would often be an occasion for Dr. Wintrobe to say goodbye to those staff members and fellows going off to start or continue their careers elsewhere. I recall Dr. Wintrobe announcing each departure and saying something to the effect that Doctor so-and-so was going to such-and-such a place "to show them how it's done." He no doubt kept in mind the words of Johns Hopkins President Isaiah Bowman over twenty-five years before about the responsibility for Hopkins men to "plant the seeds" elsewhere. Dr. Wintrobe has indeed "planted many seeds" throughout the world.

Today Dr. Wintrobe is still active in a variety of hematological and educational pursuits, his range of activity and physical vigor belying his years. I missed seeing him on that visit to Utah I mentioned in the Introduction—he was off on another junket—but I managed to catch up with him some months later in Paris where he was attending an international symposium on blood disease.

Before this trip I had taken the opportunity to view a videotape on *Leaders in American Medicine* in which he was interviewed by another former cardiology fellow from Utah, Alexander ("Mac") Schmidt. I told Dr. Wintrobe when I saw him that although all the facts seemed to be there, somehow the end result struck me—to use Dr. Wintrobe's own terminology—as somewhat microcytic and hypochromic. Perhaps it was the inhibiting effect of all those television lights. As we sat and chatted in a quiet corner of a hotel lobby in Paris one afternoon, I trust we were somewhat more successful.

■ In 1846 Brigham Young looked down on what was to become Salt Lake City and said, "This is the place." Almost one hundred years later Max Wintrobe, in a somewhat different context, apparently made the same decision. How did this come about?

I was at Hopkins and, because of my Canadian upbringing, hardly knew where Utah was when, in 1942 or 1943, I received a letter from Phil Price, who had recently become head of the Department of Surgery at the proposed four-year medical school at the University of Utah. We had become acquainted when he was at Hopkins doing experimental surgery. He asked me if I would be interested in coming out to Utah to head the Department of Medicine.

This was during the war, and there was a good deal of concern at the time about the future need for more doctors. Utah had a two-year school and sent its students to other schools for the clinical years. I had noticed two or three of them at Hopkins, and those I met seemed quite nice and good student material. That's about all I knew about Utah and its people until then.

The dean at Utah's medical school was Cyril Callister, a Harvard graduate. He was an active surgeon in the community and a very determined and energetic person. He and a few other influential medical people in Salt Lake City had decided that this was an opportune time to expand the school to a four-year program. He had gone to school with Alan Gregg[b] of the Rockefeller Foundation, and it was Gregg who had suggested my name to him.

I showed the letter from Dr. Price to my wife that evening,

and her first questions were, "Where is Utah? *What* is Utah?" We had seen the movie, *Brigham Young,* and that was the extent of the knowledge we had of Utah. So we went to the local library and looked up Utah in the *Encyclopaedia Britannica* and learned what we could. Although I did not take the offer too seriously, we decided that I should go out and see what it was all about. When I met Callister, he took me to dinner at the country club and made sure that I sat where I could get a very good view of the mountains and the green lawns and the golf course. It was obviously beautiful country, but all he had to offer me were a lot of promises and nothing really tangible regarding the future of the medical school. They then had a two-year school on the campus of the University of Utah, and had made arrangements with the county commissioners to use the old Salt Lake County Hospital, a dilapidated institution run by politicians, as the "University Hospital."

When I returned to Baltimore, I asked various people for their opinions. The most important advice, the one that clinched my decision, came from Isaiah Bowman, who was then president of Johns Hopkins University. He said, "I know you have talked to various people, but perhaps there is one point of view that I might bring to your attention, and that others may not have raised. You know that I am a geographer by profession, and what strikes me about Utah is that this is the last frontier of medicine in this country."

I was a little startled at this comment. He continued, "Do you realize that there is no medical school between Denver and the Pacific Coast and the Canadian and Mexican borders? And even on the Pacific Coast there is only Oregon, Stanford, the University of California in San Francisco, and the University of Southern California. So in an area representing almost a third of the area of the entire United States there is no full-fledged medical school. That is why it strikes me as the last frontier."

He told me, "We are in the midst of a war now, and you were asked to remain here at Hopkins to help run the department and hospital while many of our people went off to their units. We need you here, but we also have another mission: that is to develop people who will 'plant the seeds' elsewhere. Consequently, while we would like you to stay, on the other hand you really should look at this offer from the standpoint of whether this is an opportunity that deserves to be taken." My wife and I thought about it and decided to go.

Our trip to Utah was somewhat arduous and our arrival quite depressing. We drove across the country in our old Chevrolet: my wife, who was pregnant with our second child, our six-year-old daughter, and myself. The trip through the Rocky Mountain National Park was very lovely, but then we headed through the desert toward Vernal, Utah. As we approached Vernal I said to my wife, "Look, Dinosaur National Monument is near here. Shouldn't we stop and see it?" She said, "I can see dinosaurs all around here! The country looks as if there was a geological upheaval the day before yesterday. Let's get out of here."

When we stopped for lunch at a restaurant in a little "jerkwater" town whose name I don't remember, there was a noisy jukebox there but no food. We tried another place nearby where they had food, but also the biggest swarm of flies we had ever seen. They also had a Utah newspaper with a headline reading "Polio Epidemic Raging in Salt Lake City." And here we were with a six-year-old child and my wife pregnant. From that point on she was in tears.

When we arrived in Salt Lake City we spent our first night with the Prices. The next day we found quarters in a motel that was far removed from the nice home we had in Baltimore. Coal-burning trains ran through Salt Lake City then, and the window sills as well as the curtains were black with soot. We remained there for six weeks. That was the discouraging beginning at Utah. Now, fortunately, things have changed, and we see only beauty in our surroundings.

■ The arrangements to use the County Hospital, I take it, were to be only temporary, awaiting the end of the war. How long did you wait for your real university hospital?

Twenty-two years.

■ Now that we have you in Utah, may we go back to your earlier days? You were in born in Halifax, Nova Scotia, and then moved to Winnipeg.

Yes. My parents immigrated to Canada from Austria, and I was the only child. My father was in the furniture business, never doing too well. As I grew older he frequently suggested that I should consider taking a job to earn a living. I did earn a few dollars by doing a great variety of jobs, but my mother had something "academic" in her blood, although, as far as I know, there was no tradition of scholarship in the family before. She urged me to continue my studies and to work hard at them. I entered the University of Manitoba in Winnipeg a month before my sixteenth birthday and got my bachelor's degree in 1921, majoring in French and political economy.

After I started medical school at the University of Manitoba, I became interested in medical history and in the people who had contributed to medicine. I particularly remember reading about Johns Hopkins, and I was anxious to transfer there. In my second year at Manitoba I made some inquiries, but it was obvious that it would be too costly. The tuition was $600 a year at Hopkins compared to $150 where I was. Then there would be the additional costs of living away from home. But Hopkins was always in the back of my mind. Cushing's[b] *Life of Osler* made a great impression on me, and Osler became my hero and role model.

■ What happened after medical school?

The one thing I was convinced of when I graduated was that I really knew very, very little. My ignorance was enormous. I felt I couldn't go into practice because I didn't know enough to do a decent job. I took a protracted internship lasting about fifteen months and then was offered a fellowship that had just been established in honor of the retiring dean, Gordon Bell.

This happened to be at the time that Minot's and Murphy's work about the liver treatment of pernicious anemia had just appeared, and it was a very exciting period in clinical medicine and medical research. I accepted the fellowship totally inexperienced in research and, without any guidance, began to do some experimental work in dogs, trying to produce a model of pernicious anemia by destroying the gastric mucosa. We had just been through the great age of bacteriology, and we were all full of Koch's[b] postulates at the time—in order to understand a disease you must be able to reproduce it in an animal. While I was unsuccessfully making these attempts in dogs, the professor of medicine at Manitoba suggested that I compare the gastric contents of the inhabitants of the town of Holland, Manitoba, where pernicious anemia seemed to be relatively common, with those of the residents of Stonewall, where few cases had developed. I went to these towns and got all sorts of people to submit to my doing gastric analyses and checking for achlorhydria.*

While carrying on these studies I began to make plans for the future. At one point I thought I might like to go to the Mayo Clinic. Rochester, Minnesota, was not far from Winnipeg, and attracted all kinds of patients. So I thought that if I could get a fellowship in surgery there I would become a surgeon and earn a lot of money. Crass motivation! I don't suppose I really had my heart in it, though. They interviewed me and offered me a fellowship in pediatrics. I turned that down because I had read an advertisement in the *JAMA* [*Journal of the American Medical Association*] for an assistant in medicine [the rank below instructor] at Tulane in New Orleans. I

---

*Absence of hydrochloric acid in the stomach, characteristic of pernicious anemia patients.

applied for this job and was accepted. That is how my career really started.

■ You spent three years, 1927–30, at Tulane and then went to Hopkins. How did you spend those years?

When I got to New Orleans I groped around for something to do in research. Tulane had a stimulating full-time Department of Medicine; the whole school was stimulating, and the clinical material at Charity Hospital was superb. The dean, C. C. Bass, was a very fine person. He was interested in research and took an interest in me. The professor of medicine was John Musser, Jr., whose father had been the famous professor of medicine in Philadelphia.

It was the dean who had hired me while Musser was away in Europe for the summer. When Musser returned he noted that I had worked in pernicious anemia in Winnipeg and said, "Since you have already started work on the blood, why don't you continue?" He told me that there was a question that would be interesting for me to explore. "It is said that there is an anemia of the South; that normal blood values in the South are lower than those in the North. Why don't you look into that?"

So I proceeded to do this.* But as I read up on the literature concerning the blood, I soon discovered that there were no reliable normal blood values. What was called "normal" was based on only a few counts that had been made in the nineteenth century. So I proceeded to collect normal blood values. Others elsewhere, also mindful of this deficiency, were beginning to do the same. A major problem, however, was methodology, and this was what led me to devise the hematocrit as a simple and accurate means of quantitating blood. I began to accumulate considerable material, and in view of the fact that Tulane offered a Ph.D. in medicine, I decided to register

*This was found by Dr. Wintrobe not to be so.

for this degree, using my research on the red blood cell for my thesis. The document I prepared was fairly substantial and ultimately published under the title, "The Erythrocyte in Man."

It was in the process of preparing my thesis that I recognized the need for a knowledge of statistics so as to present adequately the data I was collecting. My interest in statistics led me to Raymond Pearl who, in turn, led me to Johns Hopkins.

Pearl was a biometrician at Hopkins who had written a book called *Biometry in Medicine*. His book was not only instructive but was written with a sense of humor that occasionally had me burst out in laughter as I read it. Nonetheless, I had some difficulties in understanding parts of it. I wrote him about these, and Dr. Pearl suggested that I visit him in Baltimore so that we might go over my data together. As I was reading Dr. Pearl's letter, Dean Bass happened by and inquired, as was his custom, how I was getting along. When he learned of Dr. Pearl's offer he said, "Why don't you go?" I replied that it was a long trip and expensive. And he said, "Oh, we'll pay for it." I hadn't dreamed that any institution would pay for a member of its staff to travel so far. This was a very new idea to me.

When I got to Baltimore, in the course of seeing Professor Pearl, I told him how I had always wanted to go to Hopkins. He arranged for me to meet Alan Chesney,[b] the dean of the medical school, and I told Chesney of my interest. Unfortunately, there were no openings at the time. However, Chesney was editor of the journal, *Medicine*, and, not long after our conversation, read my manuscript on the erythrocyte because *Medicine* was the logical place in which to publish it. Meanwhile, Duke University was organizing its medical school and drawing away a number of people from Hopkins. When a vacancy developed in the Clinical Microscopy Division of the Department of Medicine, Dr. Chesney offered me a position as an instructor of medicine at Hopkins.

The salary was to be twenty-seven hundred dollars a year, three hundred dollars more than I was getting at Tulane. That looked pretty good, because I had been recently married and I was also helping my parents. I told Dr. Musser of the Hopkins offer, and he raised my salary at Tulane to three thousand dollars. For me this was a significant amount, and I had to write Hopkins that I couldn't turn this down. They came back with a telegram: "We'll give you $3000." So I went to Hopkins.

■ I read your paper from 1930 on the simple and accurate hematocrit. This must have been before you met Pearl because the very last sentence reads, "A long experience with this instrument has convinced me of its uniform accuracy." There are no statistics, no tabulations, no patient data, and, as for your "long experience," you were all of twenty-eight years old. If you submitted such a paper today I suspect you might have some trouble getting it accepted.

Well, it was a very short paper. But I can see how funny that "long experience" must have sounded. It certainly does now.

■ To get into something else now, you went into academic medicine when it was essentially a WASP preserve, usually very well-heeled WASPs as well. How was it for the son of poor Austrian immigrants to venture into that territory as you did?

Baltimore was an uncomfortable place to live in because it was segregated in so many ways. However, I was there to learn and to work, and that was what really mattered.

■ You were at Hopkins for thirteen years. Did you feel you might never reach the top because of your background? Was this what made you leave finally?

My wife urged me to leave Hopkins when the opportunity came to go to Utah. "You will become an 'old fogy' here," she said. And it was obvious that I would never get a top job. I hoped that, perhaps, I would reach the rank of associate professor. That was my goal. But I was satisfied in the sense that I was able to work. The atmosphere was excellent; the standards of medical care were "tops"; and the people were very good. Everything there encouraged research and inquiry. It was a splendid place to work.

■ What was the status of hematology when you began your work?

There was no such discipline as hematology then. There were a few people known to be interested in the heart, but the subspecialties as such were not yet recognized. Until 1926 hematology consisted mostly of counting cells and looking at blood smears. That was the impact of Ehrlich[b] who had introduced stains for blood cells. But in 1926 Whipple,[b] Minot,[b] and Murphy opened the way to a new era in the study of blood diseases and, for that matter, clinical investigation.

■ The emphasis in early hematology seemed to be on the effects of nutrition primarily. Why the emphasis on this?

Partly because Minot was a very severe diabetic, and he was very concerned with his own diet and that of his patients. The focus of his thinking was: What influence will specific diets have on patients? We were ignorant about such things in those days. After all, the word "vitamin" was not coined until 1912. We spoke of "B complex vitamins" at the time, but didn't really know of what they consisted.

■ You did an awful lot of work with pigs when you got to Baltimore. Why was this so?

I was still trying to produce pernicious anemia. I and others had unsuccessfully tried to produce an animal model in dogs, rabbits, and guinea pigs. Then, in reviewing Ehrlich's work, I found that he had said that the fetus possesses red cells just like the abnormal large red cells seen in pernicious anemia [megaloblasts]. So I thought a possibility was that the unborn fetus was in a state resembling pernicious anemia and that this changed by the time of birth when normal red cell production takes place. I was anxious to study the blood of fetuses to confirm what Ehrlich had said. Fortunately, there was a slaughterhouse near Hopkins where I was able to obtain many pig fetuses. Each sow that was slaughtered had between eight and twelve fetuses, so my technician and I would go there and collect the day's slaughter to examine the blood of fetuses of different ages. I was able to show that, in the youngest, the red cells are very large like megaloblasts, although few in number; but as the fetus ages the red cells become smaller and more numerous, just as in the pernicious anemia patient who is treated successfully.

That was encouraging, so I thought I would try to produce pernicious anemia in newborn pigs by withholding Castle's[b] "extrinsic factor" from their diet. The choice of the pig was fortunate because they grow rapidly, and the effects of any dietary deficiency on the blood appears very quickly.

But it was quite a job to get this under way. I made arrangements with the Department of Agriculture to get newborn pigs from them. I also managed to get a "big" research grant of five thousand dollars from the Parke-Davis Company to support the research. This, incidentally, was frowned upon as "dirty money" by some of the people at Hopkins. Accepting money from a pharmaceutical house had never been done there before.

At any rate, in order to feed these piglets, we prepared artificial teats attached to warm bags in which we put the artificial milk. We were afraid that the piglets would not suckle anything but a live sow. The great day came when we got hold of some pigs only about two weeks old. As we began to try to feed them, my technician, who was all keyed up about it, spilled some of the milk on the floor. I thought a minor disaster was in the making, but what did the piglets do? They simply drank it up right off the floor. So all our elaborate preparations to feed them had been unnecessary.

These pig-feeding experiments were important in demonstrating the essential role of a number of B vitamins in erythropoiesis [red cell production], and we still are using that animal in Utah. An unexpected finding was that the brewer's yeast we were giving to the pigs as a source of B vitamins was a potent antianemic agent in pernicious anemia. Although it altered the blood picture, it had no effect on the spinal cord, the neurological changes. Later it became apparent that the active agent in yeast that accounted for this was folic acid.

■ You once wrote an article called "Anemia, Serendipity and Science" in which you recounted the story of sickle-cell anemia. I like to recall that a man noted for his contributions to heart disease, James B. Herrick,[b] was the first to describe these cells, but a chance occurrence between you and a student really put us on the right track about what was causing this. I would like to hear the story directly from you.

While I was at Hopkins teaching clinical microscopy, I was approached by a bright student, Irving Sherman, who told me about his interest in genetics, and wondered about doing some research with me. I was happy to encourage this sort of thing and suggested to him that he might like to try and confirm the findings of Hahn and Gillespie, who had reported changes in the shape of the sickle cell as it was exposed to different gas mixtures. So he started off on this project and confirmed their observations. In addition, in examining the red cells that were deprived of oxygen with appropriate microscope oculars, he observed that they were birefringent [refracting light in two slightly different directions so as to split a single ray into two]. I confirmed his observation but could not figure out what it meant. Neither could the physical chemists we consulted at the school.

Sherman was about to omit this finding from his report because of our inability to explain it, but fortunately I insisted that he include it. We had both seen it, and even if we did not know what it meant, it was a fact and it should be recorded, I argued. And so it was included in the *Bulletin* of the Johns Hopkins Hospital in 1940. "Bill" Castle read the paper and was as intrigued about this as I was, and his fellow, Bill Harris, confirmed our observation.

The problem continued to occupy his mind, and one day

while riding on the same train as Linus Pauling[b] he mentioned it to Pauling. Pauling immediately saw the possible explanation and investigated the problem. In 1949 he published his now famous paper in *Science* about sickle-cell anemia as a molecular disease.

■ And so did molecular biology get a big lift. Whatever happened to the budding hematologist-geneticist Sherman?

They had a symposium on hematology at the centennial celebration at Hopkins a few years ago, and Irving Sherman was there. He is a successful practicing neurosurgeon in Connecticut, and, as far as I know, that was the only research he ever did—in hematology or in any other field.

■ Before you left Hopkins you also discovered that Cooley's or Mediterranean anemia (thalassemia) was not necessarily always a severe and fatal disease. This too had genetic implications, did it not?

When Cooley first described the disease in 1925, it was not realized that there was a minor, less serious form. We now know that the severe form represents the homozygous* form of the disease, and the less severe disease, Thalassemia minor, the heterozygous form of the disease. But then we knew nothing of the genetics of this condition. Today it seems almost incomprehensible that, when Cooley studied his patients and recognized that their brothers and sisters might have the same condition, he never thought of looking at the parents.

I came into this again through a side door. A practice I established in the outpatient clinic was to have a blood smear made on every patient who came in. Whenever my technician came across anything unusual, she would bring it to my attention. One day a patient came in complaining of a headache, and my technician noted stippling of his red cells. There was no apparent explanation. Soon afterwards, I saw two more patients with unexplained stippling of the red cells, and all

*Homozygous is when the gene is carried by both parents and transmitted to the child; heterozygous is when the gene is carried by one one parent.

three were Italians. Then a sixteen-year-old boy was admitted to the wards, and he was found to have a microcytic hypochromic anemia resembling that of iron deficiency anemia but was resistant to iron therapy. He, too, had stippling. We ultimately reported these unusual cases as examples of a condition resembling Cooley's anemia but milder in degree. We later learned that in Europe two years earlier similar findings had been reported by a Greek investigator, Caminopetros. Shortly after our paper had been written a child with the severe form of Cooley's anemia was admitted to the Pediatric Service at Hopkins. I was asked to see him, and this gave me the opportunity of also examining the blood of his parents. They had the same stippling we had seen in the Italian adolescents and adults we were in the process of reporting. I added a footnote to the paper in which I mentioned this finding. That was in 1940. The full details of the whole homozygous/heterozygous state were later worked out by Jim Neel and Bill Valentine at Rochester, where many cases of thalassemia were available. We had anticipated their findings by several years.*

■ Speaking of your book, *Clinical Hematology,* I must say as a non-hematologist that it is a model of clarity and organization. Is there any special quality in yourself to which you attribute this?

I don't know. I remember that in my first year in college I had to write an essay which I entitled "Straining at a Rat," I believe. I was complimented on this by my professor, and I suppose that was the first time I realized I could write.

As for my work habits, I strongly believe it is unwise to try to work when you are fatigued. One only wastes time that way. So I rarely work beyond ten-thirty or eleven at night.

*The same sort of situation applies to sickle-cell anemia. If only one abnormal gene is inherited from a parent the patient is heterozygous and said to have sickle-cell trait. Such individuals have no symptoms. When both parents are carriers of the trait and the child receives an abnormal gene from each of them, he is homozygous for this and is affected by the disease. At one time there was a furor over excluding some young black men as air cadets when it was found that they had the trait, for this was really not scientifically valid.

There again is the influence of my hero, Osler. He made it a habit of putting aside his medical work at ten in the evening, and then he read anything but medicine. One practice I did develop, though, was to keep paper and pencil beside me when I went to bed because I found that an idea might come to me in the middle of the night. Unless I was able to get it down on paper it might have escaped me by the following morning. The idea of calculating the mean corpuscular volume (MCV), mean corpuscular hemoglobin (MCH), and mean corpuscular hemoglobin concentration (MCHC) came to me in this way.

■ Hematology, as you have known and practiced it, seems to be changing. With the solution of many of the problems of anemia and nutrition that occupied you and your contemporaries, it seems that most hematologists today are doing as much cancer work as they are hematology. Is the hematologist-oncologist the thing of the future?

I have always followed the principle that if you do what you want to do and do it well, you will be successful. If I were starting all over today, and interested in something connected with the blood, I'd still go at it. I think what is happening with hematology-oncology is an unfortunate situation. The chemotherapy which we and others developed in the late forties and in the fifties through our interest in leukemia and Hodgkin's disease has grown to such an extent that what I would consider an offshoot of hematology [oncology] has now become so time-consuming that it has come to overshadow hematology, itself, and as a consequence has drawn away potential investigation in hematology. Research in hematology has suffered because most of the hematology staff spends the bulk of its time doing oncology.

This is particularly sad because of what so many of the oncologists are doing: most of them are contributing relatively little in the search for new knowledge. Many are just using "cookbook" formulas to treat different malignant diseases, looking for the best "recipe" for each disease. That, of course, is worth finding out, but what is far more important is finding out *why* people develop Hodgkin's disease; *why* they develop leukemia. What are the fundamental differences between different forms of leukemia? We are spending a disproportionate amount of effort on "recipes" and application of what we already know, and far too little on studying basic mechanisms. We have made great progress in the treatment of some of the leukemias and lymphomas, but too little effort is being made in getting down to the "nitty-gritty."

■ In all the reviews you have written about the work you have done in hematology, you have always been generous in acknowledging the contributions of those who worked with you: George Cartwright,[b] Jack Athens, Dane Boggs, and others. Looking back on it all, what did you, personally, find the most satisfying?

This is difficult to answer because one gets satisfaction from so many things. At a commencement in Utah last week, one of my earlier students, John Dixon,[b] received an honorary doctor of science degree, and in receiving it acknowledged my help. Homer Warner,[b] whom you knew when you were in Utah, received a similar honor and also acknowledged my encouragement. Many of our former fellows now hold important positions elsewhere. I am pleased with that, naturally. And the reaction to my book, *Clinical Hematology,* certainly has given me great pleasure. It is satisfying to know that all the effort that the writing of the book entailed has been found worthwhile.

I have been very fortunate in having been able to pursue my objectives and do all the things I wanted to do. I have tried to do them as well as I could. And if they happened to work out well, all the better!

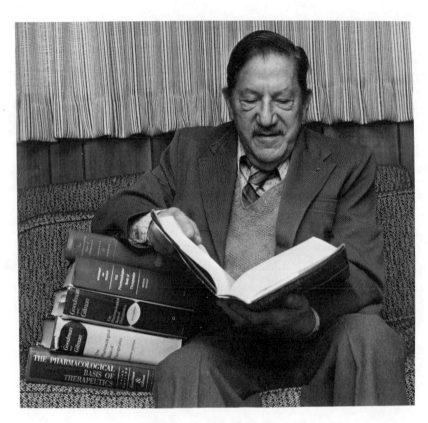

Louis S. Goodman, M.A., M.D.

CHAPTER 6

Louis S. Goodman, M.A., M.D.
(1906–   )

ASIDE FROM a rewarding glimpse of the man, himself, the inclusion of Louis Goodman among this collection of interviews provides an opportunity to view several other important aspects of the growth of American medicine. Dr. Goodman's reflections on the University of Utah complement those of Dr. Wintrobe on the building of a modern medical center. As a pharmacologist, Dr. Goodman was a pioneer in the last of the so-called basic sciences to be recognized as an indispensable ingredient in the training of our doctors. Finally, as an already prominent member of the medical research community at the end of World War II, Dr. Goodman was a major witness of, and participant in, what has already come to be called the golden age of American medical research: the entry of the federal government as a major funder of research in the postwar years.

As a result of the Flexner Report and other developments we have previously discussed, as early as the first decade of the century it became apparent that apprenticeships and the attendance of a series of lectures by clinicians could hardly prepare one for the rigors of medical practice. From our European counterparts we learned that such disciplines as chemistry and physiology would be required in the training of physicians. The enforcement of such requirements helped lead to the dissolution or reform of the many propietary medical schools (those run for profit by private investors). The cost of laboratories and basic science laboratories and equipment precluded easy profits, and the resources of private or state universities were usually needed to establish such facilities.

As early as 1870, when the University of Iowa established its state-supported medical school, the curriculum included anatomy, physiology, microscopic anatomy, and chemistry. But pharmacology as such was poorly developed, and courses such as materia medica dealt with the preparation and use of the crude medicinals that were then available.

Although a number of valuable drugs were introduced before and during the nineteenth century (morphine, digitalis, colchicine, quinine, caffeine), it was only after 1930 with the introduction of the sulfas and vitamins, and then in the 1940s with the advent of antibiotics and antihypertensive agents, among others, that the true flowering of effective pharmaceuticals came about. Previously, physicians often resorted to concoctions of dubious value, being sure to prescribe in Latin to convince their patients, and perhaps themselves to some degree, of the efficacy of their potions. The high alcohol content of many of these at least assured some relief of pain and sedation, although the same effect could have been obtained from a whiskey bottle—and often was. Today we need not mask our medicinals in Latin, and with a truly effective medical armamentarium we may safely prescribe in English.

The accelerating advance in the availability of all kinds of drugs since World War II can perhaps best be illustrated by a single case in point. When President Franklin D. Roosevelt died from a massive brain hemorrhage in 1945, it was the end result of long-standing and severe high blood pressure. The only medication then available to the first citizen of this rich and powerful country was phenobarbital, a mild sedative with minimal antihypertensive properties. Today there are about a dozen *classes* of effective antihypertensive agents available, with dozens upon dozens of varieties to suit the particular needs of each patient. The hypertensive patient who cannot be controlled with a combination of two or three of these when a single drug is ineffective is rare indeed.

Despite the advances in pharmacology over the last fifty years, as late as 1954, when this writer attended medical school, there was no pharmacology department at his institution. The subject was taught by members of the Department of Physiology. This was not unusual at a number of schools even at that late date; but now, thanks to the efforts of Dr. Goodman and his confreres, this situation has been remedied.

Louis S. Goodman was born in Portland, Oregon, and received his bachelor's degree from Reed College in 1928. He received a master's degree and medical degree from the University of Oregon and then spent a year (1932–33) as an intern at the Johns Hopkins Hospital in Baltimore. The next ten years were spent on the faculty at Yale Medical School; then, after a year at the University of Vermont, Dr. Goodman accepted the chairmanship of the Department of Pharmacology at the University of Utah College of Medicine in 1943. He has remained there ever since.

Although responsible for important basic research such as the development of anticonvulsants, Dr. Goodman is most recognized for achieving recognition for pharmacology as an independent scientific discipline through the many editions of his textbook and the many generations of pharmacologists who trained under him at Utah. The excitement and accomplishment of those nearly forty years are, I think, well captured in his remarks that follow.

Salt Lake City, Utah
March 2, 1978

■ Pharmacology at one time had a fairly low position among the basic scientific disciplines.

Yes. It used to be part of a physiology or biochemistry department or in materia medica or relatively ignored altogether in the medical curriculum. When I first came to Yale in 1934, the students there would argue with the students at Harvard as to (a) which school had the worst football team and (b) which school had the worst department of pharmacology. Pharmacology was in great disrepute, but Alfred Gilman[b] and I worked very hard to change that. The first edition of our book, which came out in 1941, helped to transform the entire field, to make pharmacology "respectable" and attract a number of good people to the field.

■ I don't suppose there have been many textbooks with as long and widespread success as Goodman and Gilman. Although you must have heard this a thousand times, I must say the literary quality is exceptional: it doesn't read at all like a textbook.

Well, even when we went to a multiauthored work, Gilman and I selected our own people. These were either former students or associates of ours, and we made sure that the style and cohesiveness of the book were as finely polished as we could make it.

It has been a very gratifying success to us. It has been translated into many languages, even Japanese and Romanian. Can you imagine—Romanian? When that edition came across my desk I had forgotten it was going to be translated into Romanian, and at first glance I thought it was the Italian edition, which was about to come out. I found I could read it and then remembered that Romania was the penal colony of the Roman Empire. So they took Latin with them, and some Slavic words were intermingled. You can read Romanian, particularly scientific Romanian, if you know a bit of Latin. There are also translations into Spanish, Portuguese . . .

■ While we are on the subject of "The Blue Bible" I would like you to clarify something if you will. When I was a student in the mid-fifties there was a rumor going around that you and Gilman had a sort of Gilbert and Sullivan relationship. You know, the original Savoyards never spoke to each other during the latter years of their association, despite their continued public success. Was it ever the same with you and Dr. Gilman?

That story is absolutely false. Gilman and I have been close friends since 1933 at Yale. Our families have been close. His son's middle name is "Goodman."*

The story got started in the early fifties when the second edition of our book was delayed, and it didn't finally come out until 1955. There were good reasons for this delay. Gilman and I were both very much involved in building up our respective departments, he at Columbia, where he had gone from Edgewood Arsenal after the war, and I at Salt Lake. We started revising the book about 1946–47, but enormous advances in pharmacology had come along, and these resulted in repeated revising as we attempted to update the material. While we were involved with this, Drill and his associates at Yale came out with their textbook, and somehow the story went out that although there might not be another Goodman and Gilman (that is, perhaps we were not getting along well), the Drill textbook could be relied upon to come out in subsequent editions and keep everyone up to date.

Well, when we came out in 1955 with our second edition, it swept Drill off the market. Drill sold something like 10,000 copies in its first edition, which came out a year or two before our second edition, which sold 120,000 before our third edi-

*And the principal editor of the latest (sixth) edition (1980) of the textbook.

tion came out in 1965. The reviews of our book were superb. When Modell reviewed our book and compared it with Drill he said, "Chapter for chapter my money is on Goodman and Gilman."

■ **You have spent most of your professional life here in Utah. What made you come here?**

I was at Vermont at the time I was invited to come out for a visit in 1944 by the newly appointed dean of the new four-year medical school, Cyril Callister. He was a very impressive person and very convincing. He was traveling around the East recruiting people for the school and told me that some very prominent professors were in Utah already, people like Wintrobe whom I had known from my Hopkins days. So in July of that year I came out for a visit and was given the "royal treatment." And there were very exciting people here. Wintrobe, for instance, had a stable of aggressive teachers and research workers: Yager, Cartwright,[b] Hecht,[b] and a number of others in the Department of Medicine. The basic sciences, however, were pretty dismal, and that's what Callister was trying to improve. He was trying to get rid of the "dead wood" that had been here at the two-year school, and he showed me documents from the American Medical Association about what needed to be done at the school. He agreed that the facilities were pretty minimal but said he would be able to get funds for remodeling the Pharmacology Department and building a student laboratory. He did get funds from the Latter-Day Saints Church.

But Callister lied to all of us. It came out later that he had told all of us individually that Utah had set aside funds for a new medical school and as soon as the war was over and the restrictions on steel were lifted there would be a brand-new medical school and university hospital. He was a terrific salesman, and none of us was suspicious enough to go to the state authorities or other prominent people in the community to see if this was really so. It wasn't.

What other reasons brought me here? I had come from the West originally, and this was an attraction to me. Unlike older established schools, there were no fixed traditions at Utah to interfere with what plans I might have for teaching and re-search in the department. And innovation was to be the thing. My acceptance of the chairmanship would include the option of bringing along some top people I had with me, which I did. All these were very exciting features, so I came.

When I speak of pharmacology here, there was really noth-ing before we began. When I arrived I looked at the requisition book, and there had been only two orders in the previous six months: one was for six pencils and one was for two guinea pigs. By the end of the first year we were spending nearly one hundred thousand dollars a year (not counting salaries), and that grew so that by the time I gave up the chairmanship in 1971 we were operating at close to half a million dollars a year. Only a small portion of this ever came from the state; it was federal research and industrial money that enabled us to grow.

Shortly after World War II the Office of Scientific Research and Development was replaced by the granting system oper-ated through the National Institutes of Health. We were in at the very start of that. The surgeon-general was trying to estab-lish a few key grants that would set the pattern for the future; he wanted one that would have great appeal in a regional area. Leo Marshall was a professor at the medical school here and reaching retirement at the time. He occasionally would serve as acting dean. He had been in the Public Health Service and was well known to the officials in Washington. He pointed out to them that, thanks to the Latter-Day Saints Church's in-tense interest in genealogy and its detailed family records of multiple marriages with numerous children, Utah would be an ideal place for the study of hereditary diseases. A type of muscular dystrophy, for example, is very common in these parts.

As a result of these efforts, the Department of Medicine here received Public Health Service Grant No. 1, which was the Metabolic and Hereditary Disease Research Program. It was started with a hundred thousand dollars, which is "peanuts" today, but in 1945–46 this was one of the largest grants ever. I was responsible for bringing Emil Smith out to head the biochemical aspects of that project, and a committee of four was set up to attract additional staff. Wintrobe was chairman, and Leo Samuels, Horace Davenport, and I were on it. The new staff was assembled in tarpaper shacks, and you may remember a news story about it in *Time* magazine.

■ What do you see as your major accomplishments in the department here?

I think the main things were our teaching program and our research programs. We had some awfully good people with us, and they went on to become professors at other institutions or chairmen—Toman, Nickerson,[b] Borison, Esplin, Sayers. We brought out some exciting new drugs; the alpha adrenergic blocking drugs, for example, were discovered here at Utah by Nickerson and me.

On the teaching level, you may not realize it, but our department was one of the first in the country to have all sophomore medical students do original research. And for a period of three or four years, from 1946 to close to 1950, we made our mark in the field by reporting on this program at national meetings, about how it worked, and what was necessary to make it work well.

There were some restrictions. Pharmacology was a two-term course, and we could only allow the students to work in areas in which we had the necessary expertise and equipment with which to help them. All this was also expensive, but we could use categorical funds from industry and federal government grants, provided the projects the students selected were germane to them. Once a project was approved, the students were released from formal work so that they could work on original research, first under instruction, and then independently. At the end of the second term they would report on their projects to the rest of the class and to the staff, and the more outstanding students were invited to present their work either at the Federation meetings [Federation of American Societies for Experimental Biology] or the fall Pharmacology meetings. This was quite a source of kudos for them. We spent thousands of dollars in sending these students to present their research, rehearsing them, preparing slide material for them, helping them work up the data for publication.

I'll never forget one year in Chicago when we had a presenting student by the name of Fairbanks who, incidentally, came from a prominent Mormon family with many outstanding members. He had worked with Borison on the nodose ganglion of the vagus as a chemoreceptor area for veratrum alkaloids. He had beautiful proof of this with marvelous colored slides, most of which we made ourselves or taught the artist to make. When the time came for the paper to be presented, we had to move to a larger hall because people were standing outside the original room selected, trying to get in. After the delay and then the presentation, people began asking questions, and everybody kept calling him "Doctor Fairbanks." Finally he said, "I'm not a doctor. I'm a sophomore student in Dr. Goodman's department in Utah."

If you look through our department publication file, some of the outstanding senior authors were medical students at the time, and surveys that were later made among alumni showed that these experiences in pharmacology were among the most motivating and exciting that they had in medical school.

This particular student program finally came to an end. The head of biochemistry, Leo Samuels, saw what we were doing in pharmacology and decided to do the same in biochemistry.

Well, these programs took an enormous amount of time, and once the students were confronted with the same sort of thing in two of the basic sciences they were absolutely strapped for time, and it became impractical to continue them. Another reason that sticks in my mind for ending the program was the growing conviction that if a student was interested in research, why should he have to work on one of our departmentally assigned problems and be limited by what we had to offer? Why shouldn't he go to *any* department that could give him the appropriate instruction? About this time the NIH came out with summer fellowships for medical students and post-sophomore year fellowships, and this helped us to decide to discontinue our own program. But a number of students profited from it, and we learned a good deal from it.

■ These must have been very exciting days, indeed. There was the general impression—correct me if I am wrong—that the medical school in Utah was pretty much the fiefdom of Wintrobe and Goodman at the time.

Nothing could be further from the truth. There is no question we ran our own departments. But we were very keen that other departments be strong and the school as a whole be strong and that all its education and research problems be far above par. This idea that we ran the school is nonsense. We finally shook down the administration of the school so that we had an executive committee on which every departmental chairman sat, each with an equal vote. Max and I frequently voted on opposite sides for various reasons; we often voted on the same side. But each of us, I am sure, voted for what we thought was best for the school. Let me give you an example.

I had come to Utah to head a joint Department of Physiology-Pharmacology but with assurance that I could split them into separate departments as soon as I could find an appropriate candidate for physiology. I recruited Horace Davenport, a superb man who stayed with us about eight or nine years and then left for Michigan. We searched and searched for a replacement, and although a number of distinguished people visited us, the facilities weren't too good and we were having some difficulty in finding the right person. We finally became very keen about Carlton Hunt, who had been at Johns Hopkins and then spent time at the Rockefeller Institute as well as at the Albert Einstein School of Medicine. We offered him the job, but he wanted a salary at least equal to what he was getting, which was about fifteen thousand dollars per year. Such a "large" sum was unknown to us at the time; even the president of the University, Olpin, wasn't getting that. Max and I were getting about twelve thousand dollars. We recommended to President Olpin that he give Hunt the salary he was asking for, and the president said, "Do you realize that you're recommending a salary higher than you own?" We said, "Of course. You don't understand the market. If we want an awfully good man we have to pay what the traffic requires and hope that eventually our own salaries will come up to that as well."

There was never any question of any jealousy among us as we attempted to build the school. There were a number of people, I believe, who thought that this was becoming a synagogue because Max and I were Jewish, but nothing was further from the truth. A fellow in my department by the name of Toman was thought to be Jewish by many, but he was actually a Catholic, or at least raised as one. People frequently took Leo Samuels, the head of biochemistry, to be Jewish because of his last name and because he was religious and wouldn't teach on Saturdays. Leo Samuels was a Seventh-Day Adventist, and as you know, their Sabbath is Saturday, not Sunday. I think the only Jewish person I had in my department was a very distinguished, internationally known pharmacologist, Walter Loewe, who was a refugee from the Nazis. The university gave him the title of Distinguished Research Professor but never paid a penny of his salary. We handled this from our own funds for the remaining seventeen years of his life, and we profited greatly from having had him here.

■ There are a number of denominational medical schools, mostly Catholic, and one, quite naturally I suppose, is accustomed to seeing a large number of people of that faith on the staff. In a certain sense, this being Mormon country, I always wondered why there were not more Latter-Day Saints people in high posts at the medical school.

Well, the only available Mormons were those who had been clinicians in the two-year school, teaching Physical Diagnosis, Introduction to Medicine, and making rounds at the County Hospital. They weren't academic people, and it was firmly decided when we all came here that there would be full-time department heads and staff in all the clinical as well as basic science areas. These would be people primarily interested in teaching and research. There were some awfully good private practitioners in the community, many of whom became very staunch defenders of the medical school. There were a few very good surgeons. Many of these people were given clinical appointments, but a number expected to become full-time professors and were disappointed.

But no one was recruited with the denominational consideration in mind one way or the other. There was enough of that in the past. Back at Yale I recall one dean, a former Jew himself, who made it his business to know the religious background of every applicant in order to make sure too many Jews did not get in. But we're living in an entirely different climate now, and all of this has changed in the wake of the Holocaust, the civil rights movement, and so on.

■ Looking back on your years in Utah, you have had so many successes: How about your disappointments? Did you ever regret going into a basic science discipline rather than clinical medicine, which you could have done as an M.D.?

I came to medicine through psychology. While I was at Reed College my older brother was in medical school and told me, "You're going to have to learn a lot about the nervous system and physiology before you can get anywhere in psychology." This led to a shift in my plans, and I went to medical school at the University of Oregon. I had a wonderful experience in research there over a three-year period with the late William Fitch Allen, a world-famous experimental neurologist who was responsible for our concepts regarding the reticular formation of the brain. He was a sort of scientific father to me for years and helped in orienting my thinking toward research and teaching.

We have had a good life here, my family and I. We were a little isolated in the early days, but what with air travel and phones, we became a Mecca! You yourself came out here to study. We, of course, were frustrated with the slowness with which the new, long-promised medical center came about. But on the whole I think we accomplished what we set out to do.

As for your own aims in your book, I warn you that oral history is only as good as the memory of the individual, and that can fade with time and become distorted. A case in point. A book was published in about 1975 called *Pathways of Discovery in the Neurosciences*. It consisted of personal reminiscences of a number of prominent people, one of them Herbert Jasper.[b] We were at Reed College together in the late 1920s, and he went into experimental psychology and was one of the first to play around with the electroencephalograph. He describes his years at Reed College with "Lewis" Goodman (my first name was misspelled) and how he was more interested in the biochemical basis of behavior and I more interested in psychoanalysis and how the two of us were almost kicked out of Reed for experimenting with hallucinogenic drugs.

I hadn't seen him for years, and when I read this story I wrote to Jasper, "Look, you and I overlapped only one year. I never experimented with drugs at Reed. I was never on the verge of being expelled and your memory is doing you a disservice." He wrote back terribly upset about his gaffe and wanted to know how I would like to have him correct it in the literature. He had been ill with laryngeal cancer and had undergone surgery prior to dictating that story and wondered whether that accounted for the fault in his memory. There were three pages of apology in his letter.

I wrote back and told him to forget about the whole thing and that if anyone read about me in this way I would be happy for them to think that I was sufficiently adventurous as a student to do something so illegal and immoral as to almost get kicked out. So oral history can be a dangerous thing, and you have to be extremely careful.

■ I'll try my best.

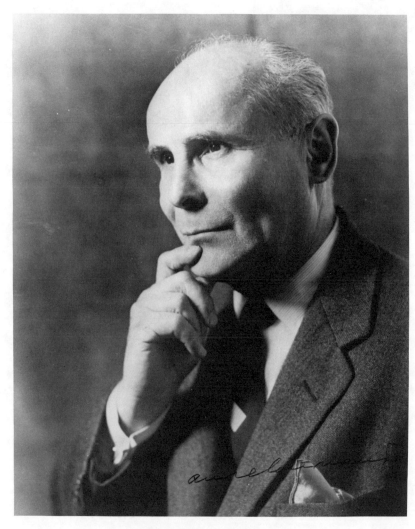

André Cournand, M.D.
(Courtesy of The National Library of Medicine)

CHAPTER 7

André Cournand, M.D.
(1895–   )

When I first gave my mind to . . . discovering the motion and uses of the heart . . . I found the task so truly arduous and full of difficulties that I was almost tempted to think . . . that the motion of the heart was only to be comprehended by God.

William Harvey (1578–1657)

T O UNDERSTAND the nature and importance of Dr. Cournand's contribution to the study of the heart through the technique of cardiac catheterization, one must first reflect on earlier periods of history. The heart, the traditional romantic source of human passion, has fired the imagination of mankind throughout all time. One of the high points in the study of the heart was William Harvey's discovery of the circulation of the blood, a revelation that had an incalculable impact upon our future understanding in that it overturned some major misconceptions about the heart that had been propagated by another great scientist, the Greco-Roman physician Galen, and that had persisted unchallenged for fourteen centuries.

Other important discoveries about the circulation were, of course, made from Harvey's time until the present century— Marcello Malpighi's discovery with the microscope of the capillary system that had eluded Harvey a few years earlier, for example—but it was the role of chemistry, more than any other branch of science, that may have spurred this work on. Since antiquity the relation between the air and the blood that courses through us was well recognized. It was finally the experiments on the nature of air, culminating in the discovery of oxygen by Joseph Priestley and Antoine Lavoisier in the eighteenth century, that provided a thrust toward the development of heart catheterization techniques.

How was this so? By the time of the mid-nineteenth century a controversy had arisen as to the source of the heat generated in the bodies of mammals. Lavoisier had suggested that animal heat was produced by "combustion" in the lungs when oxygen combined with carbon to form carbon dioxide and with hydrogen to form water. The heat of the body was provided by the calories generated by these two chemical reactions. This view was accepted as dogma by many until 1837, when Gustav Magnus proposed another theory to account for body heat. He proposed that the heat was generated in the tissues of the body rather than in the lung and based this conviction on the experimental finding that venous blood coming from the tissues had a higher carbon dioxide content and lower oxygen content than blood coming from the lungs.

Enter Claude Bernard, the great French physiologist at the Sorbonne. He reasoned that if combustion were occurring in the tissues of the body, then the blood returning to the right heart chambers would be warmer than that found in the left heart chambers. If combustion were occurring in the lung, which empties its blood into the left heart chambers, then the opposite would be the case. He performed his initial studies in the horse, advancing mercury thermometers from the jugular vein to the right heart, and from the carotid artery to the left heart. He found the temperatures on the right slightly higher than those on the left and concluded that Magnus had been correct. He repeated this finding many times and in different species. He also introduced the measurement of pressures in the heart through catheterization.

What about measuring blood flow through the heart? For this we are indebted to a German physician-physiologist, Adolf Fick (1829–1901) who, in a single-paged communication presented before the Society of Physiology and Medicine in the university town of Würzburg in 1870, stated the principle upon which almost all subsequent methods of measuring cardiac output have been based. Think of a "black box" with fluid-filled tubes feeding to, and draining from, it.

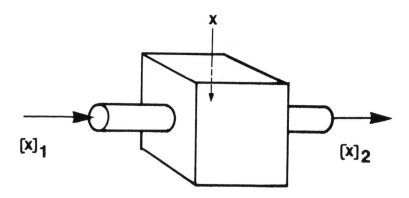

Let us assume that the fluid contains a substance, x, as it enters the box and that more of this is added to the fluid as it passes through the box. Therefore, the concentration in the exiting fluid $[x]_2$ is greater over a period of time than when it entered, $[x]_1$. By simple mathematics one can see that if we know three of the unknowns involved, the two concentrations of x and the amount of x added to the fluid while in the box, we can easily solve for the fourth, the flow through the box, because:

total x added = (change in concentration x) (flow per minute)
per minute

Rearranging:

$$\text{flow per minute} = \frac{x \text{ added per minute}}{[x]_2 - [x]_1}$$

If we now reveal that the box is the lung and x is oxygen, then:

pulmonary blood flow per minute =

$$\frac{\text{oxygen consumption per minute}}{\text{oxygen content difference between}}$$
$$\text{arterial and venous blood}$$

A similar equation can be derived for carbon dioxide (except that in this case, the substance is removed rather than added in the lungs) or any artificial tracer such as dyes added to the circulation. The so-called direct Fick determination involves obtaining blood from the right heart before it goes to the lung and then blood from the left heart or an artery after it has been oxygenated. The amount of oxygen added is determined by having the patient expire into a tank and by measuring the volume and oxygen concentration of the expired mixture and comparing it with room air.

Interestingly enough, Dr. Fick never performed a Fick determination. He was content to describe the principle involved and let it stand on the basis of its own incisive logic. The first direct Fick determinations validating the method were made in dogs sixteen years later. Seventy-one years would pass before Dr. Cournand would perform the first direct Fick determination in man.

If one could measure pressures in the heart and determine to what degree its pumping action might be impaired by various heart diseases, why was the method not adopted earlier than the mid-twentieth century? There were a number of reasons. The state of the medical art was limited at the time. One could not predict what might happen in man if a catheter were passed into his heart. And then, even if one could characterize various heart diseases by the effects they might have on pressures and flow, what good would it do? There was no corrective surgery available for heart disease, nor would there be until almost the mid-twentieth century. Even in the physiology laboratory the method did not achieve popularity, largely because of another innovation. In 1914 the brilliant physiologist at the University College in London, Ernest H. Starling, developed a heart-lung preparation in the dog to study the functions of the heart. Although this provided many insights into cardiac function for physiologists and physicians alike, it involved considerable surgery and disruption of the normal environment of the heart within the intact animal. The preparations tended to deteriorate after a few hours, and despite the knowledge gained from them, they were clearly inferior to catheterization studies later performed in closed-chest animals and man.

In 1929, however, the feasibility of cardiac catheterization in man was brought sharply to light. Werner Forssmann, a twenty-five-year-old surgical house officer in Eberswalde, near Berlin, demonstrated that a catheter could be safely passed from an arm vein into the human heart without danger. Although opposed by the senior physicians at his clinic, Forssmann managed to deceive a nurse into thinking *she* would be the subject so that he could gain access to the sterile surgical instruments he needed. He persuaded the nurse to allow herself to be tied down on the procedure table, but then anesthetized his own antecubital fossa (the inner aspect of the elbow) and passed a ureteral catheter from a vein to the heart. He then climbed several flights of stairs to the X-ray department to document his success with a chest film. He repeated the procedure on himself several times thereafter to convince others of the safety of the procedure.

Forssmann's rationale for the use of heart catheterization was for the safe and rapid delivery of life-saving drugs into the heart without risking damage to the heart wall or coronary arteries by sticking needles through the chest wall and into the heart, which might also result in punctures of the heart wall through which blood could accumulate and compress the heart in its own sac (cardiac tamponade). When he came to the Charité Hospital in Berlin, he tried to convince the chief surgeon there, Ernst Sauerbruch, of the safety and potential value of the procedure, but failed. Forssmann, discouraged by the consistent and overwhelming opposition he found to his ideas, ultimately gave up in his attempts to popularize them and was all but forgotten for much of his later life. In 1949, after cardiac catheterization had become a well-accepted procedure, Benatt in the British journal, *Lancet*, wrote about the early history of cardiac catheterization. He noted that by that time over 10,000 catheterizations had been performed throughout the world and wondered about the fate of that obscure German house officer, Forssmann, who had somehow faded from the medical scene.

Forssmann was rescued from oblivion in 1956 when he was included in the Nobel Prize for medicine that was awarded to André Cournand and Dickinson Richards for their work on catheterization of the heart.

Cournand and Richards "got into" the heart by way of the lungs. They were chest physicians, that is, primarily interested in lung diseases such as tuberculosis and emphysema, and were attempting to study the relationship of these to cardiac function, as well as the results of certain types of treatment for these diseases upon cardiopulmonary function. When they began working together in 1932, measurement of blood flow by the direct Fick method was almost unthinkable. There was no problem in obtaining arterial blood by puncture in order to obtain a sample to analyze for its gas content. The problem was obtaining the gas content in the venous blood returning to the heart from the tissues. They began by using a carbon dioxide rebreathing method, with the patient breathing into a collecting bag; estimates were made of venous blood carbon dioxide content from this. They soon found that the method was of no use in patients with lung disease and were impelled toward the direct method of obtaining venous blood from the right heart. The rest, as they say, is history.

Soon after Cournand and Richards demonstrated the feasibility of obtaining pressures and flows safely in intact patients, surgeons found that they could ligate a patent ductus and correct other extracardiac malformations of the circulation; Charles Bailey and others found that they could open up tight heart valves and later repair or replace those that would not close properly; the development of the pump-oxygenator allowed, for the first time, the repair of intracardiac abnormalities such as congenital defects (e.g., holes between the heart chambers). All this stimulated and was stimulated in turn by advances in the diagnosis of various heart diseases and estimation of their severity through the use of cardiac catheterization. Even in lung disease, where surgery plays a much less prominent role, Cournand and Richards were able to use catheterization techniques to show how the state of well-being could be improved in such patients by nonsurgical means, and how their lives might be prolonged. Studies in shock and artificial ventilation techniques also fell within their range of study. It is for all these accomplishments that André Cournand and Dickinson Richards with their associates have been so honored.

The author, early in his own career, had a revealing personal encounter with Dr. Cournand. I had just finished a fellowship in cardiovascular disease at the University of Utah, and was looking for a junior position at another institution. Like most young men at this stage of my life, I was not quite sure about what I wished to do, and was still trying to find a proper area of research to which I could devote my efforts. I visited Dr. Cournand in his office at Bellevue and approached the great man at his desk. I recall an immense street map of Paris filling an entire wall of his office behind him. He soon asked me about what I wanted to study, and although I really had nothing definite in mind, I expressed a certain interest in determining the effects of potassium depletion on the heart. Dr. Cournand then proceeded to inquire about all the details of the "proposed investigation," none of which I was equipped to supply at the time. I emerged from his office thinking to my-self, What was all that about?

In the last twenty years I think I have learned something of what that was all about. During our more recent conversation I mentioned this episode to Dr. Cournand, who naturally had forgotten it among the thousands of others he had conducted with budding young scientists. He was concerned about how I had been intimidated:

"Was I polite with you?"

"Very polite."

"Good."

". . . but very rigorous, intellectually rigorous"—as he was and has remained with himself, as with all others, throughout a very brilliant, fruitful, and rewarding career.

New York, New York
December 11, 1979

■ One tends to think that catheterization of the heart is a rather recent innovation to medicine, but you have pointed out that it has a considerable history.

It is very important to recognize that a lot of work had been done on catheterization of the heart in experimental medicine in the past. The term "heart catheterism" was actually coined by Claude Bernard[b] in 1847, and in 1876, after over twenty years of animal experiments, he published a book recapitulating a series of twenty-two lectures he had given at the Collège de France. In the fifth lecture he described the technique of right heart catheterization and left heart catheterization essentially as it is performed today. There is not a word to change. So even before 1900 everything had been done—in animals, of course—but then Starling[b] came along with his heart-lung preparation, and for a while, even though it was a great advance, this competed with the use of the catheter in studying the heart in the intact animal.

■ Once something is well accepted in society or science, it is difficult for people to imagine the amount of resistance that might have met it when it was initially presented. John McMichael[b] writes that when Werner Forssmann approached the surgeon Sauerbruch[b] about using catheterization in treating their patients in Berlin, the reaction was that "he ran a clinic, not a circus!"

There was great resistance to this. At the time one did not ordinarily pass tubes into the heart. It was unfortunate for Forssmann to have started something and then see others develop the technique. I first met him in 1952 when I was visiting Heidelberg. He was practicing urology in a small town nearby, and the professor of pharmacology at the university invited him over for me so that we could spend a Sunday afternoon together. Now, Forssmann was a very intelligent man and wrote extremely well in German, as is reflected in the English translations of his writings. Like many physicians of his time, he was well prepared in the humanities before he began the study of medicine. But he was obviously not a scientist. What did strike him was the important idea that if heart catheterization could be performed safely in animals, it could also be safely performed in man. He also was the first to have the idea that if you injected a radiopaque substance into the heart, you could get better visualization on X rays of the cardiac structures and pulmonary vessels. But he worked alone; he didn't collaborate with a good radiologist in order to get good pictures, and he didn't get reproducible pictures either on himself or animals. You see, he was not prepared to work with other people, and I think that was his main trouble. When he was working in Berlin and tried to interest Sauerbruch in the possible advantages of heart catheterization in introducing drugs directly into the right atrium, Forssmann probably didn't get support from some key people he needed because of some personal differences between them.

■   My former chief, Hans Hecht,[b] at one time carried on an extended correspondence with Forssmann and got the impression that, despite his major contribution in demonstrating the feasibility of heart catheterization in man, he may have overstepped himself later in claiming credit for all the advances it led to.

Professor Eric Berglund once showed me a letter from Forssmann claiming that he had the idea for every development published later on by others in the literature. This is what I call "cryptomnesia," that is, "secret memory." It is a term introduced by Robert Merton, and refers to the situation in which you read something somewhere and later forget the origin and come to think that the thought was your own. Forssmann deserves great credit for introducing the catheter into his own right atrium and suggesting the later use of angiography with the injection of radiopaque substances for X-ray pictures. The reason for his use of catheterization, stated in his first paper, was to introduce drugs directly into a heart chamber rather than risk cardiac tamponade by inserting a needle into the heart through the chest wall. He vaguely referred to "heart function," but he never mentioned the study of the physiology of the circulation. When he died a few months ago, I regret to say that in the article published in the *New York Times* scientific section, the writer attributed to him all the work that was initiated by our group during and after the Second World War in New York.

■ Forssmann first catheterized himself in 1929. The following year you arrived in New York from France, and in 1932 you had already formed an alliance with Dickinson Richards to study the circulation. How did this come about?

I started my studies in the Faculty of Medicine at the Sorbonne in Paris in 1914. The war had started, and except for a few of the older professors, most of the faculty had gone off to serve in the army. After about four or five months I decided to volunteer myself, and first went into an infantry regiment. I was then assigned as a medical student to an advanced ambulance service and later as an auxiliary battalion surgeon. We were taught to stabilize fractures and perform a number of other first-aid procedures before shipping the wounded back behind the front lines. There were a tremendous number of casualties among physicians in the army on the front, so that is the reason they put us students there. I was wounded and gassed on the eighth of August 1918 and spent the whole of the winter in Paris before starting in at the beginning to study medicine again in the spring of 1919.

I had a long period of training as a student, intern, and resident. By 1930 I had written my thesis for my M.D. "Acute Disseminated Sclerosis" and was about to start as an assistant in medicine at a hospital in Paris. Before beginning this, I

decided that I would like to spend a year in the United States. I
had already more or less decided to practice hospital medicine
rather than go into private practice in an office setting. The
chief of the Chest Disease Service at my hospital in Paris was
a friend of Dr. James Alexander Miller at Bellevue Hospital in
New York and arranged with him to have me come here. Although I had had thorough training in internal medicine and
chest diseases in France, it was decided that I spend my first
three months at Trudeau Sanatorium in upper New York State
in order to improve my English before moving on to Bellevue.

■ Did you intend at that time to return to France?

Yes. But while at Bellevue I published with Oswald Jones a
paper on the shrunken middle lobe of the right lung in bronchiectasis. Then Dr. Miller offered me the opportunity to stay
on in a full-time research position. "If you succeed," he said,
"maybe we'll make something of it. Are you willing to take a
chance?" And I agreed. I was thirty-five years of age at the
time.

I already had a wife and two children in France and had to
arrange to get them settled accordingly.

I started as a fellow in medicine and was supported by a
chemical foundation. In 1933 I became chief medical resident
of the Columbia Division at Bellevue. At about this time I
began my association with Dickinson Richards, who was then
an assistant attending physician at the Columbia-Presbyterian
Hospital uptown in Washington Heights.

■ There are two schools of thought about the conduct of scientific research.
The popular one, I suppose, is that the scientist plans precisely in advance what
he is going to do and then does it. This, at least, is what we all try to imply in
our research grant applications, although Albert Szent György,[b] one of the
people I admire most, once admitted, "When I go into the laboratory I'm
never quite sure what I'm going to do."

Now I would like to quote you directly. "In February 1932 Dickinson Richards
and I began a collaboration that was to persist until February 1973. . . . At the

start of our collaboration we agreed on a systematic and comprehensive examination of cardiopulmonary function both in normal patients and patients with chronic pulmonary disease." You were both thirty-seven at the time and still fairly early in your careers. Did you really have your whole plan thought out so systematically at that time? The question intrigues me.

Let me tell you how all this came about. When Dr. J. Alexander Miller, who was head of the Chest Service at Bellevue, asked me to stay, he inquired if I would be interested in doing some work with Dickinson Richards on the following subject: Why is it that some patients undergoing thoracoplasty [a therapeutic collapse of the lung, usually performed for tuberculosis at the time] die and others do not? What makes the difference in the result?

Richards and I recognized that unless you could study the function of the lung, the chest cage, and the circulation (that is, the heart) the answer would not be forthcoming. You must realize that Richards was superbly prepared to approach such studies. While he was working for his medical degree at Columbia he also earned a master's degree in physiology. He was greatly influenced by the work of Harvard's Lawrence J. Henderson on the physiology of the blood and respiratory gases. His earliest work, prior to our collaboration, dealt with the effects of anemia on the circulation and the oxyhemoglobin dissociation curve of the blood; he also studied the effects of oxygen therapy in heart failure and pulmonary disease. He spent a year in London with Henry Dale, later Sir Henry Dale, studying the hepatic circulation. So that by the time we got together in 1932 we had a clear idea of what had to be done. We prepared an exhibit for the New York Academy of Medicine in 1933, outlining the problems to be studied, and we constantly referred to it. (It was reproduced years later—1938—in the *Journal of Thoracic and Cardiovascular Surgery.*) In it we delineated all the structures involved in circulatory and respiratory function (the chest wall, the muscles, the lung, the heart, the blood, the arteries and veins and tissue, et cetera), the function of each of these (ventilation, gas transport, energy exchange, et cetera), and the techniques of measurements involved (ventilation, blood gas content, blood pressure, cardiac output, and so on).

These were all the considerations that we had in regard to studying, first pulmonary collapse therapy, then prevalent in the treatment of pulmonary tuberculosis, and later chronic fibrosis of the lung and emphysema. Still later on, the methods became applicable to a wide variety of lung and heart diseases.

■   What specifically got you into catheterizing the heart?

A popular method for measuring cardiac output at the time was the "indirect Fick" method using a rebreathing technique and measuring carbon dioxide in the expired gases. This is an indirect way to find out the concentration of the gas in the blood coming into the right heart from all parts of the body: the mixed venous blood. But in patients with pulmonary disease one could not predict this from the rebreathing method because of the different blood flow and gas distributions through different parts of the lung, normal and abnormal. We realized that we would have to get venous blood samples directly from the right heart in order to get accurate values of gas concentrations to compare with the arterial blood gas concentrations that we could easily get by sticking a brachial or radial artery. Using the difference between the two, we could directly apply the Fick principle.

In 1936 I returned to Paris on a visit with one of my former teachers, Dr. G. Ameuille, who had completed pulmonary angiography in a hundred patients. I spoke with him and reviewed all the cases that had been presented at the Société Medicale des Hopitaux. His work on this when published, incidentally, had been received very critically by the great cardiologists of the time who told him it was "monstrous to do such a thing as introduce a tube into the heart of a patient."

But what impressed me was that he had had no complications. The patients had tolerated the procedure very well. So I brought back with me to the United States some ureteral catheters, which at that time were manufactured only in France, and also some large needles with which to introduce them into veins through the skin. Between 1936 and 1940 we studied dogs exclusively, developing the techniques for manipulating the catheters. On one occasion we also had the opportunity to study a chimpanzee. George Wright, who was a resident on the Chest Service, offered to advance ureteral catheters under fluoroscopic control into the right atrium of human cadavers in order to determine necessary catheter lengths for human studies, and establish external reference points for measuring intracardiac pressure.

It was not until 1940 that Dr. Walter Palmer, chairman of the Department of Medicine, gave us permission to attempt a direct Fick determination of cardiac output in a patient, but he insisted that we choose a very ill patient. Unfortunately, the subject, who had cancer, had extensive metastases to the lymph nodes in the axilla, and Dick Richards was unable to get the catheter past them and into the right atrium. Our next opportunity came at Bellevue where Dr. Herbert Chasis and his associates were interested in measuring cardiac output in hypertensive patients using the ballistocardiograph, the method introduced by Isaac Starr.[b] But they needed a reliable independent method to calibrate the ballistocardiograph before they could make their measurements. They were part of a group directed by Homer Smith,[b] the great kidney physiologist; and they were the first ones to have emphasized the importance of blood flow to the kidney in systemic hypertension. I went to the dining room in the Nurses' Home, where all of us at Bellevue ate at the time, and sat down with Homer Smith, who started talking with me about measuring cardiac output. I told him the best way of getting a good Fick cardiac output was by passing a catheter to the right atrium as had been done by Forssmann and others. Smith said, "If that's the best method, why not do it?" and he arranged with the head of his department of medicine to allow us to study some of his hypertensive patients. This led to our first report on the direct Fick method for cardiac output, published in 1941. Between 1941 and 1945 we improved the technique to include the measurement of heart pressures, develop better catheters and needles, provide electrocardiographic monitoring during the procedure, and so forth.

■ We know of the resistance that Forssmann and Ameuille met to the procedure of heart catheterization. What was your own experience after you made your initial reports?

Something happened in December 1941, December 7th, to be precise, that resulted in the total absence of resistance to the development of cardiac catheterization in this country. This, of course, was the attack on Pearl Harbor and the beginning of World War II for the United States. Immediately after Pearl Harbor there was a meeting of the American Thoracic Surgical Society in New Orleans, and I met there with the surgeon Alfred Blalock.[b] I showed him what we could do with the catheter, because we already had experience measuring cardiac output and pressures, and indicated that there was also the possibility of now measuring blood volume with the methods being developed by Gregersen, the professor of physiology at Columbia. Blalock at that time was chairman of the "Shock Committee" in Washington, and I told him that we might be able to contribute greatly to the study of shock by the use of these new methods. He said, "You have your grant," because this was precisely what he was interested in, what with the war casualties coming on and all. We were lucky to have a man like Blalock to deal with, a surgeon who was an investigator and had studied shock in dogs, but realized that the situation might be quite different in man.

So we studied all kinds of shock in 125 cases: traumatic

shock, hemorrhagic shock, burn shock, ruptured viscus [bowel] leading to shock. We studied all kinds of treatment: plasma, whole blood, saline, gelatin, drugs. In New York City for the first two years of the war there were still a number of automobile vehicles in operation, and we arranged to have all severe traffic injuries studied by us. We had a very good team, with a surgical resident on call twenty-four hours a day. I had my technicians in contact with me by phone, and as soon as a surgical resident had a case, he would call me and I would go to the hospital to see the patient with him. I could then call in my technicians at any time, the middle of the day or night, to study these patients and evaluate their treatment. When traffic decreased (with gas rationing) and the number of traumatic cases were reduced, we turned to the study of shock in burns and the other situations I mentioned.

Once the procedure of heart catheterization became well accepted for these cases, and it was realized how well it was tolerated, we were able to turn our attention to the study of a wide variety of pulmonary and heart diseases.

There was another interesting development as a result of the war. In 1944 I was asked by the air corps if I would take on with me a captain assigned to study pressure breathing. At that time they were very anxious to find out the best way to assist breathing in personnel who were wounded in the air, and were perhaps in shock or going into shock. Which type of pressure breathing might be the best in terms of effect on the cardiac output?

Bennett was the first engineer with whom we worked, and before the final model was constructed, we had a special instrument prepared in which we could control every aspect of pressure breathing: the curve of pressure, the type of release of pressure (sudden or gradual) from peak inspiration to expiration, the volume of each respiration, the rate of respiration, et cetera. We worked on this for almost two years to develop the best system. This resulted in the prototype of all the kinds of ventilation-assisting devices that are now used in hospitals by anesthesiologists and others.

■   You spent just about your entire career at Bellevue. The popular concep-
tion of it used to be that it was just a place they sent mentally deranged people,
picked up off the streets of the city. What was it really like?

I have always been a Bellevue-Columbia man. From the time of the early thirties when I began there, Bellevue's reputation constantly improved because Columbia, New York University, and Cornell each had their divisions there. Now, there was a fourth division early on that was later taken over by New York University, and that was one that might have been called the "political division." The physicians there were not of the same caliber as those on the university divisions. There were always these large wards on Bellevue, each with at least twenty-five beds, and sometimes additional cots were put up in the middle of the ward, so that material conditions were not the best. But the nursing care was excellent, and the attending staff and house staff provided the finest medical care for their patients. I would also emphasize that, although there were three university services, this did not affect cooperation among us. Homer Smith, for example, was a New York University man and I was with Columbia, but that did not prevent our groups from working together. On the shock work all three university services were involved.

■   The medical circles during the years in which you worked were not often
very hospitable to women, but one cannot help noting the number of women
who have always circulated around you—Ferrer, Harvey[b] . . .

You're speaking of the women who worked with me? For a moment I thought you wanted to know about the women "in my life"!

■   No, I didn't want to get that personal.

I don't know if it has anything to do with my being a Frenchman, but at Bellevue, from a very early time onward, I was always in favor of using the best talent I could find regardless of race, religion, or sex. Throughout my life this has never made any difference to me. I had the first black secretary at Bellevue and then an Oriental secretary. I worked with Janet Baldwin because she was a pediatrician interested in congenital heart disease and was interested in applying our method to the diagnosis of that kind of problem. We worked with Eleanor Baldwin, who contributed to many other types of studies. Réjane Harvey and Irené Ferrer were interested in acquired heart disease and the influence of pulmonary disease on the circulation and worked with us along those lines.

■ Speaking of your French background, I have always wondered if you ever felt some special affinity for Alexis Carrel[b] who also came from France and, as you know, was the first "American" to win the Nobel Prize in medicine for his work on experimental vascular surgery and organ transplants. Was he a hero of yours?

I knew of his work, of course, but I wouldn't say that he was a hero of mine. Incidentally, Carrel's wife seldom came to the United States; she preferred France. And when I was unable to bring my little family with me when I first began working in New York, they remained for a time in the same village in Brittany where the wife of Carrel lived.

■ Do you have any regrets about your career?

Oh, yes. I have missed many things. For instance, I was probably the first one to go into the coronary sinus* from the right atrium. I realized where I was but didn't take advantage of it to study the metabolism of the heart. I should have written a book on clinical shock but never did. You see, I prepared over forty reports for the committee on shock: monthly reports, semiannual reports, annual reports, biannual reports. By

---

*The main vein draining the heart itself.

1945, when we prepared our final report, I was so fed up with reports that I never wrote the book, although we did sum up our findings in four or five papers that went into the literature.

Then I began to feel the pressure of other groups of investigators who were going ahead with the study of all kinds of heart disease. We realized that we could study cardiac failure, congenital heart disease, rheumatic heart disease, the pulmonary circulation. But you couldn't do everything. We had to go ahead and prepare papers as the technique was developing, and in order to "remain liquid" in financing, I had to continuously prepare grant applications, et cetera.

■ Who were the people who influenced you most in your life?

You asked me if I had a hero in my life. I have written a number of things about Dick Richards. With Robert Debré, a world-renowned pediatrician who was my chief in Paris, Richards was one of the two greatest men I have been in close contact with in my life. He was a humanist; he was a Hellenist; he was a scientist; he was a superb clinician; and he was an outstanding gentleman. I have never met another man as remarkable as he. We had a most unusual collaboration. Initially he taught me many of the techniques we would have to use for our research, and we worked together at Columbia and Bellevue from 1932 to 1973, the year of his death. A collaboration of forty-one years.

■ Did you ever have arguments?

A lot of arguments, but always "nice" arguments in which we respected one another.

Richard Riley, who was Dickinson Richards's brother-in-law, once compared the two of us when he presented the Trudeau Medal to me. We were the same age but totally different people. He was very solid, admirably organized, while I was more prone to go off on a tangent and imagine things. Riley suggested that perhaps I had a bit more imagination than

Richards but that he had a much more solid scientific background than I.

■ It sounds like a good combination. It certainly worked.

It was a perfect combination.

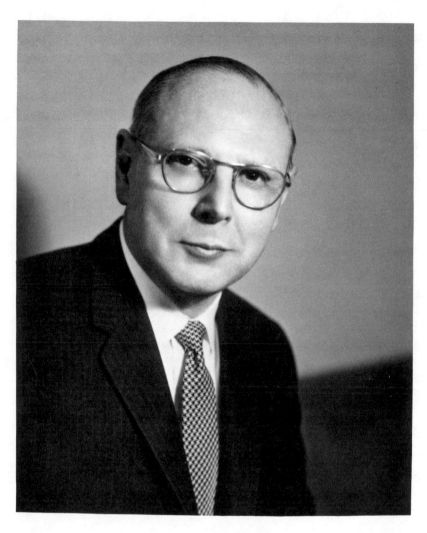

Charles P. Bailey, M.D., Sc.D., J.D.

CHAPTER 8

Charles P. Bailey, M.D., Sc.D., J.D. (1910–   )

IF, DURING THE 1940s, Horatio Alger was still writing stories about poor boys who rose from rags to riches, he could well have based one of his tales on the career of Charles P. Bailey. Born in a small town in New Jersey and growing up in poverty with only a widowed mother to care for him, Dr. Bailey has nonetheless achieved, if not riches, the peak of fame and appreciation for his contributions to heart surgery.

Rheumatic fever is related to a preceding infection with a common type of bacterium, a streptococcus, following which, in susceptible individuals, a type of autoimmune reaction takes place, damaging the heart valves and resulting in what we call rheumatic heart disease. At the time Dr. Bailey began his work on surgery of the mitral valve, rheumatic heart disease was still a major problem in this country. Since the introduction of the free use of antibiotics in the United States, the incidence of rheumatic fever and subsequent rheumatic heart disease had markedly decreased. The beta-hemolytic streptococcus is very sensitive to many antibiotics. However, some cases of rheumatic heart disease continue to occur in the United States, and in undeveloped countries where access to antibiotics is restricted it remains a major cause of cardiac incapacity and death.

As a result of rheumatic scarring a valve may become narrowed (stenotic) or fail to close properly (regurgitate). The mitral valve (so called because its two cusps were felt by anatomists to resemble a bishop's miter) is the most common valve to be involved in rheumatic heart disease. Mitral stenosis is the most common problem that involves this valve, which separates the left atrium from the left ventricle.

Initial surgical attempts at correcting mitral stenosis were made before the development of pump-oxygenators and open-heart surgery. The surgeon had to work on the beating heart blindly, by touch. Dr. Bailey was not the first to attempt to relieve mitral stenosis in this manner. In 1924 Dr. Elliot Cutler in Boston, assisted by Drs. Claude Beck and Samuel Levine, as noted by Dr. Bailey, reported attempts to treat mitral stenosis surgically. Dr. Cutler's approach was from the ventricular side of the valve using an instrument he devised called a cardiovalvulotome. This tube contained a cutting mechanism; it was passed through the ventricular wall and through the valve into the left atrium. The cutting device was used to remove a piece of the valve and thus reduce the degree of obstruction between the two chambers. The instrument was difficult to use; mortality was high; and with removal of part of the valve substance a case of severe mitral stenosis could be converted into a problem of severe regurgitation.

Bailey's contribution was to show that an atrial approach to the valve was preferable and that the surgeon's finger was perfectly adequate as an instrument. Instead of cutting off a piece of the valve, he inserted his finger in the stenotic opening between the two cusps of the valve and, by pressing in one direction and then the other, he widened the commissure so as to restore the valve opening to a more normal state. There was less chance of regurgitation developing after this than in the Cutler procedure, but it did occur, as did restenosis in later years. Nonetheless, it was an excellent palliative operation until the development of bypass procedures, which made routine visualization of the valve possible along with the option of replacing it entirely with a manufactured valve prosthesis.

Besides his work on the mitral commissurotomy operation, Dr. Bailey made many other contributions to cardiac surgery. In 1954 he was the first to excise successfully a postinfarction left ventricular aneurysm. In 1956 he carried out the first retrograde coronary endarterectomy. (This was before the development of coronary bypass surgery, of course.) He also contributed to the development of techniques for treatment of aortic valve disease, closure of septal defects, and solution to the problems related to the use of prosthetic heart valves, which still are far from perfected.

Dr. Bailey attended Hahnemann Medical College in Philadelphia and in that city between 1948 and 1958 did the bulk of his work. Between 1959 and 1962 he headed the Department of Surgery at the New York Medical College; and following that, for a period of ten years he headed the Section of Thoracic Surgery at St. Barnabas Hospital in the Bronx.

Toward the end of his medical career, Dr. Bailey did a complete turnabout. He went to Fordham Law School, from which he obtained a degree in 1973. Although he continues to see some "old patients," he is now essentially a lawyer and serves as a legal counsel to physicians in a New York Law firm. His remarks on medical-legal problems, although unnerving, are delivered with the expertise of someone who has acquired great knowledge from addressing both aspects of the question, and I therefore have included many of them.

New York, New York
August 28, 1979

■ Could you tell me about the development of the closed mitral commissurotomy operation for mitral stenosis?

When you talk about either me, or Dwight Harken,[b] or Russell Brock,[b] you really have to talk about the other two as well
because, within a three-month period, entirely independently,
each of us came out with the same ideas, both as to concept
and as to a technique of surgery, for mitral valve disease. And
this technique proved to be sound and satisfactory, at least
until the time when direct vision surgery became possible
because of the development of the heart-lung machine. Later,
when plastic valves became acceptable as prosthetic replace-
ments, an even broader therapeutic horizon opened up. I have
often said that if any two of us had died the remaining one
would have kept right on and would have brought out exactly
the same final product. It's still a very valuable procedure in
undeveloped countries where open-heart surgery is not yet
feasible and where plastic valves may be too expensive. And it
does enable one to do a very good job on about half of all cases
of mitral stenosis and a fair job on another quarter, so that, in
the sense of logistics, it is still a very valuable method. I just
happened to be lucky enough to do the first operation, on June
10, 1948. That lady is still alive and still pretty healthy after all
these years. Dr. Harken did a similar procedure within a week
of that date, and Russell Brock did another one within three
months. Neither Harken nor I had published our work at the
time that he did it.

The reasons I was able to make a contribution to mitral
surgery were threefold:

1. I had long been an amateur photographer and was used to working in the darkroom guided by the sense of touch. This helped with a closed procedure where you could not actually look at what you were doing.
2. I had made an extensive study of the anatomy of both the normal and the diseased mitral valve from autopsy material and also in the animal laboratory.
3. Having sold ladies' underwear to earn my way as a medical student, I had a good knowledge of such things, and was early on impressed by the similarity of the mitral valve structure to the old-fashioned feminine girdle. Perhaps this is what suggested the mitral commissurotomy operation to me.

■ The history of heart surgery is fascinating. In 1895 Billroth,[b] who was no mean surgical innovator himself, wrote a monograph on trauma of the heart in which he stated: "No surgeon who wishes to preserve the respect of his colleagues would ever attempt to suture a wound of the heart." As late as 1945, when you published a textbook of thoracic surgery, you never even referred to intracardiac surgery. Three years later you and Harken and Brock were doing precisely that! What was Smithy's role in this?

First off I would point out that, despite what Billroth wrote, Rehn in 1896 did successfully suture a wound of the heart. As for Smithy, his work was entirely independent of ours. He was from South Carolina, and it was his survivals with the old Cutler[b] operation for mitral stenosis that really stimulated me to finally do that first successful case.

In the Cutler operation for mitral stenosis they performed a punch-excision of part of the valve itself (rather than widening the mitral orifice that had become narrowed because of the disease).

■ I reviewed your paper and I was amazed. I know surgeons must have courage to introduce something new, but I wondered reading it what kind of a man, or woman for that matter, can take five patients, have four of them die, have one succeed, and then say, "This looks very promising."

Obviously, I felt there were irrelevant reasons for the loss of the first four patients and that the principle was entirely sound and could be developed, but just needed further effort. These other cardiac surgeons I mentioned had some unsuccessful cases, too. All of us had had a considerable background of animal work before this and, of course, had operated on dead human hearts, so that we were not unfamiliar with the pathology. Finally, however, you have to face the "moment of truth," and the poignancy is so great that I can't really express it. You know that almost all the world is against it; you know that you have a great personal stake and might even lose your medical license or at least your hospital privileges if you persist. In fact, the thought crosses your mind that maybe you really *are* crazy. And yet you feel that it has to be done and that it has to be right. At the time I did the last of those five operations, the finally successful one, I was sure that I was, at the very least, in danger of losing all of my hospital operating privileges.

■ Was that at Hahnemann?

No, that was at the Episcopal Hospital; I had already lost my privileges to do this kind of surgery at Hahnemann because two of the four previous patients had died at Hahnemann. The professor of cardiology there, Dr. George Goeckeler, who later became my very good friend, was at that time so bitterly opposed to any further such efforts that he formally invited me to come down to his office to discuss the whole thing with him. First, he allowed me the privilege of the floor, which took up practically all of the interview. Then, after I had finished telling him what I thought could be done, and why, he pulled out a previously typewritten sheet of paper on which he had methodically explained that, as an ethical physician, it was one's Hippocratic duty not to do harm when he could do no good. He ended up telling me that it was his Christian duty to keep me from doing any more of these operations.

Dr. Goeckeler was a great, sincere, and dedicated physician, and he really felt he was preventing me from committing manslaughter in this fashion.

Realizing that "the jury had been out before the court had been called into session," I responded with some heat. I told him that I believed in this operation, that I was sure I was right, that I knew the results of medical treatment for this condition were so poor as to be almost worthless, and proclaimed that it was *my* Christian duty to continue with this effort and to make it successful, and that I was prepared to spend the rest of my life in that effort. We shook hands and parted.

■ There was a feeling among many cardiologists in the past that rheumatic heart disease was mainly a disease of the muscle and that the valves, narrowed or widened by the process, had little to do with the clinical manifestations.

Yes, and that was why Dr. Samuel Levine[b] was chided by some experts in the nineteen-twenties for letting Dr. Elliot Cutler of Boston attempt this type of operation on his patients. You see how even the brightest people can be wrong.

■ There is always the question of priority. Was there any feeling of competition among you and Harken and Brock?

Well, of course there was. It was mainly, I think, between Harken and myself. Brock had more of the dispassionate view of the Englishman, and he always maintained good relations with both of us. But I should tell you about Horace Smithy.

At a meeting at which I reported these five cases of mitral stenosis with the one survival, Smithy had already operated on eight cases, and it is my recollection that five of them had survived surgery. He was called upon to discuss my paper. I hesitate to think of what would have happened if Dr. Harken had been the discussant and had Smithy's record with which to "clobber" me, but Smithy was devoid of that competitive feeling. Although he had a much better "batting average" than I had at the time, he was most gentlemanly and considerate in mentioning his own work. He didn't present it very fully, so that he didn't "steal the show." He merely said that he had used the method of Cutler but acknowledged that this converted the stenosis [narrowing] essentially into a regurgitation [leak]; and then this wonderful man, who could have outshone me and "stolen the day," said, "But I think Dr. Bailey's technique (which was essentially converting the small opening into a Halloween pumpkin type of smiling mouth) is a much more physiological method, and that is the one I am going to use from now on."

■ His generosity was admirable—especially for a surgeon, I must venture to say.

Well, there are some wonderful people in surgery, but there are no more egotistical and more competitive people than surgeons. But Smithy was not only a "Southern gentleman," he was a true gentleman or he would have been unable to resist the temptation to capitalize on the position he was in at that time. After the public session at that meeting I had a good long talk with him in private, and you can imagine how warmly I have always felt toward him.

I learned that he, himself, was driven to develop cardiac surgery because he hoped to develop a method applicable to his own case because he was running out of life. He had me listen to his own heart, and I heard the terrible rumble of aortic stenosis [narrowing of the valve leading from the left ventricle to the main blood vessel, the aorta]. I had to admit to him that I hadn't worked on or considered that problem as yet, so I was not able to offer him any hope or much encouragement, in fact. Probably because of this he subsequently went to Dr. Alfred Blalock,[b] who wasn't at all willing to operate on Dr. Smithy with his knowledge at that time, which, I suppose was not much better than mine. There was no pump-oxygenator yet, so this was before open-heart surgery had arrived. Any attempt would have had to have been made by a closed method, as with the mitral valve work which we were doing.

Dr. Smithy subsequently found a patient with aortic stenosis and brought him to Baltimore where at Hopkins he and Dr. Blalock attempted to operate him for this condition. Unhappily, the patient died on the operating table, and I'm sure this deterred Dr. Blalock from any further efforts in that direction. It also disappointed Dr. Smithy beyond all belief because with this man's death his chances, however remote, of persuading Dr. Blalock to attempt something on him had gone into the grave with the patient. Smithy died of his aortic stenosis in the fall of 1948. I had met him the preceding spring; he was only thirty-four.

■ What was the source of the friction between you and Dr. Harken?

Well, my mother was redheaded; my daughter is redheaded. I never was, but *Harken* was—that is, until he became gray. And there is an old saying in India that you never find two tigers on the same hill. What they really mean is you don't find two *male* tigers on the same hill: one always drives the other off. And at that time Harken and I had no idea that there was a whole mountain range that would be occupied by heart surgeons in the future, so we just tore at each other with the classical vigor of redheaded people.

■ There may be another connection. Early in his career Dr. Harken spent several months in New Jersey at the old Pollak Chest Disease Hospital in Jersey City. What about your own early days?

I was born and raised within two miles of Fitkin Hospital in Neptune, New Jersey, and my mother had something to do with my going there for an internship after I finished medical school at Hahnemann. My mother wasn't Jewish, but she was what you might call a "Jewish mother" type in that I was destined to be a doctor before I was born. She thought that was the kind of son she should have. And she brainwashed me so thoroughly that I never thought of being anything but a doctor for the first forty years of my life. She wanted me to intern at the local hospital because I think she had some idea that she might become a member of the board of trustees there and have some influence on the health and medical care of her neighbors. There was another factor important to me: they paid twenty-five dollars a month in wages to interns at Fitkin, whereas at Hahnemann and at Philadelphia General or any other place where I might have been interested in interning, they paid nothing.

■ Your mother sounds like a pretty strong character. What about your father?

Well, I don't think I ever heard him express himself on the subject, but I'm sure he didn't object. My father was a banker, but at a relatively early age he left banking, and I guess you'd say he became a stock market manipulator. The trouble is that one day *he* got manipulated and lost all his money. From then on he had a series of different jobs. He died when I was only twelve, and when I saw him coughing up blood into a basin as my mother tried to soothe him I just stared at this awful exhibition of how mitral stenosis can terminate a young man's life. He was only forty-two. I was already scheduled to be a doctor but was going to go into cancer research up to that time. At that very moment I changed my entire medical direction, and my mother was never able to persuade me otherwise. Indeed, it seemed to me a much simpler job to solve the mechanical problems of valvular heart disease than the chemical and biological problems of neoplastic development.

■ Are you saying that, as a boy, you were already thinking of what kind of specialty you were going to do as a physician?

Oh, my mother had made up my mind for me before I was five; maybe before I was three!

■ Did any of your teachers encourage you along the lines of cardiac surgery?

No, it was the shock of my father's death and the sober realization that the heart was only a mechanical pump which certainly would be responsive to the physical laws that all mechanical pumps would be subject to. The fact that this idea hadn't been developed or, perhaps, even expressed very much did not deter me. I just thought that nobody had thought of it yet. When I was a freshman in medical school, I drew a diagram of a proposed heart-lung machine with these principles in mind and presented it to Dr. John Scott, the professor of physiology there. It was not dissimilar in design to the diagrammatic pattern of our current heart-lung machines. And Dr. Scott did encourage me.

■ Let's get back to the progress of your career. After your internship you went into private practice in Lakewood, New Jersey, for about five years, then took two years' training in thoracic surgery at Sea View Hospital in Staten Island.

Yes, but first I went to the graduate school at the University of Pennsylvania for an academic year. There they encouraged us, based upon the anticipated coming of the certifying boards in the various specialties, to take additional residency training on top of the postgraduate training. My thesis was "Extraperiosteal Pneumothorax for Tuberculosis," for which I received my master's degree in medical science in 1943. I was a lecturer in thoracic surgery at Hahnemann from 1940 to 1948, and professor and head of the Department of Thoracic Surgery there from 1948 to 1958. In 1955 I received a doctor's degree in medical science—Sc.D. (Med)—also from the University of Pennsylvania.

■ Those must have been pretty heady years, what with the mitral surgery and all that rapid professional advancement.

Actually, the academic rank did not disturb my sense of balance. The fact that I could more or less run my own show was, of course, a great comfort. But I could see that this new field was an entirely uncharted area, and it was up to me to develop it in all respects that I could, and that was really exciting. People from all over the country and even all over the world visited me at Hahnemann, and I was a speaker on a great many medical programs. I turned out to be a pretty good medical writer and speaker. I was invited to lecture in Europe, South America, Canada, Mexico—and what I had to present was usually something new and different from anything they had had before.

■   What led you to break with Hahnemann? You were there for over eighteen years.

Well, a few things happened. One was that we obtained a new professor of surgery, and under the new regime all the surgical subspecialties were to be reincorporated under the General Department of Surgery with the two exceptions of gynecology and thoracic surgery (which included heart surgery).

Despite these arrangements, I soon found that the new professor and chairman of surgery had been given the right to give all the lectures on thoracic surgery to the students. My teaching would be limited to the residents. Furthermore, since that chairman had been certified by the American Board of Thoracic Surgery, he would be allowed to do his own private chest surgery, and his initial results in this did not bode well for his and my future.

I was upset about this and complained to the dean, and when he left for Europe in the spring of the year, I turned to the chairman of the board of trustees, but I received no satisfaction. Lacking any positive response, I decided to resign my academic position at least until the fall when everyone would be back and perhaps things could be straightened out. In the meantime, I recommended that my next in command, a Dr. Henry Nichols, be made the acting director of thoracic surgery. I continued to operate at the hospital under my junior's direction, so to speak, but would not be part of the faculty, at least temporarily.

I had reason to believe that there might be some discomforting conferences and discussions in the fall, so I took certain precautions. I went to the medical school where the new professor of surgery had been before he had come to Hahnemann, and I met the new dean down there. It seems that there had been a real scandalous situation there, ending up with the resignations of two department heads, one of them our newly arrived professor, and the firing of a third.

While there I met one wonderful man who was a physician but also the scion of a tobacco company family. He met me in his office and explained that he had never practiced medicine for money because he had been born wealthy. But he had run the Surgical Department of the City Hospital for many years and had always been on the teaching faculty of the medical school. As a member of the board of trustees of the Teaching Hospital and medical school, he had been one of those who had selected this young man to head the Department of Surgery. But, in his own words, he didn't think the latter had been "rightly brought up." Suddenly this new professor of surgery was making rounds at the City Hospital at six-thirty in the morning and calling the old doctor from the hospital and demanding: "I am making rounds and I expect all my staff to be with me. Why aren't you with me?"

To which the old man replied, "Ah cain't rightly accumulate myself until nine or ten in the mornin'. But from nine to ten in the mornin' until midnight *I'm your man*. But I just cain't get down there at six-thirty in the mornin'."

The new professor then informed him, "Well, then, I can't use you. You're fired!"

The old surgeon was shocked. He sat around awhile and then called the president of the board of trustees. "Say, do you know what? That new young professor of surgery just fired me." To which the president of the board replied, "You're wrong. He cain't fire you. *You're his boss!*"

The old surgeon concluded, "It was a very 'unhappy situation' after that."

Well, the dean gave me copies of newspaper after newspaper with crayon-outlined articles about the scandal, and I had an armful of these when we reconvened at Hahnemann in the fall. I also had another newspaper item with me. Franklin Roosevelt had just swept a previously strongly Republican part of southeastern Pennsylvania and had carried in with him a number of people who would otherwise never have been elected. In Bucks County they had an individual named John Brown running for tax collector on the Democratic ticket. But, since there were not too many Democrats in Bucks County, they had simply put the name of a donkey, "John Brown," on the ballot. After Election Day, in the newspaper here was this picture of the winning candidate with his ears sticking out through this straw hat. My defense to the combined council of the faculty and staff was: "You fellows have done the dumbest thing in the world by electing this kind of 'tax collector' for chairman of the department. If only I had been on the selection committee for a new professor of surgery I would surely have found out all about this in advance." And I passed around the newspaper.

■ It's amazing how often this happens. Some "new guy" appears on the scene to head a major department or division, and he is heralded as the greatest thing that ever happened to the faculty. Within a year you find out he is a real "yo-yo" and wonder how they ever could have hired someone like this. You then go back to where he was before and learn all sorts of awful things about him from the people he really worked with at his former institution. It's unbelievable, but I suppose Santayana was right: those who cannot remember the past are condemned to repeat it.

In my "autumn years" I've become somewhat of a history buff, and I will swear that's the truth.

■   What finally happened?

Well, they were shocked and asked me what I suggested. I told them I would go "into limbo" and remain there until they were ready for a new professor of surgery. I told them that it would be about two years before everyone realized that this "John Brown" couldn't even collect taxes and that they would have to replace him. "When you want a new professor of surgery you will know where you can find me." How about that for telling off the board of trustees, the dean, and the administration?

But it didn't happen that way. The new professor had been in the Korean War and had made friends with a lot of the "brass" who were now in a position to help get him grants. Hahnemann had always been shy of grant money. I soon realized that, despite his past, it would be longer than two years before his exodus. I also realized that I was in no way qualified to head a general surgical department. I'd have to learn.

I had received an invitation from the New York Medical College to become the chairman of its Department of Surgery. They were in pretty poor shape at that time, and I thought that if I went there I would do my best and would at least learn "on the job." In any event, I expected that, were I to leave after a few years, at least I'd leave the department in a lot better condition than when I arrived there.

The dean of Hahnemann tried to dissuade me, but I still went to New York and did get wonderful on-the-job experience in running a surgical department. I believe I improved the place, and I think I was responsible for the development and maturation of some fine doctors there. However, the dean at New York Medical College was a true tyrant with autocratic powers such as you don't usually see in these modern times. I soon realized that those people who had come before me had gone through a "honeymoon" period and then had gotten into a period of what I called "slavery"—and it was! I told my wife before the first year was out to get prepared for another move, and by the end of the 1961–62 academic year l had left.

I had made no prior preparations for the future. I had a number of associations offered to me. I contacted a couple of the new medical schools that were developing at that time. However, I had had a "bellyful" of the machinations of high-level academic life, and I thought I'd like to be a free practitioner of medicine. What I wanted was a hospital where I could develop my specialty of cardiovascular surgery without being tied to a medical school. This I found at St. Barnabas Hospital in the Bronx where I was active for more than ten years.

■ This brings us up to 1973, and we seem to be getting into the legal phase of your career. How did this happen?

While I was in the Philadelphia area I had been sued three times for medical malpractice. None of the charges were valid and I managed to get a defense verdict each time. But neither my lawyers nor my doctor colleagues could tell me just what was going on. This opened my eyes to a new world, and I made up my mind then that someday, when I had more time, I would go to law school, because this was too complicated a problem to be resolved simply by the reading of a book or two.

When I came to New York there was still another malpractice case carrying over from my Philadelphia days, but which had to be fought out in the New York courts. Again there was no justification for the case, but my very excellent defense lawyer from Philadelphia was terribly hamstrung by the differing rules in New York (which hampered his style), and it was necessary for me to bring in a number of extra medical witnesses to finally get a defense verdict. One of them was Dr. Dwight Harken, who is now one of my dearest friends!

Well, the time came that I finally did go to Fordham Law School (at night), and I graduated in 1973. But I still did not have the answers to my questions. Law school teaches one how to pass the bar examinations. It doesn't answer fundamental questions such as: Why are there so many medical malpractice cases? Of course, you might also say that medical school only teaches one how to pass the state licensure examinations. It, too, doesn't address some of the philosophical questions which may have caused one to enter medical school.

So I became a dilettante at law.

Then two years ago (1977) a case that was absolutely phony was brought up against me eleven years after its occurrence. It was tried in Newark, New Jersey, in a federal court. This time the plaintiff got a verdict for thirty-five thousand dollars in a two-million-dollar law suit.

The truth is that the diagnosis had been absolutely right: she did have a fistula [an abnormal channel] between the right coronary artery and the right atrium. I did operate it properly and up to all recognized standards and had adequate medical testimony to that effect. And she suffered no injury from the operation except the scar. But she had been terribly psychoneurotic and, in fact, had been complaining of chest pains from the age of twenty-two, even though the fistula was asymptomatic. It often takes to middle age for these fistulae to produce heart failure. Her nonspecific chest complaints had led to her being sent to me for a coronary arteriogram, which had disclosed this abnormal communication. Now, after the admittedly purely prophylactic surgery, she was still terribly psychoneurotic, but that was mainly because she had married the wrong man. Now, I didn't feel any responsibility for her having married the wrong man; she married him before she had ever met me, and she never indicated to me that it was the wrong man, so I never gave her any advice about that. She still had the wrong man after the surgery.

After some years she finally went to a doctor in New Jersey, and he got the idea that maybe she had never had this fistula at all before surgery. So he sent for the preoperative diagnostic movie films, the cineangiograms. And the "dum-dum" hospital, without saying a word either to me or the fellow in charge of the heart catheterization laboratory, sent out the only copy of the film in existence. The doctor in New Jersey, who happened to be a psychiatrist, turned them over to a cardiologist who was supposed to take it up to another hospital and view it on a suitable projector. On the way there, he claimed his car was burglarized and the film stolen. Now, I cannot believe that a theft of that kind would occur. Why would anyone want to steal a medical movie film? Maybe the plaintiff's lawyer destroyed it, but even if he did, it seems to me that that was the responsibility of the patient or her agents or her doctors; it certainly wasn't mine.

And yet, without the film, our proof of the preoperative diagnosis was gone. Now, I'm convinced that justice often does not exist with the jury system. The jury is an anachronism abandoned by most other countries. Plaintiffs' lawyers will argue vigorously about this and shout "Preserve the jury system!" but that is because they are making their money out of it, not because it is right.

Long ago, before this ever happened, I had declared that if I was ever found guilty of malpractice I would never operate again. So I am finished with surgery, having done my last case in April 1979. Now I am a practicing defense lawyer.

■ You're sixty-eight now. What happens to aging surgeons that don't become lawyers?

Well, if they get tremors or Parkinsonism, of course, they have to quit. If their brains are not functioning sharply they ought to quit. Usually hospitals and medical schools retire you at sixty-five. You lose your chiefship, and once you do, you usually find it's hard to go back and become just "one of the boys" again. From then on the residents may help you, but they don't give you the kind of respect that they give the fellow who is chief—and from whom they will have to get their certification and recommendations. They may try to convert you to using the new chief's methods, or often have ideas of their own and begin to argue with you about them. It's not as much fun doing surgery after you have reached sixty-five.

There are some other things missing when you get to be an older surgeon, too: the joy of living, "joie de vivre." I used to look forward with anticipation and excitement to doing an operation. Well, these things seem to take longer as you get older; my kind of operation often takes eight hours. So you no longer get that old thrill. And you worry more as you grow more conservative. You think, My God, there's a twenty-five percent chance he'll die. You used to think, There's a seventy-five percent chance he'll live and get better. However, with the change in medical practice and the increasing threat of malpractice suits where anything new is "dangerous," you don't rush ahead as readily as you once did.

■ You edit the monograph, *Cardiovascular Advances*, and when the first volume came out I was amazed to see that the legal section, which you wrote, constituted almost ten percent of the book's four hundred pages. Just to summarize the reasons you said we live in such a litigious society: disappointment in the results realized by the patient or a misunderstanding between doctor and patient; a patient's desire to punish the doctor he doesn't like; avarice of the patient; and frequently all this is complicated by a jury deciding to punish a physician or just to compensate a very unfortunate person even if the doctor was blameless, because they feel they ought to give the injured patient something, anyway.

You see, that last one is a "sneaker." Every time you read a medical or surgical textbook about a given disease, particularly things that you treat surgically, they'll give you the figures: such-and-such a chance the patient will survive, such-and-such a chance he will die, such-and-such a chance that he will be *better*. The last is not the same as the number that will survive. It never is. And there are varying degrees of improvement; not everybody gets entirely better, and the reasons are

many. There may have been too much preexisting disease to
correct it entirely. It may be that other tissue and organs have
deteriorated secondary to the primary disease or in association with it. Or it may be that the patient has a psychoneurotic element in his symptomatology, and this is not going to go
away postoperatively. And all that means is that among the
survivors perhaps only twenty-five to seventy-five percent, depending on what their problems are, will have a "perfect" or at
least a good result. Furthermore, in a recent California study
of twenty-one thousand hospital admissions, Mills, Rubsa-
man, and Boyden* found that nearly five percent suffered
some medically related injury associated with their hospitalization. Modern medicine is dangerous. In only seventeen percent of these injuries among those twenty-one thousand
patients was there any provider fault, but the question is
raised: Shouldn't all of these innocent victims receive some
compensation?

So, the jury lumps it all together. They feel that these people
ought to have some kind of compensation. Now, the doctor
doesn't live who can always get ideal results: he can only get
up to the level that is reasonably possible. Doctors, if they
only understood, would realize that they are in a "catch 22"
situation. They can't win; they have to lose. In our fault-based
compensation system the plaintiff's lawyers may try to "cook
up" a spurious case of fault whenever the result is not perfect,
and the jury may be disposed to "buy it."

■ Have modern doctors in any way themselves contributed to this problem?
As compared with the old-timers?

I don't think doctors are all that different today. We are all
basically part of an imperfect species. I look back on the physicians I knew during my youth, and there were some real
sons of bitches. But there were great and kindly ones, too.

*D. H. Mills, D. Rubsamen, and J. S. Boyden, "Report on the Medical Insurance Feasibility
Study," California Medical Association and California Hospital Association, 1977.

There were some guys who would chew their patients out and say, "Never come back and darken my doorway again; I'll never treat you again." There were patients who would say, "That goddammed doctor; he set my leg wrong and look at the crook I've now got in that bone!" I think we all make a variety of mistakes, but there was an overall feeling among the public that the doctor had some godly touch, that he was like a priest, or minister, or rabbi—and you don't sue them. And they didn't sue doctors in those days except in very rare and unusual cases.

Today's doctors are more successful financially than they were in the past. To that extent patients envy us and don't feel sorry for us as they did when every other patient didn't pay us—and everybody knew this. I suppose the fact that most doctors don't come out at nighttime or do house calls anymore may bother them a little. I think that specialization in modern medicine, where you get a whole team working on you instead of just one doctor who is in charge, must depersonalize the medical attention. And some doctors treat their patients as diagnoses instead of as sick people.

The world has changed, and our position with respect to litigation proneness is infinitely more vulnerable. We could easily strengthen that position by group and individual personal actions, but so far we haven't done anything for ourselves except to complain and act paranoid. We ask the Legislature for "tort reform"! There are some individual physicians who have done what I have done. They won't operate anymore, and some won't even practice medicine. But until doctors are willing to do this in concert the overall problem will remain.

I've thought long and hard about this, and I can tell you what they could do. First of all, they'd have to be organized into a great unified group. Call it a union if you like. It would have to be organized technically as a union, or else legally they would not be able to invoke their rights as citizens in a group. But presently doctors are so prejudiced against unions that I don't see them joining the equivalent of a union in the foreseeable future. But if they suffer a little more, maybe they will. At any rate, they would have to agree to follow their own leadership. Now, in any state, or preferably nationally, that leadership could very simply declare a strike. They would set up emergency centers at hospitals and clinics here and there, as was done in New York City in 1976, so that no patient would suffer from an acute emergency without medical help. But no postponable medical services would be provided until the legislature changed its rules.

The legislature in two weeks, maybe four, would change the rules because of public pressure, and the new rules could be fair and reasonable. Let me ask you: Who can judge best whether an orthopedic surgeon has done the right thing in a given case?

■   I would say another well-qualified orthopedic surgeon.

I would prefer three orthopedic surgeons. That would tend to eliminate personal bias. Oh, yes, they have these so-called medical malpractice panels now. But in New York, for instance, they are composed of a judge, a lawyer, and a doctor of the same discipline as the "defendant." You and I, even though we're doctors, wouldn't be too good at judging the work of an orthopedic surgeon. How could two medically laypeople, a lawyer and a judge, ever be expected to know what a medical case would be all about?

■   Having a panel consisting solely of doctors judging another doctor may lay them open to the charge of protecting their own. We always hear complaints about lawyers not being able to get doctors to testify against doctors.

Every member of a hospital staff knows there is no one harsher than a doctor in judging another doctor when he thinks the son of a bitch did something wrong—or "conned" the patient! And there could be safeguards against any kind of prejudice either way on the part of an all-doctor panel. The doctor panels would be organized in such a way that each year an expert (unpaid) could sit on a panel for, let us say, two weeks. They would only serve in areas very distant from their own, so that none of the problems of local relationships would interfere. They could be disqualified for any proper reason. By having a panel of several doctors instead of only one, any personal bias that might sway one would be counterbalanced by the other doctors. In this way I think you would have real justice.

■ It must be terrible to be sued. I've been lucky, I suppose. I've never been sued.

Well, the "law of averages" is warping against you all the time!*

■ Did you have any great disappointments in your life?

I regret that I didn't have one or two of my sons go into medicine. And I have reflected on some of my past decisions. My father always seemed to have difficulty in holding onto jobs because he had a tendency to argue with his bosses and to express his own ideas so vigorously that they found it desirable to separate. I have found some trace of that characteristic in my own personality. I'm probably the only doctor you know who has told two different medical school deans where they could stick their professorships.

But I sometimes have mixed emotions about Hahnemann and regret that I left when I did. On the other hand, Hahnemann has just been through another administrative and organizational convulsion, and sooner or later I probably would have had my head "lopped off" there if I hadn't left when I did. And, I never would have gone to law school had I remained in Philadelphia. But I would have liked another ten

*In 1981 the law of averages stopped "warping" for the author when he found himself named in a suit with four other doctors at his institution.

years to work on the mitral valve problem; there's still a great need for improvement of these prosthetic valves.

■   Your career was really unique. Our own professor of surgery likes to give a lecture on the history of surgery to our medical students. In this he points out that in American surgery almost all the major figures have descended in line from one of their great forebears: Halsted, Cushing, and so on. . . . You seem to have developed pretty much on your own.

I was aware of the great things in medicine. I had done a lot of reading about these people, but I didn't come from any of the schools that are supposed to produce great people, partly because I didn't have enough money to go to these schools. I was a bright boy: I probably could have made Harvard or Hopkins if I had tried, but I would not have been able to pay the tuition. It was quite inexpensive at that time to go to Hahnemann, which was also teaching homeopathy. So at least I got two degrees out of it: doctor of medicine and doctor of homeopathic medicine.*

Anyway, I have the old-fashioned idea that in America you can do whatever you want with your life, and it never bothered me to be in a minority medical position. In fact, it may even have made me work harder.

*Homeopathy was a system of therapeutics founded by Samuel Hahnemann and based on the theory that diseases can be treated by administration of minute doses of substances that would, in healthy persons, produce the same symptoms when given in larger doses.

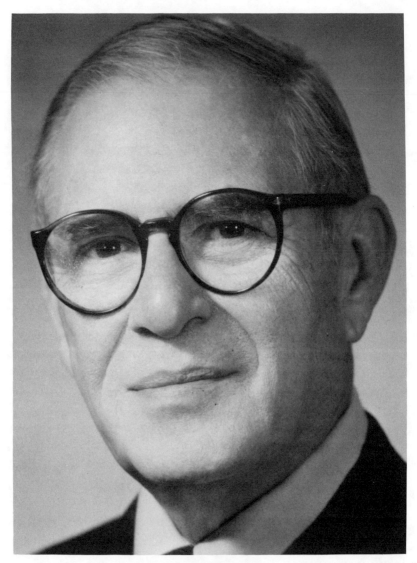

Louis Weinstein, Ph.D., M.D.
(Courtesy of Harvard University)

CHAPTER 9

Louis Weinstein, Ph.D., M.D.
(1909–   )

O NE CANNOT THINK of a group of infectious disease experts putting their heads together over a particularly baffling case without someone remarking somewhere in the course of their deliberations, "Well, Lou Weinstein would say . . ." Dr. Weinstein has been characterized by another well-recognized expert in the field as "the best intuitive infectious disease man alive today."

Louis Weinstein, in the course of a half-century in microbiology and medicine, has been encyclopedic in his coverage of infectious disease. In Boston, noted for its plethora of medical experts of all kinds, Dr. Weinstein, in one way or another, has been involved almost constantly throughout his career with all its prestigious medical schools and hospitals.

He began as a microbiologist at Yale, where he taught and did research at the medical school until 1939. He then decided to obtain a medical degree and moved to Boston, where he has remained ever since. He completed his medical studies and postgraduate training at Boston University under its renowned chairman of medicine, Chester Keefer. His first major post following this was at the Haynes Memorial, a hospital for communicable diseases, where he would remain for twelve years and gain the vast experience for which he is so respected today. In the preantibiotic era, communicable diseases posed a much greater threat to other hospitalized patients than they do now, and therefore patients with infectious disease were often sequestered in special hospitals some distance away from the rest of the hospitalized population.

It was the years at Haynes, with its thousands upon thousands of patients with a variety of infections, that shaped the young physician Louis Weinstein. In 1957, however, with antibiotics well established and the potential threat of communicable disease to other hospitalized patients diminishing, the role of the special infectious disease hospital declined. It was at this time that Dr. Weinstein shifted his activities to the Tufts New England Medical Center, where he served for the next eighteen years as chief of infectious diseases on both the Adult Medicine and Pediatric services.

The year 1975 marked his sixty-fifth birthday, but retirement was unacceptable to the still vigorous Dr. Weinstein. He moved over to Harvard's Peter Bent Brigham Hospital, his current base of operations. "As long as I can work and do a job," he maintains in his bouncy, machine-gun delivery style, "I'll never retire."

Although at any one time, nominally, a faculty member primarily of either Boston University, Tufts, or Harvard, Dr. Weinstein has made his presence felt at all three throughout his time in Boston. Similarly, he has been a frequent consultant at other hospitals such as the University Hospital and the Massachusetts General, Evans Memorial, and West Roxbury Veterans Administration hospitals.

Dr. Weinstein has been, throughout his career, a "triple-threat man" in medicine. His clinical acumen is legendary. His teaching ability is unexcelled, and besides the many students and house staff that have profited from his guidance, over one hundred specialists in infectious disease have trained with him. Many of these now occupy important positions in the field throughout the country. Finally, as a researcher, from the time of his studies on hormone effects on the bacterial flora of the vagina (still frequently referred to in obstetrical circles), he has continued to contribute to our knowledge and understanding in all aspects of infectious disease.

Among the over five hundred papers that have emanated from his laboratory are landmark studies pointing to the beneficial effects of certain antibiotics, as well as the first clear demonstration of "superinfection," the problem of developing a second infection while on antibiotics for the initial one. He has made important contributions on the postrheumatic fever effects on the kidney and the importance of host factors (characteristics of the patients, themselves) affecting the course and outcome of infectious diseases.

There have been other outstanding infectious disease specialists during this era, people such as Max Finland at Boston City Hospital, Paul Beeson, and others who have made fundamental discoveries in the field. Yet none have had quite the unique personal impact of Dr. Weinstein as a teacher and a healer. It is for this reason that, when other medical experts fall ill in his community, it is to Louis Weinstein that they often turn as personal physician. No greater compliment can be paid by one doctor to another.

Boston has been fortunate in having Dr. Weinstein around for the last forty years because, although they may be relative rarities now, the infectious scourges of the past—scarlet fever, diphtheria, polio—are well known to him and, from time to time, are apt once againt to raise their ugly heads. He can also discuss maladies like cholera and anthrax, entities that, in modern America, we can read about only in a book—one very likely to have been written by Louis Weinstein.

■ Right from the time you finished your medical residency in 1945 you went to an infectious disease hospital in Boston, where you spent the better part of the next twelve years of your life. I suppose that was the basis of your broad experience in infectious diseases.

That was the Haynes Memorial Hospital. It had 150 beds and served as the main communicable disease hospital for southeastern Massachusetts. This was the Infectious Disease Division of the Department of Medicine of Boston University, with the rest of the department situated at the Massachusetts Memorial Hospital [now the University Hospital], about six or seven miles distant from it. I think I learned more per day at Haynes about all of medicine than I've since learned in a week or perhaps a month.

When I went there I had only two house officers to assist me. No medical students were assigned at first, because they did not believe the place was running right at the time. The residents and I worked literally twenty hours a day. Every night I would sit down with the charts of a hundred patients, look over every record, and tell the two house officers what I wanted them to do on the following day. I had an unusual opportunity to see a wide variety of infectious diseases. I saw about eight thousand cases of scarlet fever while I was there; between 1946 and 1950 I saw about six hundred cases of diph-theria; I also saw a great deal of rheumatic fever. A few years ago I added up my total experience with poliomyelitis both at the Haynes and Massachusetts General Hospital, Boston City Hospital and Quincy City Hospital. This came to a total of thirty-five hundred cases. We had two large epidemics of this disease, in 1949 and 1955, as you know.

■ In the past they used to say that syphilis was the great teacher. If you knew syphilis you knew medicine. In your experience, you might claim the same for polio.

I certainly agree. I've always said that if one really wanted to find out how good an internist he was, he should take care of some patients with paralytic poliomyelitis. They had all kinds of problems. They had electrolyte and fluid problems. Because they were under such high stress, they had multiple-stress ulcers from the fundus of the stomach right down to the rectum, so we had problems with gastrointestinal bleeding. I saw three or four patients who, while very quietly lying in their respirators, ruptured the esophagus and were found to have large stress ulcers postmortem. About a third, at least, of the adults had paralyzed bladders, so we got into all sorts of trouble with urinary tract infections and kidney stones. Since they were lying in respirators, and could not ventilate well, we saw pneumonias in very large numbers. The psychiatric problems were innumerable, so that, in fact, we had an attending psychiatrist coming each day to visit the patients, especially during the 1955 epidemic.

■ I once saw a photograph of the Haynes during that time, and it looked like the engine room of the *Queen Elizabeth*, what with all the "iron lungs" lined up. You had one hair-raising experience with this at the time, did you not?

There are certain episodes that happen in your life that you never forget, even though you may not have been in any personal danger. I recall the circumstances of this episode very clearly. I had been pleading with the administrators of Haynes to get our own generator for the hospital, since we had so many people on electrically powered respirators in 1955, and had to rely on outside current for supply. We had no backup in case of power failure outside. Well, like all hospitals at the time, they were in a bit of financial trouble and just could not come up with the funds for this. One morning, after it had been raining for several days, I was sitting in my office at about eleven A.M. with the administrator of the hospital and my chief resident, making plans for the influx of patients we expected during the day. We often saw as many as thirty-five suspected cases a day, and admitted twenty with polio, so there was always the problem of where we could put them with only a total of 150 beds in the entire hospital. While we were discussing this, the lights in my office suddenly went off. I knew that if the lights in my office were off then there was no electricity anywhere in the hospital, since we were supplied by a single line. I ran over to the respirator ward, and here were twenty-four respirators standing still. If you ever want to experience a frightening situation, this was it. Fortunately, we had mainly the Emerson respirators, and they had a long handle on the front which you could use to work them manually. Well, we got the nurses in, we called in some garage workers from the back of the hospital, and the cooks, and in a few minutes we had all twenty-four respirators being pumped by hand. But this was strenuous work; you couldn't do it for more than ten or fifteen minutes without a rest. There was a group of ministers not far from us who were undergoing medical training for hospital work, and I called them and got them in to help.

The fright of the patients was unimaginable. They knew that they could not survive without those respirators going. By early afternoon I had gotten in touch with the army people at Fort Devens, and had them send down one of their portable generators. We hooked it up, turned on the machines, and the generator shut off. It was clear that we had overloaded it. We tried a couple of more generators, and finally, by eight o'clock in the evening, we had a big enough one in working order to run the respirators. This was after nine hours of constant hand pumping, but not a single patient got into trouble; all survived. That was the last big polio epidemic, and the hospital finally bought its own emergency generator.

■ Tell me something about your experience with scarlet fever as a result of streptococcal infection. I don't believe I've seen half a dozen cases, and you've seen thousands.

This was the most common disease in the hospital; we used to admit about twelve hundred cases a year. Scarlet fever, as we saw it when sulfonamide was the only treatment, was a very different disease from what one saw after the introduction of penicillin. The numbers of complications and the types of complication were fantastic. There were huge numbers of otitis media [middle ear infections]. We used to make ear rounds every morning and evening, and if we had a hundred cases of scarlet fever on the service, we might pick up twenty red ears in the morning. These would be draining in the evening, because this was typical of streptococcal otitis. Sulfonamides would not prevent the development of mastoiditis [infection of the bone behind the ear], so maybe, of these twenty with otitis, ten or twelve would have the infection progress to mastoiditis. All these suppurative complications of scarlet fever—sinusitis, rhinitis, skin infections, vulvovaginitis in children, mastoiditis, and occasionally bacteremias—were just fantastic. Very often these children would be hospitalized six, seven, eight weeks. I once calculated the average stay for a large group of patients, and this came to forty days.

Penicillin changed all that; we now know that the streptococcus is gone in forty-eight to ninety-six hours, and you can send patients home. Mastoiditis became so uncommon that we got rid of all our instruments with which mastoidectomies, the only treatment we had for this complication, were performed. We also had frontal bone osteomyelitis develop in some of these patients, and the old treatment used to be to whittle away at the frontal bone, but practically none of these patients survived prepenicillin. Dr. Leighton Johnson was the chief of otolaryngology [ear, nose, and throat] at Boston University, and I was involved with him in curing the first case of this without surgery. We had this little boy come in on a Sunday night with the typical so-called Pott's puffy tumor, with cool pale edema [swelling] over the forehead. We recognized osteomyelitis of the frontal bone, and that night I prepared two little pieces of ureteral catheter, which we inserted into the frontal sinuses at surgery Monday morning. After Dr. Johnson sewed the catheters in place, we gave this child five thousand units of penicillin intravenously every three hours, because this was all we had. And every two hours for the next two weeks, I pushed one thousand units of penicillin through the catheter into each sinus, and finally achieved a cure. Today we think little of giving fifty or sixty million units of penicillin a day, but it was in short supply at the beginning.

I had all kinds of experience at Haynes. I delivered a fair number of babies there, because the obstetricians were afraid to come out there during the polio epidemics. We had a surgeon assigned to the Haynes, and any patient that developed acute appendicitis, for example, during a contagious disease of childhood would not be accepted by any other hospital. So I scrubbed on these with the surgeon on the average of once a week for years. During my first year alone at Haynes, I scrubbed with the otolaryngologist on forty-five mastoidectomies. I think I learned to be a pretty good practitioner of medicine there.

■ Is it still active?

No. The Haynes Memorial closed one year after I left, in 1957. That was the summer of 1958. Infectious diseases were coming under better control and could be handled in general hospitals. The census at Haynes had been falling, and the population had been getting so low that, during its last seven or eight years, we converted half of the 150 beds there to a tuberculosis sanitarium. So I then had the opportunity to get a lot of experience with tuberculosis as well. But it was clear that that type of hospital was going out of vogue, and I don't believe there are any left. I had always preferred that infectious disease be included in a general medical department, and that these patients should not be sitting out somewhere distant from the rest of the medical population. You should have a patient with chicken pox in one room and another with myocardial infarction in the next for the best system. Of course, on pediatrics you still need some segregation because of the high risk of contagion.

■ Let's talk about the early years. You were born in Bridgeport, Connecticut, and originally went into microbiology before medicine.

My whole family lived in Bridgeport. At the time we were the only Weinsteins in Bridgeport. My grandfather's brother came there from Russia, and brought over all his nephews and nieces, and made sure that we all settled on Wallace Street.

I had some early problems with career choices. I had been a professional musician, having learned to play jazz violin, which very few people could do, apparently. I had been working with orchestras from the age of fourteen or fifteen, playing dance music. At the time I went off to Yale, I wasn't sure that I didn't want to stay in music, and worked as a musician all through my time there and in graduate school.

My second choice, after music, was initially medicine. But at Yale, when I took my first course in microbiology, it was under Leo Rettger, who had set up the department at Yale. He convinced me that the brightest people did not go into medicine and that I should stay in microbiology, so I switched my major from premedical to biological sciences. I got my Ph.D. in microbiology at Yale in 1931 and spent the next eight years there in microbiology at the medical school.

■ What turned you toward medicine?

There were two considerations that influenced me. While at Yale I was interested in the role of endocrine function on the vaginal bacterial flora. To carry out this investigation I worked in a gynecological clinic in Bridgeport where I could see a great many more patients than at Yale, and while I was there, an obstetrician with whom I worked urged me to get a medical degree and come back to join his practice. This was a field in which I had some basic scientific interest, and was attractive to me. The second consideration was that I was already married, and realized that there were restrictions for people of my ethnic background in getting academic appointments. When I got my Ph.D. at the age of twenty-two, I thought I had done very well, but when I received job offers these were all from commercial institutions. Then, as I scanned the microbiology departments around the country, it was pretty clear that Jews were far from the favored people as far as appointments were concerned. At Yale, if I remember correctly, there was not a single Jew teaching in the undergraduate school. Louis Goodman, Abraham White, Alfred Gilman, and Harry Zimmerman, I think, were the only Jews with real academic rank in the medical school. I had been put up for assistant professor at Yale by my chief, but it was made clear to me that that was far as I would ever be going to go there. I decided that if I was going to depend on my Ph.D. for a livelihood, I would always have to be dependent on someone else's good graces. This would not be the case if I could practice private medicine. I had credit for the first two years of medical school from my work at Yale, and then arranged to go to Boston University to get my M.D. I chose Boston University because I had become interested in immunology; and Sanford Hooker, one of the best immunologists in the country, was there at the time. I wanted to study the possible role of immune mechanisms in the problem of eclampsia [a form of high blood pressure in pregnancy with brain and kidney complications].

While at Boston University I came to Chester Keefer's[b] attention when I worked in his laboratory one summer with Rammelcamp[b] between the junior and senior years. I had been told I could have an internship at Boston City Hospital if I wished, but I had decided that I would prefer to get my training in a smaller hospital. I applied to a number of these and asked Keefer for his recommendation. He said, "What do you want to do?" And I said, "I am going into obstetrics and gynecology." And then he said, "What? You want to be a midwife?"

That sort of struck me square between the eyes, and at that moment I decided to go into internal medicine instead and have never regretted it.

■ Tell me about Keefer. I met him briefly only once, many years ago.

Chester Keefer was, in my opinion, a very remarkable person. He has really been my model, I'm very happy to admit. I think people around the country felt that, in his day, he was probably the best clinician in the country. He was a first-rate teacher and a good scientist. He had already done excellent research work when he had been at Hopkins on the house staff. I had the greatest admiration for him and still have. At least once a week I still teach something I learned from Chester Keefer.

He was a very tough man, very demanding, and nothing short of perfection satisfied him, but I didn't mind that. He was very rough on students and house officers, and if you missed a physical finding you had your head torn off! And he developed a sense of judgment in you in a way that could be very uncomfortable. I remember once he was making teaching rounds on a patient who was on my service at the time. I had suggested that the patient be cystoscoped, but when Keefer saw the case he disagreed. He asked me why I wanted the patient cystoscoped and was still not convinced. I said that I still thought the patient should be cystoscoped, and he said, "Okay, young fella, you want the patient to be cystoscoped? You get cystoscoped first."

■ Did you get cystoscoped?

No! And the patient did not get cystoscoped, you can be sure. It was an uncomfortable lesson, but I learned it.

He was a very hardworking man and demanding of himself. For example, one of the things I noticed about him and admired greatly was the so-called clinic he gave for third-year students every Saturday at noon. No one was permitted to see him Saturday morning, because he would be busy preparing that lecture. I thought this most unusual for a man with his teaching ability to spend two or three hours in the morning each week in preparation for a discussion with medical students on a topic he had probably presented twenty-five times before. But when he gave that lecture, you knew that it was up to date, that whatever had appeared in the literature within the previous week would be included.

He was upset with me when I left Haynes Memorial and Boston University to go to Tufts in 1957. He was very jealous about keeping the people he had in his department. But this passed, and we became very close friends. I was his family doctor, and I took care of him, his wife, and his daughter when they were ill. I enjoyed my association over the years with Keefer and owe him an awful lot.

■ When you describe Dr. Keefer, about his being such a hard taskmaster, some people might think you are describing yourself. Are you as tough as he with your staff?

I confess that many of us who worked intimately with Keefer have modeled ourselves after him. But the teaching of infectious disease to students and house staff today is different from the past. More than is generally recognized, the old infections continue to pop up. Diphtheria is still around the country and has been endemic [continuously present] in the skid row people in Seattle. But young people have not seen a lot of these diseases and often fail to recognize them.

When I first came to my present position at the Brigham,

the first cases of scarlet fever were missed. As a matter of fact, I was very impressed when at Tufts to discover that young people had so little experience with the common contagious diseases. Not their fault; they just had not seen enough. I was called one day by the house staff to come see a patient with dengue ["breakbone fever," a viral infection usually seen in the tropics causing pain in the back and extremities]. Now, this lady lived in Concord, Massachusetts, and it was the month of January. There has never been a case of dengue in Concord, and you don't see dengue in January. The lady had scarlet fever. Several months later the house staff were excited over a case of "measles" that turned out to be a classical chicken pox. Another case of "drug rash" turned out to be measles. A case of diphtheria was missed. A woman was brought in with "infectious polyneuritis," and she had the most classical poliomyelitis you would ever want to see.

What complicates the matter is that many of these diseases have changed their character over the years. The rash in scarlet fever can be so fleeting that it may be missed by the time the patient gets to the hospital. Rheumatic fever, I believe, may have changed in its clinical presentation. Subacute bacterial endocarditis* certainly has, and you'll miss many cases if you insist on the presence of changing murmurs, petechiae [hemorrhagic spots], and other peripheral manifestations. I have a woman with this now who had nothing but a faint systolic heart murmur—with six positive blood cultures. Mycoplasma pneumoniae has changed: it used to be described as circumscribed in the lung, benign, in no need of treatment, and without complications. None of this is now consistently true.

■ It may be getting more and more difficult to recognize some of these infections, but it seems that it is also becoming more difficult to treat them

*An infection involving the heart valves.

with the emergence of resistant strains of organisms, and such an incredible proliferation of new antibiotics that one finds it difficult which to choose.

I have some pretty clear-cut ideas about this. I have been playing with antibiotics from the time they first arrived. There is no question that more and more organisms are becoming more and more resistant to more and more antibiotics, and this is the result of the so-called pressure of antibiotic use. It's a well-established observation that if you begin to use one antibiotic to a large degree in a hospital, within a given period of time a number of strains that were previously sensitive to that antibiotic will become resistant. So that is one problem.

The other problem is that the more and more people we expose to antibiotics, the more and more are getting sensitized. This is a problem that I don't think is being addressed as strongly as it should be. Our attention has been focused on the resistant bacteria. I'm interested in what is going on with the people who are getting these antibiotics, and I would say that fifteen percent of the people I see, either in hospital or as outpatients, give me a history of sensitivity to penicillin, if nothing else. And we have seen a number of people who have been sensitized to a multiplicity of antibiotic agents they have received for the treatment of nonexistent infection, infection not amenable to antibiotics, or fever not related to infection in the first place. What the future of this is going to be I do not know.

What about the multiplicity of antibiotics available? What bothers me is that many are "me too" drugs. For example, there are ten cephalosporins right now, all with pretty much the same spectrum of activity. There are a number of penicillins and four or five tetracyclines. But if you group all the drugs into their own classes, there are perhaps six or seven general types of antibiotics. Physicians would do well to become acquainted with one drug within each group, and use this unless specific reasons indicate otherwise.

Over the years, I have become impressed with several stages in the history of antibiotics. The first stage is the stage of hyperenthusiasm. When I first began writing on the tetracyclines in the antibiotic section of Goodman and Gilman, I reviewed all the papers on them, and I was impressed by the uniformly good reports they received during the first three or four years. They cured this and they cured that; only good things. Over the next three or four years we entered the stage of critical evaluation: now you saw papers coming out saying that the drug was not as good as we thought it was, and some side effects began to creep into the reports. The last three or four years' stage consists primarily of reports about untoward effects. So you really need nine or ten years to evaluate a new antibiotic.

The tetracyclines were introduced in 1946, but it wasn't until 1959, thirteen years later, that the dental defects were first reported. Chloramphenicol became available in 1946, and it also took thirteen years for one of its side effects to become apparent: the so-called Gray syndrome [a bluish color of skin accompanied by shock] particularly in newborns, and, unlike the tetracycline problem, this one can be lethal. Why does it take so long to find these things out? Because the reactions are relatively uncommon, and therefore it is more difficult to recognize them early. The rule should be not to accept a new antibiotic to replace an old one with which you are experienced unless you have a very specific reason.

■ I would like to raise another problem with which you have been concerned: medicine and public policy. In 1976 we had the swine influenza scare, and you wrote a very influential editorial for the *New England Journal of Medicine* recommending vaccination. Do you regret that now?

I have reflected on that a good deal. I originally wanted to make the conclusion of that editorial a bit "wishy-washy" but was pushed by the editor to make a definite yes /no stand on the issue. I was a kid during the influenza pandemic of 1918

and remembered people dying all around us, although, fortunately, my family survived. I had read all the subsequent
reports about the pandemic and was amazed to learn that the
death rates exceeded those that were experienced in London
during the Black Plague in the Middle Ages. It was awful. I
thought that since there was some evidence that the outbreak
of Fort Dix in New Jersey was due to the same virus that had
caused the 1918 pandemic, it was the better part of wisdom to
attempt to prevent the disease. No one could predict what was
about to happen, but it seemed to me that, if there was any
possibility of danger of any kind, it would be better to attempt
protection rather than wait for the tragedy to happen, and see
people dying in the course of it.

Now, who could have predicted that the Guillain-Barré syndrome [an inflammation of the peripheral nerves causing pain
and paralysis] would develop as a problem? And this was
really the only problem. We had been giving influenza vaccine
to loads of people for many years, and we had never had
Guillain-Barré develop. Secondly, we know that Guillain-
Barré develops with a variety of active viral infections, and
this was a *dead* virus we gave. It was probably a hypersensitiza-
tion phenomenon, and there is some experimental evidence
that these people get immunized to their own nervous system.

If I had to do it all over again, I would probably make a
similar recommendation but, perhaps, use amantadine rather
than the vaccine. When the question about what action to
take arose in 1976, there was a committee in Massachusetts
organized by the commissioner of health to discuss the whole
problem. I suggested that, if there was any question about
using vaccine, we might consider amantadine, an antiviral
agent which was active as prophylaxis against influenza A,
which the swine flu is, but not influenza B. This was not
received with much enthusiasm because amantadine had
been reported to be neurotoxic [damaging to nerves]. In actu-
ality, it was not significantly neurotoxic if you used it in the

right dosage, and in Parkinsonism people have taken it for some time without difficulty. So I might push hard for amantadine if the question arose today.

■   There was an interesting coda to the whole swine flu vaccine controversy. A former associate of yours, Martin Goldfield, was an official concerned with public health and infectious disease in New Jersey. He came out *against* the use of the vaccine, and when he was ultimately proved right, because the epidemic never did develop, it was rumored that he so embarrassed the higher-ups that they fired him.

The rumor is correct, because I have discussed this with Goldfield. He is one of the brightest people that I have trained, a very bright man. He discussed his stand with me long before this came out in public, and I saw his point of view. There were other people who took the same stand that there was no strong indication for mass vaccination. I think he saw my point of view as well. It was a discussion based on scientific grounds. I felt very badly to hear that he had, in fact, lost his job over this, and I didn't like it.

■   The final irony of the whole business is that New Jersey was firing Marty Goldfield for being right, while the Ford administration was firing Ted Cooper[b] for being wrong. So much for state and national politics. How about politics on the university level? Have you ever been involved in it?

I made up my mind many years ago that I would never get involved in medical politics. Unless I am called to serve on a committee or something, I stay out of them. In the first place, I don't consider myself sophisticated enough to be a politician. And secondly, this is not my interest. Thirdly, I want to devote myself to doing what I enjoy the most: seeing patients, doing research, and teaching.

■   You must have been offered a number of department chairmanships?

In 1951 I was offered the chairmanship in a very large hospital which I need not name. I went to this place and spent a week there. I was told that I had been selected from a group of people. During the week, I went around visiting and talking with various people, and on the way home I took the train, which gave me a long time to think. I realized, the more I thought about it, that this was not for me. In the first place, three quarters of that kind of job is administrative: getting money, hiring people, firing people, trying to keep everybody happy. I had been trained in microbiology, and thought I was an adequate teacher and clinician. I had administered 150 beds at Haynes, but this new place had 1,200 beds. I decided then that I was not an administrator, and to try to do this would mean giving up everything I felt I did well and enjoyed doing. From that time on, I turned down every chairmanship I was approached about—and two deanships as well.

I don't see how some of those people who run big departments can keep track of things. What has happened historically is very interesting. The prestige of being a department chairman is no longer there. When you and I were growing up in medicine, there was one professor. He was the chief with his entourage of assistants all down the line. He was the power, and often better as a physician than anybody else in the department. That's why he was made chairman.

■ Is there anything other than medicine that really interests you?

Music. For a long time I played a lot of music. Franz Ingelfinger[b] was a very good pianist, and we were very close friends. He and I played sonatas every Monday night for perhaps seven or eight years. But then we got too busy and quit. I keep track of baseball pretty carefully. I watch football, but I'm not crazy about it. My big problem is that I don't have any hobbies, and don't know which hobby to develop. My hobby is work.

■ What has given you the most satisfaction?

Everything. I was just telling this to one of my younger people last week. These youngsters are in a quandary. Should they go mainly for research or mainly for clinical medicine? I told him that I get as much boot today, after all these years, in making a diagnosis that someone else has missed, as I do out of anything I do in the research lab. On the other hand, I'm now involved in studying a new immunological phenomenon that immunologists said did not exist, but I have pictorial proof that it does. I've gotten a big boot out of every one of these experiments, and a big boot out of teaching: I love to teach. So I don't see why you have to like one thing better than another.

The fellow asked me, "How do you do all of those things?" I said, "It's very simple. I work seven days a week and twelve to fourteen hours a day." But I have a crazy definition of work. To me work is doing something I don't like. I have gone to some parties that I've considered the worst work I ever had to do. They were a bore. That's work! When I see patients—even two neurotic patients like I saw yesterday, and with whom I had to spend two hours discussing things—I might say to myself, "Gee, why am I wasting my time with this?" But thinking about it on the way home I reflect to myself, I really learned something from those people. My problem is that I enjoy everything I do. And if I work hard and I'm enjoying what I do—to me that isn't work.

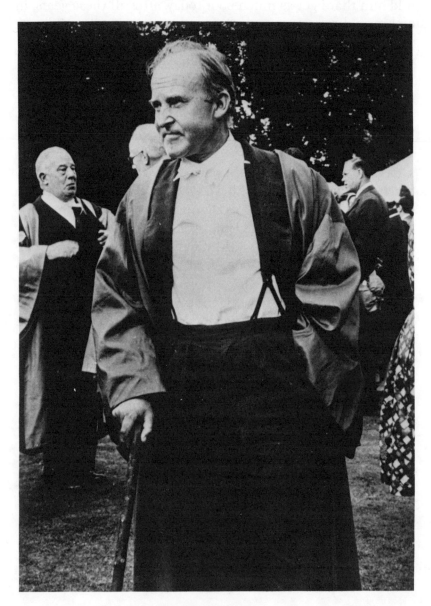
Sir George White Pickering, D.M.

CHAPTER 10

Sir George White Pickering, D.M. (1904–80)

Oh! Wad some power the giftie gie us
To see oursels as ithers see us!

Robert Burns

IN A BOOK about American medicine, why an Englishman? The ties of culture, language, and political history are obvious. In medicine as well there has been a long-standing relationship between the two countries. These were uniquely embodied in one man, William Osler, who, though born in Canada, made his medical mark in the United States and spent his final years at Oxford University as Regius Professor of Medicine. It was therefore fitting that Sir George Pickering, who assumed the same chair in 1956 and who has been a close observer of the American medical scene for many years, be called upon to contribute to this collection.

Pickering's erudition, wit, and forthrightness made him a popular guest on this side of the Atlantic, and, in the course of his career, he probably spent time as visiting professor at most of the leading medical schools in the United States. When the Josiah Macy, Jr., Foundation and the National Library of Medicine jointly produced the two-volume *Advances in American Medicine* at the time of our bicentennial, it was George Pickering to whom they turned for "The View from the United Kingdom."

Professor Pickering was educated at Dulwich College and Pembroke College, Cambridge. Among the many medical teaching posts he held was professor and director of the Medical Clinic at St. Mary's Hospital Medical School in London (1939–56), Regius Professor of Medicine at Oxford University (1956–69), and master of Pembroke College, Oxford (1969–74). Early in his career he worked with Sir Thomas Lewis (1891–1945), a major figure in following up on the work of the inventor of the modern electrocardiograph, Willem Einthoven. Among his more admirable traits, Lewis also had the reputation of a somewhat fearsome personality on occasion, and I was interested in learning from one of the current grand old men what it may have been like to work for another "leading light" in his youth.

Professor Pickering's main research interest was in the problem of high blood pressure, and to this he brought the same open-mindedness and clarity of thought that characterized all his lifetime pursuits as teacher and scientist.

Besides his books on hypertension, which are highly regarded throughout the medical world, Sir George wrote two classics of quite a different nature. In *Quest for Excellence in Medical Education. A Personal Survey* he sifted a lifetime of experience and in a slim volume presented us with his valuable insights on the subject, applicable to any modern nation today. In *Creative Malady* he analyzed how the illnesses of such diverse personalities as Charles Darwin, Florence Nightingale, Mary Baker Eddy, Sigmund Freud, Marcel Proust, and Elizabeth Barrett Browning contrived to bring about the great accomplishments of their remarkable lives. His book may have well been the creation of Professor Pickering's own malady, severe arthritis of the hips, which kept him bedridden periodically until he benefited from a total replacement of both hip joints. It is a masterful exploit in historical and psychological detective work and a tribute to Pickering's own idol, the surgeon-psychologist Sir Wilfred Trotter, whom he also discusses. Thanks to Pickering's sense of style, it is a book as readily accessible to the general reader as to the physician.

As for more recent history, Professor Pickering was present at the birth of Britain's National Health Service (NHS) and observed its development through childhood, adolescence, and middle age. As a leader of one of England's great teaching hospitals he worked intermittently under the National Health Service since its inception.

As we attempt to come to grips with the provision and financing of medical care in the United States, we have had the advantage of observing our British cousins with their National Health Service for over thirty years.

What do we know about the NHS? At the end of World War II in 1945 when a Labour government came to power in Great Britain, it had a clear and urgent agenda of priorities. The Bank of England, coal, electric power, and other institutions of national scope were quickly nationalized. The National Health Service Act was passed in 1946 and went into effect in 1948. The aim of this was to provide medical care for all regardless of ability to pay. The means of accomplishing this goal involved government ownership of all hospitals and employing all professionals involved in health care. Today this involves twenty-four hundred hospitals and approximately one million doctors, nurses, and other health workers.

There were three basic arrangements provided for under the NHS plan:

(1) Primary patient care would be provided out of hospital by general practitioners who, after signing on with the plan, would have lists of patients for whom they would be responsible.

(2) Specialists ("consultants") would be hospital-based for all their practice (inpatient and outpatient). When patients

required hospitalization, their care would be turned over
by the GPs to the consultants.

(3) Local authorities would be responsible for visiting nurses,
social workers, and other health-related service out in the
field.

Although there was some resistance on the part of physicians as they viewed the government about to assume such
awesome powers, they were somewhat mollified by the
provisions that allowed for some private practice. By 1950,
95 percent of the population were on the lists of the
NHS physicians, who constituted 88 percent of the country's
physicians.

Has it worked? There is no doubt that, on the whole, the
British public would answer a resounding yes to that question.
A chronic problem, however, has been underfinancing. Many
hospitals are outdated, and technical improvements are hard
to come by. In 1978 the cost of health care in Great Britain was
5.6 percent of the gross national product as compared to 8.5
percent in the United States. Translated into dollars, $700
were spent for each American, three times the amount spent
for each Briton.

The bureaucracy running the NHS has oftentimes seemed
on the verge of doing it in. Frequent "reforms" may have
caused more problems than improvements, as Dr. Pickering
will point out. The GPs are generally solidly behind the NHS,
although inadequately paid. The specialists have frequently
been at odds with the NHS, which, under the last Labour
government, was about to remove the remaining private beds
in the hospital system. With the current Conservative government this has not happened, and private medical insurance
and private hospitals are beginning to emerge conspicuously,
albeit on a small scale.

The number of specialists has been rigidly controlled by the
government. This the government can easily do because all
such positions are hospital posts within the NHS. In surgery

this has resulted in a shortage of surgeons or, at least, inadequate service, as demonstrated by the frequently long delays involved in awaiting elective surgery.

In 1975 there were 65,000 practicing physicians in Great Britain (exclusive of house staff), of whom only 16,000 were specialists. In the United States in the same year, among 270,000 physicians, 216,000 were specialists.

What can we learn from the British experience? First and foremost stands the fact that no one there can be driven into economic ruin as a result of illness. Too often this may not be the case in the United States, despite the large scope of the private insurance industry and associated government programs.

After this, one compares the two systems and finds excesses or shortages on both sides. We are spending too much on medical care; the British, not enough. We have too many specialists and too few GPs; chronic care of our patients is too often fragmented into organ systems. The British have too few specialists and too many GPs; it is hard to believe that a general practitioner can master all aspects of all the complicated diseases that must be managed chronically on an outpatient basis. Most of our doctors are probably overpaid, with the opposite the case in Great Britain. We perform too much surgery and the British not enough. Our medical care system may be running out of control, but the weight of the government bureaucracy may be stifling theirs.

We are unlikely to go the NHS route in this country. We are too big, distrustful of central authority, and incapable at the federal level of controlling costs, one of the "benefits" of the British system. Traditionally, the separation of the community-based GP and the hospital-based consultant is well established in the United Kingdom. This separation has not been as well ingrained here, and I, for one, am not sure it should be. We can, nonetheless, continue to follow the course of the NHS and learn as much as we can from it.

Although aware of its failings, Professor Pickering was a staunch supporter of the National Health Service and makes his case clear as the author serves as probing interrogator. Pickering was in the thick of British medical politics through his positions on such bodies as the Medical Research Council and the Council for Scientific Policy, and his knowledge was firsthand.

As for American medicine, Dr. Pickering acknowledges our technical superiority, but his remarks about some of our failings are devastating and right on the mark. These are delivered with the heartfelt conviction of a "brother" or "cousin" rather than with the malice of an ill-willed critic.

Until his death, sadly before the completion of this book, Professor Pickering continued to view the world of medicine from his own private perch in Oxford and, perhaps as well, through the eyes of two of his three daughters who practice medicine in Great Britain and a son currently at Cornell in New York City.

Sir George's own words are likely to convey the flavor of his character. In person he reminded me a bit of John Houseman in *The Paper Chase*, and, indeed, there was a slight physical resemblance. But here there was a real intelligence at work, and not just the portrayal of it; there was genuine humor and a vast expanse of humanity.

■ Winston Churchill always used to refer to the special bond between our two countries and, as a matter of fact, I have always been a great admirer of his (my son's middle name is Winston). In medicine we are certainly aware of this close, long-standing relationship.

Well, I think it's very natural because, after all, you started as us. I like to take American visitors around the college of which I used to be the master, because I like to show them the founder of the United States whose statue is in my old college at Oxford. His name was James I. Your countrymen are always surprised at that, but it's true. He was such a bad king that a lot of people left this country and emigrated to the New World to found the Colony of Virginia and the Massachusetts Bay Colony.

■ Well then, I suppose we have to be thankful to James I for that. I had not realized that he was famous for anything other than that great version of the Bible and writing the colorful polemic against the smoking of tobacco.

Oh, yes. He was a bad king and therefore they left.

■ Perhaps it was because we were once a colony of yours, but it seems that Americans tend to have an inferiority complex in some ways vis-à-vis the British.

Do you think so? I don't think they need to have. And I certainly am never conscious of any feeling between the British and the Americans other than the relationship between brothers and cousins. Then, of course, we have the great advantage that we speak the same language, and that is true of no other two great countries.

■ I am interested in what it is that made you the man you are. Were you, as they say, "to the manor born?"

If you mean rich, indeed not. I was one of those lucky people who was born a poor boy because my father died when I was three, and my mother brought me up on a very small income. We came from the far north of England. My mother was the daughter of a hill farmer in Northumberland, and she was born just about ten miles from the Scottish border. My father came from farming stock in the middle of the county of Northumberland. So I'm a farmer on both sides.

■ It must sound inane to say this, but you obviously missed having a father to guide you. Did you find any substitutes along the way?

I don't think I did, really, but I became aware that I was unfortunate in not having a father because I never learned to be a good carpenter, or a good man about the house. So I made sure that did not happen when I had my own son.

Because of our limited finances, I had had to earn part of my living while I attended medical school at St. Thomas's Hospital in London. At the same time I was visiting master in biology at Westminster School just across the river. Three times a week I had to rush out of the hospital, and board a bus, and cross Westminster Bridge, and jump off at the other side, and rush to school where I taught the sixth form. Later I then rushed back across the bridge and became a medical student again.

I was very fortunate in my teaching experiences. Westminster School is one of the great public schools in this country— what you would call a private school in the United States. I taught biology there. I later taught the medical curriculum as a university teacher, then professor, and then as a head of a college. So I have had remarkable opportunities to see the whole gamut of medical education from start to finish, and that's very unusual. And that I owe entirely to the fact that I had to earn my living.

■ When you began the practice of medicine, in England as in the United States, most of those who taught were also private practitioners. You were one of the early ones to teach full-time.

Yes, I was one of the earliest full-timers.

■ You worked for Sir Thomas Lewis[b] for about nine years. Could you tell me about him? Was he a hard taskmaster?

He was, indeed, but I was one of the few who got on really well with him. And for two reasons: I admired him tremendously, and I didn't care much what he said to me. If we disagreed, I used to stand my ground and didn't give way; but, on the other hand, I learned not to argue with him because he got very heated in an argument and would make the most ridiculous statements. He could also be extremely rude and extremely unkind, which, I am sure, he afterwards regretted. And so, what I used to do was to put forward my arguments and leave it. And it was very interesting, because, quite frequently, he would come back to me a couple of months later and put my case to me; only now it had become *his* case!

■ That seems to be an occupational disease of chiefs.

I think I was the only person in the department who played it like this, and I think I played it in this way because I had a sense of humor and I found it rather funny. But I had great admiration for Lewis because he had a first-rate mind and the most beautiful pair of hands I've ever known. He was extremely neat in his work and he was very methodical. When he started a thing he finished it, and then went on to something else. He was also, I thought, extremely fair. He never said anything bad about you behind your back unless he had said it first to your face, and that I liked.

What I learned most from him was method. I did both animal and clinical research with him, but particularly the latter. He had finished his work in the dog on atrial fibrillation [an irregularity of the heart] by the time I came to work with him, and was working in animals on cutting nerves, and allowing them to degenerate, and seeing the effects. As I said, he had an excellent pair of hands but was the master of the acute experiment rather than the chronic one. All our cats whom he tried to maintain alive went septic because he had no concept of surgical asepsis. He didn't cut tissue but tore it apart, and his watch chain used to dangle in the field, and he would sweat into the wound. In other words, his asepsis was rather elementary.

But he had the capacity for posing a question with the utmost clarity, and in such a way that it could be answered. And he was most ingenious in devising these experiments to get the answer, mostly in studies involving man. So I learned from Lewis the use of the experimental method in analyzing the phenomena of disease. There was never anybody as good as he before him, and there certainly hasn't been anybody as good after him.

■ Were there others like you who "bloomed" under Lewis's tutelage, or did he make a few wither?

Oh, he made a great lot wither, but I doubt if they were very much good as starters.

■ There sometimes are very prominent people in medical history who, by the weight of their own past accomplishments, have impeded the introduction of new ideas with which they disagreed. There is a story that has been told about Lewis resisting the introduction of cardiac catheterization; and McMichael,[b] a pioneer of these in Great Britain, in an introduction to a book on the subject in 1969, described a 1943 meeting of the Physiological Society at University College Hospital Medical School that was chaired by Lewis, and to which he made a report on his results. Referring to Lewis, McMichael wrote: "He described our opening paper as 'startling,' and at the lunch table he shook his head, hinting that we should abandon the procedure."

I know nothing about that. McMichael knew Lewis because Lewis was at the University College Hospital and McMichael worked there during his early formative period. But he did not work with Lewis then; he worked with others, although he was influenced by Lewis. He was interested in heart failure, which was, of course, an interest of Lewis's as well, but I don't think McMichael was actively discouraged by anybody. He started the catheterization work at Edinburgh and continued it at the Postgraduate Medical School at Hammersmith, and was not under Lewis's control at either of these places.

I think I can tell you, though, that Lewis would not have wanted anyone in his own department doing this work, because I think he thought it was dangerous. McMichael and others who catheterized patients became extremely unpopular with their colleagues because it was thought that they were very cold-blooded in the way they dealt with their patients, and I have a certain sympathy for the people who did not approve of it.

■ Who else besides Thomas Lewis was a major influence for you?

Joseph Barcroft[b] was; he was my professor of physiology at Cambridge. Then Wilfred Trotter[b] was. Trotter was a very remarkable man, a surgeon who became sergeant-surgeon to the monarch. He told me that the sergeant-surgeon's original function was to accompany the monarch into battle, although in more modern times he was responsible for all surgical treatment of the monarch. Trotter had, I think, the finest mind of anybody that I have ever met. Although a surgeon, he was also the finest physician, and he became a fellow of the Royal Society because of his contributions to psychology. He invented the concept of the "herd instinct." He had an enormous influence on me, and if I am a good doctor, I owe that largely to Wilfred Trotter.

■ Americans are constantly confused, sometimes bemused, but always impressed by all the titles the English have in their institutions. Now, you were Regius Professor of Medicine at Oxford. Just what does that mean?

The "Regius" chairs refer to those appointed by the Crown. The senior chair at Oxford was the Regius Chair of Divinity;

then came the Regius Chair of Medicine and Civil Law, equal; and then came the others. The chair of medicine was established in 1546, and the first to hold it was a man by the name of Warner. He was also warden of All Souls College, and I think he was a "Rev."—a doctor of divinity as well as a medical doctor.

■ It is unusual for an American to occupy a chair at Oxford. Was the American Paul Beeson[b] a Regius Professor?

Oh, no! Beeson was the Nuffield Professor, which is an upstart which began in 1936. You see, the Regius Chair of Medicine was concerned with the whole of medicine and not just clinical medicine, as is the case with the Nuffield Chair. For instance, when I came to Oxford my chair was not only the senior chair on the Faculty of Medicine, it was the senior chair in the Faculty of Biological Sciences, and the oldest scientific chair in the university. I was never called Professor Pickering; I was called "Regius."

■ Why Regius? Where did the king come in on this?

The Regius chairs were founded by Henry VIII, and the holders of these chairs are not chosen by a board of electors; they are appointed by the monarch. I had a letter somewhere which, I regret to say, I have now lost, but it went something like this: "My dear Sir: I write you concerning the vacant Regius Chair of Medicine in the University of Oxford. I write to inquire if I may recommend your name to Her Majesty, the Queen. Pray give this matter your earnest attention and oblige. Yours faithfully, Winston S. Churchill."

You see, my name was recommended to him by the university, and, on the basis of this, he recommended me to the Queen.

Now, Beeson, or any other American, could never occupy the Regius Chair because by the Act of Settlement of 1701 the monarch could appoint only subjects of the Crown. At that time the Hanoverians were about to come in, and the English were afraid that the country would fill up with Germans. And so that was the reason for that practice, and, unfortunately, the Boston Tea Party happened, so Paul Beeson wasn't born a subject of the Crown, while William Osler was. Beeson had the Nuffield Chair, while Osler, who was born in Canada, was able to be appointed to the Regius Chair.

■ You have always been interested in just what it is that makes people behave the way they do. Your book, *Creative Malady*, about Darwin, Florence Nightingale, and others fascinated me. There are occasionally great people in medicine or science who, at one point in their lives, seem to "go off the deep end." I would like your thoughts on this. What about Andrew Ivy[b] and krebiozen, the cancer "cure"?

He was an idiot. It wasn't just krebiozen; it was other things, too. I think the man had no common sense whatsoever.

■ Did he not do some good physiological work earlier in his life?

I think it was competent but dull.

■ You speak with great feeling. . . .

I speak with great feeling about Ivy, and I say he was an idiot.

■ What about Linus Pauling[b] and vitamin C?

Linus Pauling is a great man for whom I have an immense affection and respect. I know him personally but have never discussed his theories about vitamin C with him, and I don't know how he came to put forward these views or the evidence for them. But it is extraordinary how people "get bees in their bonnets."

McMichael got a "bee in his bonnet" against the use of anticoagulants at one time, but I know how that happened. He had a very distinguished scientist called Tizzard as a patient with a myocardial infarction. He gave him anticoagulants, and Tizzard died from a cerebral hemorrhage. And that really got into McMichael's system.

■   That has happened to all of us. You may do everything correctly according
to the book, and then it just ends in disaster.

Progress is sometimes hard to make, and sometimes it takes the Grim
Reaper to eliminate the old ideas and bring in the new. You have a great gift for
turning phrases, and when you were writing about how to improve
the education of doctors, you turned one that I wish I had thought of myself:
"Where there is death there is hope." I would like to get on to the National
Health Service now. Is there hope for the NHS? You have been a great booster
of this.

I'm not a "booster"; I'm a great supporter of it. It was absolutely marvelous until the bureaucrats and politicians got at it
and ruined it. I think that what happened was that the "boys"
at the headquarters of the Ministry of Health wanted to make
names for themselves, so they sat down to see how they could
improve the service. They had "working parties" [commit-
tees] on this sort of thing and the other, and the result was that
they ruined the nursing service, for one thing. That was the
result of the Salmon Report. They wanted to improve the career service for the nurses, paying special attention to the
grade "ward sister" [head nurse] and above. So they took the
ward sisters out of the wards and made them administrators.

■   The same thing has happened in the United States. The nurses are all
getting advanced degrees, going into administration, and forgetting about how
to care for patients.

It's tragic. The reorganization of the National Health Service was the greatest tragedy done by that stupid man, Keith
Joseph,[b] who thought he was an expert at management, and
who has made an absolute mess of the Service so that you
cannot get anything done. The amount of time doctors have to
waste on committees and paperwork is nobody's business.

■   Has not the National Health Service been uneconomical?

Uneconomical? It's the most economical service in the
world!

■ What about the long waiting lines for elective surgery?

They always were long but got shorter under the National Health Service. The number of canards that have been put out about the National Health Service are infinite. The worst one is that it is "socialized medicine." It was nothing of the kind, and I used to enjoy going to talk about it in the United States. I would start off by saying, "It will come as a surprise to most of you to learn that the true architect of the National Health Service in Great Britain was a man called Adolf Hitler." And it's true.

■ How is that?

Because we knew Hitler was going to wage total war against us, and we knew that we were going to be bombed as hard as he could go. So we organized an emergency medical service. On the night the war broke out, my wife and I were in Dundee, where her father was president of the British Association for the Advancement of Science. The telephone rang at two o'clock in the morning, and it was for my wife, who was being called to her post as pathologist at Hertford County Hospital in the Emergency Medical Service. So we were all "nationalized" at the beginning of the war, and all the hospitals were taken over by the Emergency Medical Service and run as a network throughout the country. All this was to provide care for air-raid casualties wherever they happened. And they took all the Work House Infirmaries and built these into hospitals as part of the Emergency Service. All this went straight into the National Health Service after the war. The Emergency Health Service and the National Health Service merged completely. So that's how it all happened.

■ You have spent the better part of your life finding out how to train good physicians. You have stressed the importance of studying things in depth, at least a few things, for any student of medicine to become a scholar as he should. Now, the backbone of the National Health Service is the general practitioner: forty percent or more of your physicians fall into this category. I cannot reconcile the two in my own mind.

You have to have standards, and the only way to have standards is to study something in depth. If you don't, you become slipshod and superficial. Now our general practitioners have four years of what you might call tutored education after they have taken their final medical examination, and they are encouraged to go on learning for the rest of their lives. That's the great change in medical education in this country—that we now have what is called "continued education," what the French call "l'éducation permanente."

■ But do you really believe that in an arrangement whereby the general practitioner sees the patients only on an outpatient basis, and then relinquishes all control of them once they are brought into the hospital for all those fascinating and complicated examinations and treatments, is good for the GPs?

It's marvelous for the patient.

■ I agree that it's probably better for the patient, but I can't see the general practitioner getting any intellectual stimulation from it.

He can still learn if he's interested.

■ Let's get mercenary for a moment. The cost of living here is not too different from that in the States. Is it true that your general practitioners earn only the equivalent of twelve thousand a year in U.S. dollars?*

Well, I honestly don't know; I was never much good at salaries. I never knew what my own was.

■ Perhaps you're an exception, and so am I to a certain extent, although one doesn't make as great a financial sacrifice going into academic medicine in the United States perhaps as in Great Britain. Another question. In our country there is always talk about "fee for service" and the doctor-patient relationship. You have always been interested in human motivation. Do you think it makes a

---

*It was actually $40,000 on the average, with a 25 percent increase planned at the time to be completed by April 1980.

difference to the physician in the way he treats his patient if he knows the patient is paying him directly?

It never did to me. Let me put it this way. I have been into this a lot in this country, and the best doctors don't mind. There was a man called Pickles who used to be the most celebrated of our general practitioners. He was an epidemiologist, and he discovered the incubation period of hepatitis. I once asked him what he thought about the National Health Service, and he said, "I'd never go back to the old system." I asked why. He said, "Because I couldn't stand sending out bills."

■ Bills also preoccupy most of our students and house officers going out into practice in the United States. By the time they get through with their schooling and training, they are so much in debt that they are anxious to get into lucrative practices. It's a vicious cycle, in a way.

Yes, I can see that, but in Great Britain medical education is subsidized. It's not entirely paid for by the government, but it is heavily subsidized. So our fees for medical students are infinitely less than yours, and that's why we don't like to take on too many foreigners, because we would be subsidizing them.

■ I am still unconvinced that under your system there are sufficient financial or intellectual rewards for the majority of the physicians you are producing. I can't see why the brightest and best of your young people would be interested in that kind of life.

But they are, and their salaries have been improved, and there's no dearth of applicants for general practice. Now my wife knows as much about it as I do. We have two daughters in general practice, and one of them was one of the brightest girls for her year. She's jolly good and enjoys it enormously. And our general practitioners are marvelous people because they've got good minds; they get very good training and they've got a splendid spirit.

■   I don't mean to give you the impression that I think the American system
is necessarily the best . . .

It's awful! It's ghastly! Do you want to know why it's
ghastly? Because you are so beastly to your patients. American medicine and surgery are technically excellent, but your
patients are hopelessly overinvestigated and treated in the
most meddlesome way. And I think it is hideously expensive
in the United States.

And I would never be ill there because I'm damned if I'll be
at the mercy of those little pipsqueaks, the residents and interns, who are totally in control, and treat their patients only
in the interest of their own advancement. When I first used to
go to Dartmouth, they had a splendid hospital there called the
Mary Hitchcock. Then Dartmouth went from a two-year to a
four-year school. The Mary Hitchcock was taken over for clinical training, and the last time I was there I thought it was a
terrible place, because it was completely run by interns and
residents who were under no control and were extremely adventurous in the management of their patients, simply in the
interest of gaining experience for themselves.

■   One does have to strike a balance . . .

But you haven't. There is no balance. The house staff at
your teaching hospitals can do what the hell they like, and
they won't go to a place for training that doesn't allow them to
do what they like. There's a chap called the "physician in
chief"* who was the most disastrous "institution" that was
ever created in the United States, and entirely due to Gilman[b]
at Hopkins, who said, "If I'm going to run an efficient hospital
I must have chiefs of the main departments who will be responsible to me just as in a department store." Now, the physician in chief sits behind a desk and never sees patients. He

*Usually the chairman of the Department of Medicine; similarly, the chairman of surgery may
serve as "surgeon in chief."

has morning report at eight o'clock, at which time his interns come in and tell him about twenty patients in a half an hour. I think it's a terrible system.

■ Don't you have the equivalent of our house staff, the registrars, who have the same function?

They do, but when I ran the service *I* ran it, and not my registrar or intern. I wouldn't allow my younger people to do the kind of things your people do. When I was a physician to St. Mary's and then the Radcliffe Infirmary, I had a certain number of beds allocated to me, and then they had my name over the top. They were *my* patients, and my registrar and intern were not responsible; I was. They were not allowed to do anything unless I approved. I didn't interfere too much, but if they did something of which I disapproved they really "got the stick."

■ This is essentially the system we are supposed to have in the United States, but it varies tremendously, depending upon the attending physician. Many of our attendings are absentee physicians, but others—and I have always prided myself on this—exert the kind of control you described.

I've never met it, and I've been visiting professor in every medical school in the United States.

■ I must admit I am swimming against the tide. To get back to George Pickering again, I have always been fascinated by names. Dickens, in his novels, always picked just the right ones for his characters, and these occur in real life. It always seemed appropriate that we should have a Doctor Dock, and in your own writing I came across a "Henry Tidy" whom you quoted Lord Moran as calling "The Queen Mary of Medicine." I couldn't think of a more appropriate name for a very fastidious person.

I know William Dock extremely well. I used to get letters from him which began "Dear Prof Pick" and were signed "Doc Dock."

Henry Tidy[b] was a terrible doctor, one of the worst that I have ever come across. He was one of my teachers, and he had an enormous reputation because he wrote a book called *Es-*

sentials of Medicine, which was the equivalent of an abbreviated version of Osler's book. All the students used to buy it to prepare for examinations. He had no humanity at all; he was a most wretched and unkind man.

■ If you had it all to do over, would you do anything differently? Do you have any regrets?

I don't think much about the past. I'm not a person who goes in much for regrets. It's not a question that interests me very much. I would like to answer it in that way.

■ How do you account for your success? Cardiology always seem to have been full of "tough" characters, and you have such a sanguine disposition. Did you know Paul Wood,[b] by the way? He was said to be a particularly "tough" character as people described him.

Yes, he was. We came together at a meeting in Montreal, and someone was comparing us there. He said Paul Wood could get away with murder but George Pickering wouldn't even try.

As for whatever success I have had, I work very hard. I think I am not afraid of expressing my opinions; I'm not afraid of being a minority of one. On the whole I'm reasonably honest, so people trust me. I'm reasonably intelligent, so that when I do a job I usually do a fairly good job. And therefore people ask me to do other jobs. I think that's why.

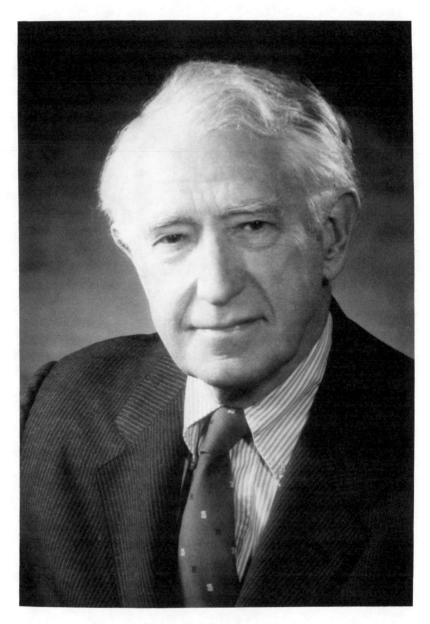

Francis Daniels Moore, M.D.

CHAPTER 11

Francis Daniels Moore, M.D.
(1913–   )

I F TEXAS can claim to have "invented" the cattle baron and
the City of Brotherly Love the "Philadelphia lawyer," then
Boston must be credited as the progenitor of the greatest collection of physicians and medical institutions in the nation.

With three outstanding medical schools—Harvard, Tufts,
Boston University—and a number of superb hospitals, including the Massachusetts General, the Peter Bent Brigham, Beth
Israel, and Children's Hospital, Boston has created a milieu of
medical excellence that has become world renowned. This
influence beyond the environs of the Charles River has extended in many ways, not least of which have been the year or
two in Boston that countless American and foreign-born physicians have acquired to give them that final "polish."

Within the very center of this island of extraordinary medical excellence, Dr. Francis Moore occupies a very special place.
He has been called "the thinking man's surgeon," and it is a
reputation that is well deserved. After completing his undergraduate and medical school years at Harvard, his next step
was not unusual: he became a surgical intern. But then he did
something that was very unusual. Instead of immersing himself in clinical surgery and collecting as many appendecto-
mies, gallbladders, and gastric resections as he could, as most
aspiring young surgeons might do throughout the course of a
surgical house officeship, Dr. Moore was drawn into a very

new and "unsurgical" area of interest. He began experimenting with newly available radioactive isotopes that could be
injected into patients and then, through blood and urine samples, be used to predict just how much water there was in the
body, or other constituents such as sodium or potassium.

This work led him directly into the determination of how
these different body constituents might be altered in patients
undergoing a variety of surgical operations. The results of all
this were his landmark contributions in understanding and
treating all kinds of metabolic derangements in surgical patients, as well as in other patients with traumatic injuries or
burns.

Although his contributions in this field alone would have
sufficed to make him a memorable major figure, his interests
and contributions have been far-reaching beyond this: peptic
ulcer, breast cancer, endocrine surgery, tissue transplantation,
and on into the training of surgeons, the history and economics of surgery, and health-care delivery. In over four hundred
publications, most of them in which Dr. Moore, himself, was
the prime or one of the prime participants, Dr. Moore has
earned a place in the front ranks of medicine.

After completing his first stint in concentrated laboratory
work as a National Research Council Fellow in 1942, Dr.
Moore completed his surgical residency training. Within six
years, in 1948 at the age of thirty-five, Dr. Moore was made
surgeon in chief at the Peter Bent Brigham Hospital and
Moseley Professor of Surgery at Harvard Medical School, a
rise that must be unprecedented in the history of modern
American surgery.

He stepped down as surgeon in chief in 1978 and currently
is Elliott Carr Cutler Professor of Surgery at Harvard. He continues in a consulting capacity as surgeon at the Peter Bent
Brigham Hospital and the Sidney Farber Cancer Institute, as
well as in a variety of other medical pursuits involving Boston,
Washington, and elsewhere.

Dr. Moore was interviewed only a few months after Dr. Pickering, and, although it was not planned, I was struck by the similar ground they covered—and in such strikingly different ways. This involved mainly the respective roles of medicine and surgery and, most particularly, the search for methods to care for our patients in the best possible way, an issue of paramount importance for us all. The temptation to contrast the two men was irresistible, the similarities and differences being as marked and, at times, paradoxical, as they were.

Both were at the top of their profession, of course. Pickering was a medical man, Moore a surgeon. Pickering, a ruddy-faced somewhat portly gentleman, "born a poor boy" into a highly structured society, had been knighted by the Crown and spoke with the authority and eloquence of the average American vision of a cultured English lord. He nonetheless turned out to be the spokesman for the National Health Service, the least elite expression of medical practice—for better or worse—that modern times have evolved.

Moore, product of a "classless" society, is no less the patrician, but of a typically American kind: upper-crust Boston and Chicago, Andover, Harvard, MIT, and Bryn Mawr run through the family like precious embroidery through a finely made tapestry. He is tall, elegant, tweedy, with distinguished patches of gray in the hair above the horn-rimmed glasses. The manner is simultaneously self-assured and self-effacing. His knowledge and recall are remarkable, and no one could put forth better than he the case for American medicine as he sees it.

■ You are not a native Bostonian.

No, I don't claim to be an old Boston "baked bean," but I didn't feel very strange when I first came here with my new wife from Winnetka, Illinois, a Chicago suburb. My father's family come from Boston, and many of my mother's family went to school there. My father, after graduating from MIT [Massachusetts Institute of Technology] in 1901, moved to Chicago where he met my mother. They were married in Evanston in 1909.

■ Do you come from a medical family?

No, I was the first doctor on either side way, way back. My mother was very interested in medicine, and my maternal grandfather was an amateur scientist. But there were no physicians on either side of the family.

When I was an undergraduate student at Harvard I had no idea, at first, that I would be going into medicine. My family had some very good friends among the prominent physicians in Chicago. They were wonderful people (and I was a patient several times) who set a very high standard. As I entered college in 1931, I expected to go either into music, since I had done a lot of music, or into ranching, because we had a ranch in Wyoming, or into business, because my father was a businessman. He was in the railway supply business, which was then centered in Chicago, the "Crossroads of the World."

■ What kind of music interested you?

To begin with, I played a number of different instruments, although my main interest was the piano. The thing I especially enjoyed was writing music, and in 1934 I wrote a musical for the theatrical club at Harvard, the Hasty Pudding Club. The show was called *Hades, the Ladies,* and it was based on the then ludicrous parlor joke going around that women would soon be admitted to Harvard. By the time of our twenty-fifth reunion we realized how prophetic that show turned out to be. I have continued to enjoy playing the piano, although I'm no good at it, and I have written three other musicals, two of them for a theatrical club here in Boston.

It was about midway through my sophomore year that I decided to go into medicine, and I can't say exactly why. I was concentrating on physical anthropology, so it was easy to work in the premedical courses, although I also included courses in philosophy, music, literature—and lots of socializing. I had a very nice time in college with that kind of curriculum, but I don't imagine I could have "made it" into medical school today with it. Although I graduated cum laude, that was nothing much, and I didn't work all that hard with all those outside activities.

Because of my association with Chicago, I originally hoped to go to medical school at the University of Chicago, but I found that they had a ridiculous language requirement at the time. They absolutely required a reading knowledge of both French and German. This might have been a good rule in 1910, but by the middle thirties there were very few German texts that weren't translated into English, and what with Hitler getting started, German medicine was already on the decline. I wrote the University of Chicago a long letter telling them that I wanted to go there, but could not read German and saw no point in learning it. They informed me of their refusal to alter this in an equally long letter to me, so I went to Harvard Medical School. The next year I was amused to learn that the University of Chicago had dropped this requirement.

■ What made you decide on surgery?

I had decided on surgery by the end of my third year in

medical school. Having played the piano all my life, I used my hands a lot. I'm very mechanically inclined—I like to do carpentry and similar things—and I was just much more excited by the interventional aspects of surgery than the other, more contemplative aspects of medicine. I was much influenced by the surgeons who were around Harvard Medical School at the time. They were a spectacular group. There was Elliott Cutler,[b] a dynamic, attractive, able man with a great deal of personal charm. He was professor of surgery at the Brigham. Then "Pete" [Edward D.] Churchill,[b] a real thinker and scientist, was professor of surgery at the Massachusetts General Hospital. Oliver Cope[b] worked with Churchill and Robert Zollinger,[b] who had been with Cutler. There was Dick Sweet[b] and Joe Meigs,[b] and Bob Gross[b] was just getting going on heart surgery as I was finishing medical school. It was a kind of golden era of surgery there at the time. There were thirty people, I believe, in our graduating class who went into surgery, and eighteen of them have become professors of surgery. It was the most "surgical" class that ever graduated from Harvard—or so we were quite certain!

■   Even if you did go into surgery you have, nonetheless, developed a reputation for being a different kind of surgeon from most. There's the old story I'm sure you know about the different specialists. The internists know everything and do nothing, the surgeons know nothing and do everything, and the psychiatrists know nothing and do nothing. Your career certainly gives the lie to the first two thirds of that, anyway.

People are kind enough to say that. I like to point out that there are many surgeons who did a lot of thinking and a lot of remarkable work. I don't mean to compare myself to them, but John Hunter[b] and Harvey Cushing,[b] just to cite two examples that come immediately to mind, certainly did a lot of thinking. I think it's just a matter of self-image. Internists like to think of themselves as terribly, terribly thoughtful, which indeed many of them are, while surgeons think of themselves as men of action, which many of them are. But there is a great deal of overlap between the two personality types.

It's very interesting that medical students have been shown to perceive the two types of specialists as very different. They think of surgeons as short-haired, athletic, politically conservative, a little more apt to be Anglo-Saxon WASPs. They think of internists as more likely to be thoughtful, beard-stroking types, politically a little far to the left, a little more apt to be Jewish, perhaps, and a little more apt to be scientific. They also have their ideas about pediatricians and psychiatrists, but there is a good deal of overlap. I know a lot of excellent internists who would make marvelous surgeons.

As for myself, I have to tell you a funny story. Surgeons, as a whole, think of me as a Harvard professor: "He must be a left-winger and in with the Kennedys." The sociologists that I have worked with on medical care delivery think: "He's a surgeon, he cuts his hair short; he's an Anglo-Saxon WASP Unitarian; he's a *right-winger!*" All I can say is that it's fun to be considered a left-winger by one group and a right-winger by the other. Actually, I don't consider myself as having any particular political stripe. I am delighted they are so confused.

■ Whatever they call you, you certainly seem to have benefited from the cross-fertilization between medicine and surgery, perhaps with some sociology thrown in, and this is reflected in your writings and lectures. In 1976 you gave a lecture before the second annual meeting of transplant surgeons, and it was entitled: "Lessons We Have Learned from the Transplantation Experience." In it you listed the seven major advances of the century. Here is your list:

1. Description of myocardial infarction by Herrick (1912).
2. Isolation of insulin by Banting and Best (1923).
3. Discovery of active principle in liver affecting blood formation by Whipple, Minot, and Murphy (1925).
4. The chemical configuration of DNA by Watson and Crick (1953).
5. Successful culture of the polio virus by Enders et al. (1953).
6. Development of the pump-oxygenator for cardiac bypass by Gibbon (1953).
7. Tissue transplantation by Hume, Murray, and others (1954–56).

■ It is very revealing that of the seven "happenings" you named, only the last two are surgical in nature. I think that reflects your broad interest in all aspects of medicine, and indeed, a number of nonsurgical people in medicine have worked with you.

Since I was one of the first people to work with radioactive isotopes in medicine, a number of people did come to work with us at various times. "Izzy" Edelman[b] as a young man was sent up by the Atomic Energy Commission and worked with us for three or four years. I was very proud of the fact that he was made professor of biochemistry at Columbia. It isn't every surgical laboratory that produces a professor of biochemistry. I'm also proud that the Regius Professor of Medicine at Glasgow, Graham Wilson, studied with us, as did the professor of pediatrics in Copenhagen, a professor of physiology at Harvard, and a number of people from all these other nonsurgical fields of medicine.

■ What drew you into research at the beginning?

The first real laboratory experience I had was in the second year of medical school when I went out to Chicago to do some research with William McEwen, a brilliant chemist who was only about four years older than I. This was in 1936, and he had the idea then of treating kidney failure with dialysis. He probably was unaware at the time of the work of Abel,[b] Rowntree, and Turner back in 1915 at Hopkins where they had the same idea. At any rate, we worked with dogs, dialyzing their blood with saline across a collodion membrane. By this time heparin was available, so we were able to prevent blood clotting, but the membrane we used just wasn't any good, and it was very frustrating. I'm afraid I wasn't much help. He needed a better physician on his team, and I was only a good-for-nothing medical student. About five years later, during the war, Kolff in Holland had the right membrane and succeeded where we failed. Nevertheless, I enjoyed that research experience, which in its own small way was way ahead of its time.

The next year we worked on a different problem. During pregnancy the amount of the hormone, gonadotropin, increases tremendously, and the appearance of this in the urine was actually used as a test for pregnancy. But the source of the gonadotropin was a mystery. A lot of knowledge about the endocrine glands had been obtained experimentally by removing the various organs and then seeing what effect this might have upon levels of various substances in the blood or urine. We believed that the placenta might be the organ involved in this case, and measured falls in urinary gonadotropin after delivery and removal of this organ, the placenta. We were right, but the only trouble was that, at the same time, some very experienced investigators were already preparing extracts of placenta to prove conclusively and directly that this was the source of the gonadotropin. So we never published the work, as nice as it was.

I enjoyed research but was still not serious about it until I was in my internship. At about that time, E. O. Lawrence in California had invented the cyclotron and in 1938 received the Nobel Prize in physics for this accomplishment. Now we had isotopes that could potentially be used for diagnosis and treatment in medicine. Means[b] and Lerman had used radioactive iodine in the treatment of hyperthyroidism, and people were doing some work with radioactive phosphorous.

I interrupted my clinical surgical training and became a National Research Council Fellow. The idea I had was that if we could incorporate a radioactive atom into a dye molecule, trypan blue, this could be injected intravenously and used to localize, by its radioactivity, internal abscesses that would be otherwise undetectable. A young chemist, Lester Tobin, came to work with me, and we succeeded in synthesizing radioactive trypan blue. We showed experimentally in rabbits how, by use of a Geiger counter, this could lead to the detection of abscesses we artificially created. This was in 1938. Interestingly enough, many physicians in nuclear medicine nowadays use very similar principles for many things. But now we have much better technology. So perhaps, again, we were too far ahead of our time for practical application.

At the end of that research three important events altered my course. This was now 1941, and within six months of this project's completion, Pearl Harbor was bombed. Secondly, I had been working at the old Huntington Laboratories, and at about this time all these facilities were moved into the Massachusetts General Hospital, making it very difficult for me to continue my work. The third event was the realization that I would now have to complete my surgical training. I was an asthmatic and declared 4-F, which I always felt badly about. I couldn't go to war, so I stayed at home and worked extremely hard in clinical surgery. When I finished my residency, I became the assistant of Dr. Leland McKittrick, who had a large practice here in Boston. I did a tremendous volume of surgery for a few years and also got my research laboratory started. It was a very hectic time in my life during the war.

■ You have done research in many areas, but I suppose your major influence has been in the use of radioactive isotopes to determine body constituents. Did this lead into the work on metabolic changes related to surgery?

The isotopic work led directly to body composition, and I guess the publication that I am proudest of is our 1946 article in *Science* on the determination of total body water and solids by isotope dilution, which was an original concept. I carried through with it for many years.

I think my research work can be divided into several different segments. There's a big chunk of it on body composition. That is why all those biochemists, pediatricians, internists, and veterinarians came to work with us. They wanted to learn how to measure body composition with isotopes: How much sodium was there in the body, how much potassium? The public is generally totally unaware that you can give this tiny injection, take a urine sample a few hours later, and then be able to tell the number of grams of sodium there is in the body—its actual weight. It's really a remarkable chemical phenomenon, that you can analyze the living body this way.

Then there is the work on the metabolism of the body with surgery, and an effort to understand convalescence postoperatively, and improve surgical care. Then I spent a long time working on duodenal ulcer. I stopped publishing on this in about 1965, but I was interested in vagotomy [cutting the vagus nerve to reduce secretion of acid in the stomach] very early in the game. I did my first vagotomy in 1943 not long after Dragstedt[b] did his.

I got started in burns with Oliver Cope. Everyone recalls that terrible fire in Boston at the Cocoanut Grove, and there is the impression that this stimulated our interest in the effect of burns on body composition. But actually we had been working on burns for eighteen months before the fire, and already had prepared one of our major papers on extracellular fluid changes with burns based on isotope dilution. The Cocoanut Grove fire was a terrible disaster and we sure learned a lot from it, but Cope's interest in burns and my own preceded this by some time. Starting in 1958 I began to work intensively on breast cancer, and I have worked consistently on this for twenty years, and have been fascinated by it. There are thousands of patients that I have treated for breast cancer, also many with duodenal ulcer, burns, and general abdominal surgical problems.

Then, on the sociology and economics area, there is something I am proud of in the historical sense. When I was a medical student, a lot of us thought that these "economic/ social" aspects of medicine were in for a revolution. At that time the American Medical Association still thought that Blue Cross and Blue Shield were communist conspiracies. The AMA was so right wing that none of the students could buy that view. So we got a young labor union organizer from MIT to meet with us once a month, and talk with us about medical economics. His name was Douglas Brown, and he was a wonderful person who later became a mediator with the national labor organizations. This aspect of medicine has been an interest of mine ever since. This was all brought into focus when the American College of Surgeons and the American Surgical Association asked me to take on the question of national surgical manpower as part of their SOSSUS [Study of Surgical Services for the United States] project in 1970.

■   I have looked into that, and it seems that we have an awful lot of surgeons in the United States. In your 1976 report you compared the number of surgeons here per 100,000 population with that in many other countries. We had 30.4 per 100,000 population compared with the United Kingdom with 14, Scandanavia with 19, and so on. Only Israel, with 32 per 100,000 had more. Does this mean we are doing too much surgery or that others are not doing enough?

Let me divide that answer into two parts: how many surgeons and how much surgery.

First of all, the main thrust of the SOSSUS Report was that we do have lots of surgeons, but, in view of the American public's appetite for medical and surgical care, I don't think we were too far out of line. Our main concern as we began this study was the number of surgeons we had *in training*: there were fears that there was going to be a terrible flood of surgeons in the near future. Starting in about 1975, the number of surgeons entering practice began to level out. They're going up a bit, but only slightly, ten to fifteen percent per year. On the other hand, internal medicine is exploding! It has trebled its annual board certification rate since 1964. Radiology is just unbelievable in the numbers that are coming out. Pediatrics is going way up. Now, of course, the number of medical students graduating in toto each year has been increasing significantly (it almost doubled between 1965 and 1980), and they have to go into *something*. So some increases are inevitable, and not particularly undesirable. I still feel uncomfortable about surgical manpower, but less so than I did five or six years ago. Still, surgeons are going to feel very crowded in 2000!

Now, for the amount of surgery. Are we doing a lot of surgery in this country, as compared to other countries? I can only say yes to that. Is it right or wrong? Well, the American public likes to be taken care of. You, as a cardiologist, know that. In England they have long waiting lines for a lot of elective and discretionary surgery. Americans don't like to wait. So I think we do perform a lot of surgery. I do not think much of it is "unnecessary" or fraudulent, except in one or two very sensitive areas. I say "sensitive" because, in appearing before various U.S. Senate hearings, especially with Teddy Kennedy, I have had some pretty rough exchanges on this matter.

It is clearly wrong to give the public the impression that the American medical profession is just a bunch of money-grubbers who do things so they can get their wives fur coats. I don't think that is a fair image. But then, Senator Kennedy throws "tonsillectomy" at me, and I have to say "Touché!" Now I, as a general surgeon, have no special interest in tonsillectomies, but it was an operation that was being seriously misused. In 1968 there were 1.3 million tonsillectomies done in this country. Unbelievable! I'm happy to say that, since that time, the number has gone down, down, down. It's probably less than a quarter of that number that are being done annually at present.

There has been no new great discovery about the tonsils or any new significant antibiotic. It's just been a better understanding of the fact that surgical operations require some thought. There were people who defended tonsillectomies, saying, "Well, no one ever died from a tonsillectomy." That's not quite true, because there were mortalities, and they were disastrous. Medicine is too sacred to "sling it around," and if an operation shouldn't be done, it just shouldn't be done. I mention tonsillectomy merely as an example. There is some evidence that surgery for low back pain and hysterectomy may also be performed in excess, but good data are awfully hard to come by.

■ I'm sure you're aware of the article that appeared in the *New England Journal* about the attitudes of surgeons toward their own families. It appeared that, considering operations, surgeons' families had more procedures done than any other group. Their wives topped the list for hysterectomies.

That's a nice study and it was done by John Bunker.[b] John is an anesthesiologist, and he did that first study showing how many more surgeons there were in the United States compared to England. He enunciated a sort of Parkinson's Law of surgery: the more surgeons there are, the more surgery will be done. Well, that's all right, but the trouble with John's article was that he didn't point out that there are also a lot more internists in the United States than in Great Britain, and a lot more "cardiac centers" and "coronary care units." There are a lot more pediatricians here than in Great Britain. They never heard of a well-baby clinic in England; they think it's a joke! And as for psychiatrists, you know that British psychiatry is only a tiny profession, whereas American psychiatry is huge. I think Bunker's article would have done a better service if he had extended his observations to these other fields instead of limiting it to surgery.

■ I find your thoughts about England interesting, because I raised some of these considerations with Sir George Pickering. You know, he thought the British system, the National Health Service, excellent, at least until the bureaucracy began messing it up.

I know George Pickering moderately well. He was a professor at St. Mary's in London when I was a visiting professor of surgery there. He and I have been on a number of panels together. He's a great person, a great individual, but he is one of the most academic of British physicians. I don't think he has any feeling for what medicine is like in the cities and towns of this country that don't have university medical schools in them. Of course, there are now a lot of affiliations between American medical schools and outlying areas, but that's not quite the same thing. I have often wanted visitors like Pickering to go to Providence, Rhode Island; or Portland, Maine; or Rockford, Illinois; or Toledeo, Ohio; or Spokane, Washington—big cities that in his years had no major medical schools but many excellent doctors. I would like him to see how medicine is really practiced throughout most of this country, because people like him really have no idea about it. The British system is very, very different. They rely on the general practitioners, and specialists—medical or surgical— are not common there outside of academia.

■ A few sparks flew when Dr. Pickering and I discussed the role of the specialist and the "primary physician" in the care of patients in Great Britain. The GPs there totally relinquish control of their patients once they enter the hospital. I simply could not see how someone's intellectual growth could continue if, every time he got an interesting case, it wound up in somebody else's hands.

That's a fascinating problem. The British have such a tradition of the family practitioner that they have locked it into the National Health Service. Each of the GPs has a panel of patients, and he is paid on a per capita basis whether he sees them or not. There's also an interesting regulation regarding surgery that is part of the NHS. No elective surgery—and that comprises over ninety percent of all surgery—can be carried out without a letter requesting the surgeon's opinion from the family doctor.

In the United States the case is totally different. Let's say a mother has her teenage son come home from a football game, and he has hurt his knee. In the first place, she's often intelligent enough to suspect something wrong with the cartilage or a meniscus herself. She is no more going to see the family doctor than fly to the moon! She is going to go right to the local orthopedist whom the family may have known for years. And when Grandpa can't see out of his left eye, chances are that Grandma will recognize that it's a cataract. They're not going to go to any family doctor; they'll be off to see the ophthalmologist who prescribed all their glasses for them.

Now several major institutions in this country are trying to convert all of American medicine to the British system of having a great majority of family practitioners. Now, you can't say this too loud (given the current medical political climate)—but they're wrong. The American public simply does not want that. Sure, they want rapid access to care, but after that access is achieved, they want the comfortable feeling of knowing that they have the best-qualified people to take care of them. Your own field is a perfect example. By golly, you go out to a little town in the middle of Wyoming—and I know Wyoming very well because I spent my childhood there—and an older person gets a pain in his chest which is accompanied by ECG changes and, dammit, he wants a cardiologist! And nothing is going to stop him.

■   What do you think about the second-opinion program in surgery—when the patient goes to a second surgeon after the first recommends an elective operation?

This was an awfully good idea, and Dr. Eugene McCarthy of Cornell really pushed it. It was a brilliant idea, and it made everybody think twice. But it does have some problems. What about a second opinion on a *negative* recommendation? Let's say a sixty-two-year-old man starts getting up a lot at night to urinate, and he has trouble starting his stream. He asks his family doctor whether he needs an operation. The family doctor does a rectal examination and, feeling only the outside of the gland, thinks the prostate is not enlarged. He says, "You don't need a prostate operation. Just don't drink so much water in the evening." Well, that patient deserves a second opinion too, because a urologist may do a cystoscopy and tell the patient, "Your whole prostate isn't very big, but it is real big in one place—right where your water comes out! You better have it fixed."

There are also nonsurgical decisions that are very important, and for which one might argue for second opinions. How
about starting someone on a lifelong course of insulin for
diabetes, or digitalis for heart disease, or electroshock therapy
in psychiatry? So I thought the idea was a good one, but perhaps it could have been focused on all of medicine, rather than
surgery alone, seeking second opinions for all major decisions.

■ To wind up the business of supply and demand in medicine, I take it you are
not overly concerned?

I think the curves are rising on the supply side, the number
of physicians, but I don't think they are out of control. They
are not rising quite so fast as some people had feared.

As for the demand side, one of the common platitudes of
sociologists in this field is that the appetite of the American
public for medical care is "insatiable." Build more hospitals,
put in more beds and doctors, and the public will simply con-
sume them, getting more and more treatment for less and less
urgent illness. That's only partly true. That may hold for
much of internal medicine, probably a fair amount of pediatrics; and fair amounts of psychiatry and radiology could be
called "insatiable." But when you get to some of the more
specialized fields of surgery, for example, "insatiability" does
not exist. The public appetite and social need is quickly
satiated.

Take urology, for instance. There are some communities in
this country where, if a young urologist wants to go into practice, the other urologists would just laugh. They wouldn't be
discouraging the new man merely to protect their own
pocketbooks. They could sincerely say, "There's simply not
enough for the rest of us to do around here, and one more
coming in will have the same problem, only worse." The reason for this is that urology is a kind of specialty that has very
clearly defined disorders. The urologist deals with the bladder,
the ureters, the prostate, the kidneys, the excretory apparatus—and there are just so many of those around to be fixed.

The same things holds for ophthalmology and neurosurgery. How many cataracts in the community? How many brain tumors? These specialties are undeniably "satiable." Enough surgeons is enough.

■   This may be true, but there are always surgical specialists trying to protect their turf by telling the newcomers how hard it is.

That's right. However, you might be surprised to know that that's not usually true in general surgery, which is a much more diffuse area, and it is certainly not true in internal medicine. In those specialties newcomers are often welcomed in to help "carry the load."

■   About the amount of surgery we do in this country, we really seem "hooked" on surgical treatment, and patients, as well as doctors, seem to accept an awful lot of it uncritically. I would like to quote a couple of things you have written that may be germane. First, you once said during a conference on ethics, "Every new operation is an experiment." At another time, in a slightly different context, you wrote: "There have been many triumphs in surgical research in this country, but there have been many unfortunate developments. Most of these have been due to the exploitation of surgical methods without an adequate scientific or ethical background. . . . Surgery lends itself to quick enthusiasm and initial exploitation." As a cardiologist, I am particularly thinking about all the coronary artery surgery, some of it unnecessary, that is being done today.

I would like to go back to those two statements. The one about every surgical operation being an experiment, I think, was first made by Halsted,[b] and the rest of it refers to it being an experiment in bacteriology. That is, maintaining an aseptic field, and every patient presents a new or different challenge to the surgeon in this regard.

As for the enthusiasm and overapplication of surgical techniques, some of them have been, of course, regrettable. Some were simply symptomatic of their time. I give you sympathectomy for hypertension. During the period of 1937 to 1952 it was probably the best treatment for certain kinds of severe hypertension in young people. Paul Dudley White,[b] among others, thought so. But then what happened? All these new and very effective drugs for the treatment of hypertension came along, and the operation was no longer necessary. As for the coronary surgery, I will grant you that there have been some institutions where the threshold for surgery has been very, very low. That is unquestionable, but I am sure you will agree that there are a number of well-defined groups now where the surgery has prolonged the lives of the patients. And, don't forget, the original purpose of the operation was to relieve angina [chest pain, due to coronary disease] and in this the surgery has been tremendously effective in improving the quality of life for these previously incapacitated people. An operation that began to improve the quality of life was then criticized for not prolonging life.

■ Fair enough. I would like to talk a little about Boston now. It has so many historic connotations for us, political as well as medical. Even here in Brookline: John F. Kennedy was born in Brookline.

Zabdiel Boylston[b] was born in Brookline, too.

■ That's just what I was going to mention. There is this fascinating story about how he started the first American inoculations* for smallpox here in Boston in 1721.

That story has been a hobby of mine for a long time, partly because Zabdiel Boylston was a member of our church. Our church is the First Parish Church of Brookline. It was founded in 1718, and it's one of the oldest churches in the United States. "Zab"—I like to call him Zab as if I knew him—Zab was a member of our church, and a prominent doctor in Boston when he started doing his inoculation work. Everybody

---

*Inoculation involved taking a small amount of fluid from the pustule of a case with smallpox, and injecting it under the skin of a susceptible person, resulting in a mild case, and conferring immunity in the future. It is to be differentiated from "vaccination" where pustule fluid from a case of cowpox (vacca = cow), a milder related disease, was used (as by Jenner in Great Britain). Later, inactivated virus that proved to be safer than inoculation became the accepted mode of prophylaxis.

turned against him, and for a few years he was very unpopular. Someone even hurled a "granado"—what we would now call a Molotov cocktail—into the home of his friend and tried to burn his house down. But then he published his marvelous book on inoculation against smallpox. The first edition was published in London in 1725, and the second edition was published in Salem, Massachusetts, in 1726. It was a lovely study, statistically, and showed conclusively that he was preventing the disease in the patients so treated.

Now, here is the story I love to tell about him, and it is one that is not generally known. Boylston was a surgeon and his father was a surgeon, and when he began inoculations, it was thought of as a surgical treatment. But later on, in just a few years it was taken over by the medical people, the physicians. One of these was Benjamin Waterhouse,[b] who was professor of medicine at Harvard Medical School. Waterhouse went to England to study under Jenner[b] who had introduced vaccination, using cowpox, and when he returned to Boston, he too began to use the vaccination to prevent smallpox. At the time two of the people in Boston who had been making their living out of inoculating people, Holyoke and Aspinwall (two good New England names), saw the results that Waterhouse was getting, and they were the first to use the phrase, "Gentlemen, this is no humbug."

Then, forty-seven years later, on October 16, 1846, John Collins Warren[b] stood in the surgical amphitheater at the Massachusetts General Hospital, and when he first saw William T. G. Morton[b] successfully administer ether anesthesia to a patient, he turned to the audience and said, "Gentlemen, this is no humbug." Now, people always associate this phrase with the introduction of anesthesia to surgery, but what Warren was doing was making a joke, because all the senior people of his time had been well aware of the vaccination story, and immediately recognized the original source of the reference, although that has been almost forgotten today.

■ Boston, of course, is just full of medical history. What is it about Boston that makes it so special? Historically, it has not always been the most temperate of cities either socially or politically, and yet, I am sure that it has had an inordinate effect upon the rest of the country. Medicine, in particular, has really been nurtured by this city. How do you account for it?

I don't know. Perhaps it is a mixture of innovation and enthusiasm. Politically, we had firebrands like John Adams and Samuel Adams at the time of the Revolutionary War, while people in Philadelphia, for example, were much more conservative. It's interesting to contrast Philadelphia and Boston during the eighteenth century. Philadelphia was a great, big, sophisticated port city. Boston was smaller, more rabid, more noisy, and people there did things in a "big way."

In medicine, they got started way ahead of us with the Medical College of Philadelphia in 1766, while Harvard did not open its medical school until 1782. And even though, for many years, Harvard was little more than a diploma factory, between 1750 and 1880 many exciting medical developments occurred in Boston, a few of which we have already talked about. Harvard did not really reform until Charles Eliot[b] became president and instituted major changes between 1869 and 1901.

The aspect of Boston that I think was most important was that it always welcomed innovation. Just today, I received a letter from an intern applicant who wants to come here because he just cannot get anything started where he is now. Here we have always had opportunities for students to do medical research. Boston has always been kindly disposed to new ideas and research. Compared to most other cities in the country, we have always been ahead in this respect. I think of New York as being medically conservative; Chicago is medically political; Boston is medically innovative.

And yet, with all the openness to new ideas and people, it's really sad to view the racial strife that is going on between blacks and whites in this city, and it is really not well covered by the press. It's worse here than almost anywhere else in the country, despite our long liberal tradition. When you think that, during the Civil War, the first black batallion was led by a Boston general, and that this was the city of William Lloyd Garrison and the abolitionist movement . . .

■   The rest of the country always thinks of Boston in *The Late George Apley* context, "Back Bay Brahmins" and all. They think of Boston as staid, when it really has always been in ferment.

There was an article that appeared in the *Atlantic Monthly*, perhaps more than thirty years ago, but I recall it well. It was called "Harvard's Heretics and Rebels." It told about the long tradition of people who toppled over old ideas and were politically inflammatory.

But the black-white confrontation here is a right-wing phenomenon; it is blacks versus the Irish; it is partly religious; and that is a peculiar thing. It is the white conservative middle class who don't want the blacks around. We have a great many Irish in Boston with many charming traits, but one of their less charming traits is that they never forget a grudge; they just can't let go. Look at Northern Ireland! And yet, who am I to comment on this? My own family has never been embattled on either side. I guess that, until you have lived in a white neighborhood that's undergoing a lot of racial change, you really don't know what it is like.

■   Like Boston, you have also had quite a past. What's in the future?

I reach my official retiring age on August 31, 1980, and at the moment I'm in the unusual position of being the most senior professor in terms of years of service of anybody at Harvard. I have been a full professor since 1948. When I do retire in 1980 I will go on doing a lot of things, but they will be different from what I have done in the past.

I have to tell you some medical history. About 1973, I noticed that I had to take my glasses off and wipe them all the time. I went to my ophthalmologist, Leo Chylack, whom I had brought to the Surgical Department at the Brigham, and said, "Leo, I think I'm having a symptom. I'm always wiping off my glasses." So I had my first cataract out in 1975, and have to have the second one out within a few years after that. For a surgeon to lose his eyesight is kind of a hard thing, so when I had my second cataract done I quit operating. I miss it, sure. I did my first operation as an intern at the Mass General in 1939; I did my first operation as professor of surgery on July 10, 1948, and still see that patient from time to time. He's now in his eighties, I guess, and doing well. So that's the way it is and—what the heck—some people just cling to the things they do, and it's not right. I know surgeons who have operated into their seventies, and they ought to quit. I stopped in 1979 at the age of sixty-six.

Surgery is an athletic event. A professional football player gets to be awful good when he's about twenty-seven or twenty-eight, I guess. A surgeon gets to be good when he's about forty-five or fifty-five. He's still young, but he has had a lot of experience. That's when he is at his peak. Maybe some surgeons drag on because they need the income. I suppose they think they can still fix an odd hernia here and there, but I have had two episodes with surgeons operating when they were too old, and I had to go in and bail them out. The patients didn't die, but I saw to it that the surgeons never operated again, and I'm happy to say that they have remained my friends.

■ What will you do in the future?

I don't think I'll do quite as much teaching. I don't think I'll do clinical work. But I have lots of hobbies, and I'm very interested in the social and distributional aspects of medicine.

I'm on the board of regents of the Uniformed Services University of the Health Sciences, and this new medical school, which will graduate its first class in 1980, will provide training for men and women who really want to devote themselves to a medical career in the Armed Services. I am proud to be a part of that.

I am also pleased about our new hospital here in Boston, Brigham and Women's Hospital. We started to dream about it in 1958, and now, over twenty years later, the building is being finished. I'm cochairman of the fund drive, and we need to raise several millions of dollars more for some of our academic programs. I look down Shattuck Street now and see that big building, eighteen stories high, and remember the medical student skits they would put on in the sixties. A student would come on stage as "Moore," and he would interview intern applicants, telling them, "Come on. You better intern at the Brigham. We're going to have a great new hospital there next year." And that was always good for bringing on howls of laughter. Well, it has happened.

■ Any regrets?

I think anybody that goes through life has some regrets. My main one is that there are only twenty-four hours in the day. Boston is the most wonderful community; it's just filled with the most fascinating people in many fields: literature, art, music. It's all within a couple of miles from where we are sitting. I know a lot of these people, but I wish I had an even wider acquaintance. But when you work hard in medicine, and you do a lot of science, and a lot of surgery, you just don't have time for a lot of socializing.

■ Do you feel that all this has also caused you to neglect your family? Successful doctors are often accused of that.

I was married the same day I graduated from Harvard College in 1935. I was twenty-one. It was unusual but not unheard of for a doctor to get married so young. It has been a happy marriage. Laurie and I have five children and twelve grandchildren. My youngest son is a surgeon, and one of my daughters is married to a surgeon, and another to the son of a surgeon. The marriages have all been to friends' families, so we are all very close, but we're not an overburdening family. We don't insist that everyone come to Thanksgiving dinner and all that kind of baloney, but we have a lot of fun together.

If Mrs. Moore came downstairs to join us now, and you asked her, I don't think she would say that I've neglected the family. But I can tell you that she has had to do a heck of a lot of work. She has been a marvelous hostess to thousands of students and house officers and colleagues. An academic career is a team operation. Women's liberation is a great thing, and I'm sure they are going to be just fine on their own, but when a wife is off doing something entirely different on her own, you can't expect a husband to accomplish all he might, as if the wife were working with him. Your expectations will have to be different.

■ Is there anything else that you would like to get into the record?

You may have read something I said about the clinical investigator in an address I made before the University Surgeons, and which has been fairly widely quoted. I used the Latin term *pontifex maximus,* which literally means "great bridge builder" and refers to the council of priests in ancient Rome who "built bridges" between the living and the dead.

Now, as I see it, the clinical investigator stands in the middle of the bridge; he is the bridge tender. At one end of the bridge there stands the pure scientist who says that this kind of a researcher is not a good enough scientist. At the other end of the bridge stands the practicing physician, the clinician, who says that this kind of researcher doesn't do enough clinical work. I have been criticized from both ends. In the last ten years I am sure that some people have said that I have not done enough clinical work. Most people were unaware of this little problem I was having with my eyes, but I'm sure I was criticized for that, despite thirty-seven years of intensive surgical operative practice. The scientist that knows my work, I think, respects it well enough, but realizes that I am no great basic scientist, and I have never claimed to be.

If there is any good advice that I can give to some ambitious young man or woman, interested in going into clinical investigation, it is that right at the beginning they should "bite the bullet," and realize that for the rest of their lives some people are going to tell them that they aren't doing enough clinical work. And, then, right after this, they'll publish a paper and the scientist will say, "You haven't got enough molecules in there," or something. The clinical investigator has to occupy that middle position "on the bridge."

■ **Well, we are a bastardized kind of profession, halfway between art and science.**

We are a bastardized profession, and everybody calls you a bastard—from both sides of the fence. The important thing to do is to work away and enjoy it, and realize that you cannot do as much clinical practice as the person who is doing only clinical practice, and you can't do quite as fancy science as the person who is doing only science. My oldest son is a distinguished scientist. He is professor of molecular genetics at Yale, and I'm very proud of him. He has a rapidly growing bibliography, and now he's studying the three-dimensional distribution of atoms in ribosomal protein molecules, using slow neutron scattering of deuterated ribosomes. I really cannot understand all of his work, but I am fascinated by it.

■ **That makes two of us!**

I don't blame you. I can just tell you that, when I look at his work and watch him at work, I realize that there is a really true scientist. But we're all different, and each of us has to go his own way. I might say that my generation of surgery, the group who got out of medical school right at the time of World War II, and who got out of college in the midst of the Great

Depression—that generation now make up the senior leaders of surgery in this country. They are a wonderful group of people, and it has been a tremendous privilege to have worked with them and known them all these years.

ADDENDUM

In the years that have passed since this interview there have been new developments dealing with medical manpower. In May 1983, Dr. Moore kindly provided this update.

The status of manpower data has made progress since the interview. The "GMENAC"* Report has confirmed the findings not only of the earlier Manpower Committee of the National Surgical Study, but also our more recently published data (*NEJM* 304 : 1078–1084, 30 April 1981). There is going to be severe overcrowding of surgeons. I am simply unable to conceive of such a problem by calculating the number of "excess" or "surplus" surgeons. I think that was an arcane mathematical exercise carried out by GMENAC. I think it is better to indicate how they will be dividing up their workload. The fact is that in the year 2000 there will be three surgeons standing on each bit of clinical turf now occupied by two surgeons, and in 1965, occupied by only one surgeon.

Escalation and overcrowding in other fields of medicine will be very evident especially in internal medicine and in specialties such as cardiology and endocrinology.

Much has been made of a recent report from the Rand Corporation showing that board-certified physicians are getting out into smaller communities; the National Surgical Study showed that this happened with surgeons within five years after the end of World War II. Board-certified surgeons went to small communities much sooner than board-certified internists and internal medical specialists.

*Graduate Medical Education National Advisory Committee.

The main impact of this entire manpower problem will be to increase the cost of medical care to the public, and there is simply no avoiding that conclusion. The average income of physicians will go down. Some conditions of medical practice might improve, and it is conceivable that physicians and surgeons will spend more time with each patient. Let's hope so. But total expense will rise.

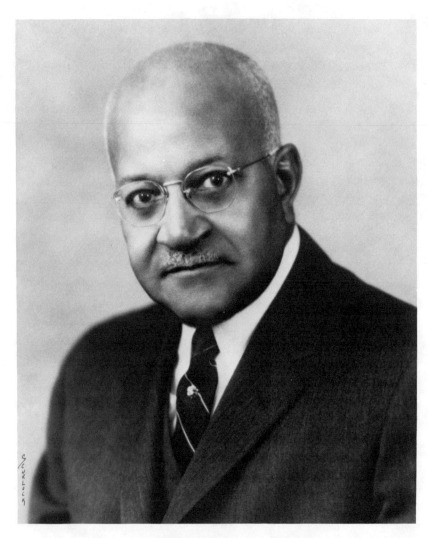

Joseph L. Johnson, M.D., Ph.D.

CHAPTER 12

Joseph L. Johnson, M.D., Ph.D.
(1895–   )

THE PERSONAL and professional life of Dr. Joseph L. Johnson can be fully appreciated only within the context of black America's medical experience.

Since the days of slavery, American blacks have been especially victimized as patients due to a variety of social and economic burdens leading to increased illness and lack of medical attention. Efforts to minister to the needs of this segment of our population have been hampered by a shortage of both black physicians and available hospital beds. Although a handful of black students were graduated from such northern schools as Harvard and Rush Medical College in the pre–Civil War years, it was not until Reconstruction that a serious attempt was made to provide training for young blacks aspiring to become physicians.

In 1866 Meharry Medical College—named for five white brothers who supplied funds for the brick building that housed it—was established in Nashville, Tennessee, solely for the training of black doctors. In 1868 Howard University College of Medicine opened in an abandoned German dance hall in Washington, D.C., and admitted both black and white students, although the former have always predominated. These two schools have accounted for the vast majority of black American physicians. As late as 1956, 63 percent of all black graduates in medicine were accounted for by Howard and Meharry, and only in the last five to ten years have a majority of black seniors been graduated from the rest of the nation's schools of medicine. During Reconstruction a half dozen other medical schools were established to increase the number of black physicians, but all of these have since gone out of existence.

Reconstruction also led to the building of hospitals that would care for black patients, as well as provide an opportunity for newly graduated black physicians to obtain necessary hospital experience as interns and residents. The Freedmen's Bureau, established in 1865, during its four and a half years of existence was responsible for setting up over a hundred hospitals and dispensaries to which black patients could come for care. Among these were the Freedmen's Hospital, constructed in Washington, D.C., on the grounds of Howard University, the Provident Hospital in Chicago, the Frederick Douglass Memorial in Philadelphia, and the Tuskegee Hospital in Alabama.

While American blacks sought improvement in their medical care through the production of more black physicians and hospital facilities, the black physicians, themselves, who were stymied in their efforts to improve the lot of their people by the racist policies of the American Medical Association at the turn of the century, established their own society, the National Medical Association, in 1895. This continues to serve the interests of its constituency through the workings of its various committees and its respected monthly journal.

We have already referred to the report that Abraham Flexner prepared for the Carnegie Foundation in 1910 and that dealt with the deficiencies in medical education in the United States and Canada at the time. Its effect on raising standards in medical training throughout the country was profound. It had a dual effect on the education of black doctors. The black medical schools, frequently the worst funded and least well equipped, were the most sorely affected by the aftermath of the report. All but Meharry and Howard were soon forced to close. Although this severely curtailed the production of black physicians, it also led to the strengthening of the academic programs at the two surviving institutions responsible for training the overwhelming majority of black American physicians, Meharry and Howard.

Howard University, in particular, has been recognized for its high standards over the past fifty years. This was in large part brought about by the appointment of key people whose devotion to excellence has been unwavering. One of these was Dr. Mordecai Johnson, who became president of the university in 1927. This efficient and forceful administrator was responsible for obtaining necessary funds from the Rockefeller Foundation and from former graduates in order to improve the physical plant of the medical school. In 1929 President Johnson appointed Dr. Numa P. G. Adams as the first black dean of the medical school. The latter would be responsible for many of the decisions leading to the current preeminence of Howard.

Adams had first been trained as a chemist, receiving his bachelor's degree at Howard before going to Columbia University in New York for his master's degree in science. He returned to Howard where he finally became chairman of the Chemistry Department, but then decided to study medicine. This he did at Rush Medical School in Chicago. Following his graduation in 1924, he established a successful practice as a cardiologist in Chicago until the call came for his return to Howard as dean of medicine.

Joseph Lealand Johnson came to the attention of Adams while they were both in Chicago. Johnson had been born in Philadelphia and had obtained a degree in agronomy at Pennsylvania State University in 1919. He taught science at high schools in Kansas for eight years before deciding to become a physician and beginning his studies in Chicago, first at the graduate school of the University of Chicago under the physiologist, A. J. Carlson, and then at the medical school. Carlson, who rose from a childhood in the United States as a penniless Swedish immigrant to the chairmanship of a major department at a great university, obviously drew parallels between his own experiences and the efforts of this young black science teacher to advance himself, and took Johnson under his wing.

Because of his work in physiology under the distinguished Carlson, Dr. Johnson received both a Ph.D. in physiology and a medical degree at the time of graduation in 1931. Adams, whose own medical career had begun in the basic sciences, recognized the ability of the newly graduated physician and offered him the chair in physiology at Howard when he decided to accept the post of dean. Dr. Johnson finally accepted the physiology position at Howard and remained in that post until Adams's untimely death at the age of fifty-five in 1940. Johnson then took over the reins of the deanship until 1955, when he returned full-time to physiology in teaching and research until his retirement in 1971.

One gathers from former students that Dr. Johnson was a quiet-spoken, somewhat formal individual, but demanding in his quest for excellence at Howard. He completely revamped the Physiology Department there—"created" might be a more accurate word—introducing modern animal facilities and providing a climate for meaningful research. His activities, as with many prominent black professionals of the period, extended beyond the classroom and the college campus. He became active in, and behind the scenes, fighting racial discrimination in the hotels, theaters, and radio stations in Washington, D.C. He has received many honors from civil rights as well as scientific societies, in both of which he has continually occupied positions of leadership.

Looking back over Dr. Johnson's long and distinguished career, I was struck by the fact that, despite many advances that we have made in civil rights, the plight of the black patient is in many ways little changed from the early part of the century. Consider that in 1910 there was 1 white physician for every 684 white patients and 1 black physician for every 2,883 black patients. In 1956 the ratios were 1:770 and 1:4,567. Today there is 1 white doctor for every 526 white patients but approximately 5,000 black patients for every black physician.

With blacks constituting approximately 10 to 12 percent of our population since the beginning of the century, the number of blacks being trained in our medical schools were only 2.0 to 2.5 percent of the total. With attempts by American medical schools to increase minority representation in the profession ten years ago, the proportion of blacks admitted in first-year classes ranged between 6 and 7 percent between 1970 and 1976. In 1980 it fell to 5.7 percent. Ironically, Howard and Meharry, which were responsible for the majority of black physicians in the past, have had a reduction in this representation in their student bodies, and in 1980 blacks constituted only 28 percent of their newly admitted students.

Throughout my interview with Dr. Johnson, as he recounted the various obstacles with which he had to contend over the years, I was reminded of the stories I have read about quadriplegics and others similarly affected: how the simple acts we all take for granted—ambulating, eating, writing a letter—are accomplished by these severely handicapped patients only with the exercise of incredible effort and determination. Similarly, in a social and economic sense, American blacks who have determined to receive their just deserts as citizens of this rich and powerful country have had to expend superhuman efforts in achieving what many of us would consider the routine accoutrements of our existence: economic security, education, a chance for employment, and good health. In Dr. Johnson's case, in particular, I was struck by the persistence of this diminutive, soft-spoken, scholarly man in reaching his lifetime goals for himself, his community, and his people.

■ You were born in Philadelphia. How did your family get there?

Both my parents were born into slavery in North Carolina. During Reconstruction my dad served in the North Carolina legislature, and during their time in North Carolina my parents had their first four children. My mother would eventually have a total of fourteen children, and I would become the youngest of the ten surviving infancy. The oldest child was a male, and he left North Carolina, came to Philadelphia, got a job, and became active in politics. He gained quite a reputation as an orator and probably got that from his association with my dad while he was in the legislature in North Carolina. After my brother got settled in Philadelphia, he prevailed upon my dad to come there, and finally the rest of the family made the move as well. They wanted to get as far away as possible from the area in which they had been held in bondage, and hoped to make a better living in Philadelphia.

■ Was the "City of Brotherly Love" very hospitable to your people then?

Not on the basis of my own experience. Brotherly love was something you had to seek and look for with a magnifying glass. It wasn't very evident.

■ What did your father and mother do to support you there?

First let me tell you that my father did not live very long after arriving in Philadelphia. He was fifty-two when he died from nephritis, I believe, and I was only two and a half at the time. So I didn't have the good fortune of his companionship, but, as far as I can learn, his first job was as a laborer in the large market down where the Reading Railroad Terminal was located. As I grew up, I did learn one interesting story about him when he worked at the market. He had a large wicker basket in which he carried produce and merchandise, and after he died that basket hung in our basement from the ceiling. I learned that every Saturday he would wrap up little bundles of meats and vegetables that he had bought in the market. Each of these bundles had the name of some person in the neighborhood who was in need, and each Saturday he would go out with this basket loaded with packages and distribute them.

Mother was quite well and active. She worked for a physician as an obstetrical nurse or, you might say, midwife. At that time, you know, there were more deliveries in the home than there were in the hospital, so the doctors had to have somebody assist them in following these patients before and during childbirth. When their time came, the patients would call my mother at the same time they called the doctor, and very often she would be there before the doctor and make the delivery herself.

■ What was it that got *you* interested in medicine?

My first interest was in the law, rather than medicine. Philadelphia was known for its lawyers—the old expression "Philadelphia lawyer"—and the courts were very well organized there. They were all in the City Hall, which still stands majestically today with William Penn up top.

When I was about ten or twelve I became fascinated with the law. So I used to cut school and go to the City Hall where I would pick out the court in which I wanted to sit. I would get there before the guards were at their stations, sit in a corner, and not dare move until recess, because if I left, I would not be able to get back in again, being just a little shaver. After awhile I got so efficient that I knew all the best lawyers, the types of cases they handled, which judges were the most interesting, and where they sat. I would get to City Hall early in the morning and see where they posted the cases, the judges and lawyers for the day, and pick out the one I wanted to sit in on.

I found the courts to be more interesting than algebra and Latin classes, but when I cut classes this created another problem: I never knew what the assignment for the next day would be and what I should study in the evening. So I spent my evenings playing basketball, in which I was also very interested. I was a member of our Sunday school team at St. Simon.

There were a lot of "ramifications" to all this. I kept getting called in by the principal because of my absences, and my mother kept getting these letters from the school, and my report cards did not show the grades that my mother and my brothers expected of me. My oldest brother was old enough to be my father, and he had a son in school with me. This boy was a very studious fellow, and would never even think about cutting classes.

An experience I had one night changed all this. I used to sleep just off the room where my mother would sit each night and often talk things over with my oldest brother. One night I heard her talking to him about how much she was worried with all the "devilment Joseph was getting into" with my cutting class and staying out late, playing basketball and all. I felt terrible when I heard her talking about how sad I was making her, so I decided to reform. I stopped cutting classes and began to behave properly. Then, a couple of months later, I heard my mother talking to my brother again: Joseph was acting in the strangest way. He was no longer cutting classes or playing basketball late into the evening. What sort of "devilment" was he up to now? So you see, no matter what I did, I managed to worry my mother.

■   I detect no interest in farming or agriculture. How is it that you took a degree in agronomy at Penn State when you left high school?

I was interested in the law, but didn't see how in the world I was going to get into law school. The University of Pennsylvania was right in Philadelphia, and that would have been the logical place for me to go if I had the money, but that was a private school and quite expensive.

Then one day our high school principal, Lemuel Whittaker, called me in to ask me what I intended to do with myself after high school.

■   Was this because you were an outstanding scholar?

Oh, no. I was a mediocre student, but he got to know me pretty well because of all the cutting of classes I had done. I told him what I wanted to do—study law—but didn't see how I could do it without any money. He suggested the possibility of my going to Penn State. The state university had a very low tuition, and also the various congressmen had scholarships to the state school that they could give out.

At that time the Vares and the Penroses were the political bosses in Philadelphia, and my older brother, who was active in politics, was an acquaintance of Bill Vare. And that's how I got to Penn State. Now, the state university was known for its agriculture program, so that's why I took up agronomy, even though this was not my interest. I knew I first had to get to college if I wanted to study law, and this was the first step.

Penn State was at the geographical center of the state, about 135 miles from Philadelphia. The train brought you to a little town, Lemont, about 10 or 15 miles from the college, and cabs and buses would carry the students from the train station to the college. I was seen off from Philadelphia by my mother; my sister; and a young lady from Camden, New Jersey, who would later become my wife. Before leaving I took her aside a moment and said, "I don't know whether I'm going to be able to make it or not, because I have only thirty-five dollars in my pocket after buying my railroad ticket this afternoon. Some help I expected did not materialize, so I'm a little disappointed. But I'm going to try, at any rate. If I can't make it on what I have, and can't get a job at Penn State immediately to

take care of my room and board, I'll go further west and won't
be back to Philadelphia until I have made it."

She said, "Where will you go?" And I told her, "Probably out
around Pittsburgh to work in the steel mills until I get enough
money to get back to Penn State."

Fortunately, as soon as I arrived at Penn State, I went to see
the president, Dr. Edwin Earl Sparks. I told him of my financial condition, and he made a few phone calls and got a room
for me to stay in a building known as the Chemistry Annex. It
seems that there had been a caretaker living there before, and
in exchange for having his old room to stay in, I would keep
the classroom on the ground floor clean and ready for use.
Then the Student Christian Association at Penn State conducted an employment bureau, and they kept a listing of all
people in the town who needed students to do work. Well, I
was out on some job every free hour I had, beating rugs, scrub-
bing floors, anything the party hiring me wanted done. So I
managed pretty well in this way.

■ **What was college like for you? How many other blacks were there on the
campus when you began?**

At the time I started there were twenty-five hundred students enrolled at Penn State, and I was one of two Negro
fellows there. The other one was much better off financially
than I. His brother-in-law was a physician in Camden, New
Jersey, and he had lived with his sister and brother-in-law
before coming to college. That other young man had had a
very active social life in Camden, but there weren't any Negro
families within twenty-five miles of Penn State, and he
couldn't take it. So, after the semester, I was the only one.

■ **World War I interrupted your stay at Penn State, did it not?**

Yes, but I spent as much time fighting the War Department
as I did the Germans. They had an ROTC unit at Penn State,
and when we got into the war the male students were being

assigned to officer training camps to be trained for commissions. But there were no officer training camps for Negroes. I wrote to the secretary of war, Newton Baker, asking why I was not being assigned to an officer training camp as were my fellow students at Penn State. The secretary of war responded stating that an officer training camp for Negroes was under consideration and, when established, I would be notified. Within a few days I received an order to report to Philadelphia for induction into the Officer Training Corps, which was being formed at Fort Des Moines, Iowa. After four months of training at Des Moines I was commissioned second Lieutenant and assigned to the 350th Field Artillery at Camp Dix, New Jersey. At the end of the war I was honorably discharged in January 1919 and immediately returned to Penn State, where I received the B.S. degree in June 1919.

■ Your first job was in Kansas. How did that come about?

As I was finishing up at Penn State, I wrote to various schools, most of them in the South, where I knew they would employ a colored man. I got a few offers from this, but then I received a response from a school that I had never heard of, in Topeka, Kansas. This was the Kansas Vocational and Industrial Institute. It included grades up to the high school level, and it was supported by the state of Kansas. It seems that someone from Tuskegee who was working in Topeka had learned of my application to his old school, and thought I might be suitable for the position in Topeka.

When I got this offer from Kansas paying big money—a hundred dollars a month—having heard of all the big farms out west, I wanted to see this area. So I accepted, and remained in Topeka one year. While there, all that time I had spent with basketball back in Philadelphia came to good use. You see, I had played for our Sunday school team, St. Simon's. The mother church was the Holy Apostles. They had a professional team, the Graystocks. The Graystocks team were so good that they pulled out of the Sunday School League and joined the professional Eastern League. I became a fan of the Graystocks and used to cut school to attend all of their games. The first thing the Graystocks players used to do when they came out on the court was to look over at midcourt to see if I was in my usual seat. I became so closely tied up with the Graystocks that I learned a good deal more about the game than the other boys back at St. Simon. Many of these boys were older than I and towered over me, so I was made coach at St. Simon, and occasionally some of the fellows from the Graystocks team would come down and help me with my coaching.

When I got to Kansas Vocational I assisted in coaching the men's team and had sole responsibility for the women's team. We used to play schools in the Missouri Valley area, and I often did officiating as well. After awhile, the people at Lincoln High School in Kansas City got to know me, because of our teams from Topeka beating them all the time. The principal at Lincoln offered me a job, and so I resigned at Topeka and moved to Kansas City.

■ It was there you decided to become a doctor.

Yes. I was teaching general science and zoology, and there was a section in Kansas City called the West Bottoms. That area was partially populated by Negroes who were very good people but very poor. I taught some of their children at the high school and made frequent visits to the West Bottoms. I got the feeling that those people were not getting the medical care that they should have because they couldn't afford it. The idea struck me that I would go away and prepare myself thoroughly in medicine, and then come back to Kansas City and serve the people in the West Bottoms. Another idea struck me, way ahead of its time, that I would organize these people and they would pay me twenty-five cents a month for their health care. There was no such thing as health insurance at the time;

I just thought that this might be a way that these people could get the care they needed and could afford. As for the more affluent people in Kansas City, if they wanted my services after I returned, they would have to pay well for it.

■ How was it that you went to the University of Chicago for your training?

To backtrack a bit, when I came to Kansas City there was a requirement that all teachers in the school system have, in addition to a bachelor's degree, so many hours of courses completed both in methods of teaching and the history of education. I had to go to summer school to get these credits completed in order to get my teaching license. There were no summer education courses offered at the University of Kansas in Lawrence, so I decided to go to the University of Chicago because I had heard of its quality.

The first summer I enrolled in these education courses, I attended about two classes in methods of education and realized that what they were teaching was what I already knew and had been teaching in the sciences. As for the history of education, that was something that I could just read on my own. So I quit those courses and took courses in science instead. In the fall I took the education examination for my teaching certificate, passed it, and got my license to teach in Kansas City.

Now, when I got this idea to study medicine, and work with the people of the West Bottoms, I talked it over with the principal of Lincoln High School. The principal had a wealthy friend, a furniture manufacturer by the name of Volcker, on the board of education, and told him about the idea. Volcker idolized the principal, and anything the principal wanted that he could supply, he would do it. Volcker agreed that it was a good idea and encouraged me. So I resigned and went to Chicago. People of the faculty with whom I was closely associated thought I was crazy, because I was making progress at the high school, and getting advanced every year, but I left anyway.

When I got to Chicago there was a long waiting period and a lot of applications for the medical school, so I registered in the graduate school. I was thinking of pathology as a specialty, and also wanted to study physiology, because I knew of the importance of physiology to medicine. In graduate school I took courses in biochemistry and almost all the courses of physiology, including the ones that the medical students were required to take. At the same time, I began research in physiology under A. J. Carlson.[b]

About a year later I entered medical school.

■ I see. That's how it is that you received a Ph.D. as well as an M.D. when you graduated. Any problems in medical school?

Before the hospitals were built on the university campus all medical students did their first two years on the University of Chicago campus. After two years of basic science at the university, the medical students would go over to Rush Medical College on the West Side for their final two years—their clinical training. While I was still in graduate school, they had just finished completing the construction of Billings Hospital, which was on the South Side. So now the students had a choice. They could either go to Rush on the West Side for their clinical training, as had been the custom, or go to Billings on the South Side. However, if you wanted to go to Billings, you had to be engaged in medical research, and a requirement for graduation would include a thesis representing some research in the medical sciences.

Because of my work with Carlson, I decided to go to Billings and continue my research for the M.D.-Ph.D. degree. In the summer preceding the beginning of the clinical training period, like all the other students, I went to the dean's Office and indicated my preference. But, lo and behold, the "old evil showed his head" again, as I had seen so many times before; it wasn't anything new to me. When I told the dean's secretary that I intended to remain on the South Side and go to Billings, she said that she "didn't know" and that I would have to see Dean Harvey.

None of the other students had to see the dean; they just indicated their preference and she put them on through, wherever they wanted to go. But I was the only black student, and they had never had a Negro at Billings Hospital. In fact, it was a lily-white institution throughout: no Negro patients, no Negro nurses, no Negro physicians—no Negro orderlies, maids, or anything else. So I saw Dean Harvey, and he said, "I don't know, Mr. Johnson. I just don't know whether Dr. McLean, the director of the University Clinics, would permit you to work over there. As far as I'm concerned, it's all right with me, but Dr. McLean would have to approve."

I said, "If Dr. McLean is the barrier, with your permission I'd like to go see Dr. McLean." The dean gave his permission, so I hiked over to the hospital to see McLean. After working my way through about three secretaries, I finally got to see him, and he told me, "I don't know, Mr. Johnson. We've never had a Negro here, and when patients are ill they are very sensitive. I don't know if they would accept you."

It was decided to put the issue before a committee of the hospital, and it turned out that my chief, Dr. Carlson, was a member of the committee. When they said they didn't know if I would "work out," he asked them if they ever had a Negro patient, doctor, nurse, or student in the hospital before. The answer was no. "How do you know, then, it would *not* work if you have never tried it?" he asked. They decided to try it, and I did my student work at Billings and stayed on a year after in a sort of internship. Dr. McLean later told me that he never for one moment had reason to regret that decision.

There were many interesting episodes while I was there, and one combined the Jewish and Negro features. I was making rounds one day with Dr. Louis Leiter, a professor of medicine and specialist in kidney disease. We stopped in the room of a woman who was obviously startled when I walked into the room, and when she saw me among all the staff men, she said, "And what are you?" Leiter, who was Jewish, jumped in and said, "He's a student doctor; what do you think he is?" When I had occasion to visit her room later, she expressed amazement at Leiter's response. "I don't know why the doctor jumped on me so harshly when I asked what you were. I didn't know. I thought you might have been a Mexican." It dawned on me then that, in her mind, it was inconceivable that a Negro could be functioning in that hospital; that I would have to have been something other than a Negro!

■ How did you get to Howard?

I became friendly with Dr. Numa P. G. Adams, who was practicing medicine in Chicago—Numa Pompelius Garfield Adams. His office was about two blocks from where I lived in Chicago. He had made quite a name for himself at the University of Chicago—Rush Medical College AOA* and all that, and was a very successful cardiologist. Numa became interested in me when he heard about me working under Carlson in physiology. As far as he knew, none of the other colored fellows had entered into research in physiology. I used to drop by his office frequently to see him.

While I was finishing up at Chicago, Adams got a call from the president of Howard University, Mordecai Johnson, to come for an interview for probable appointment as dean of the Howard University School of Medicine. They had never had a Negro dean before. At first he wasn't sure he wanted to go; he had developed a very successful practice in Chicago. Then finally he told me, "I've decided to take it. I've been down to Howard and they have offered me the deanship. But I want you to consider coming down in physiology if I give you the call." I said that I would consider it, although I didn't believe he was very serious about it at the time. Toward the end of my work

*Alpha Omega Alpha, the honorary society for scholarly achievement in medical school.

in Chicago, he wrote me and offered me the professorship in physiology. I replied that I was inclined to take it but was finishing up some work with Carlson and Dr. Russell Wilder, the chairman of the Department of Medicine at the University of Chicago at the time.

When I was ready to look into the position at Howard—I had never been there and knew nothing about what it was like—Carlson and Wilder decided that they would come down with me, and look the situation over with me. When we got back to Chicago, I asked for their opinions, and I remember Carlson's words quite well.

"Vell, Johnson, I'll tell yew. Yew can stay here at the University of Chicago and be a little fish in a big brook or you can go to Howvard University and make a real contribution. Yew've got an opportunity there to build a department of physiology vich yew won't have here. The department here is pretty vell set and functioning. That's my opinion. Yew make your decision." So I decided to go.

■ What was the Department of Physiology like at Howard before you came?

The man who was head of the Physiology Department was also head of the Department of Pharmacology, and he was also a radiologist. When Carlson came down he wanted to see the Department of Physiology and, going through the department with the man who was the nominal head at the time, he asked, "Vhere are your dog boards?"

The man gave him some tale about how he had lent them to someone in the Pharmacology Department. "Yew have loaned the boards? Don't they have any of their own in pharmacology?" Then he asked for something else that they did not have, then something else, and finally he exclaimed, "Vell, the laboratories here are too damned clean! I get the impression dere's no vork goin' on!"

So they really didn't have anything, and it was up to me to

organize the department, set up the animal section, and so forth.

■   You spent a total of seventeen years in physiology and then became a dean. What made you do this? A friend of mine, you know, once commented on an offer to become an assistant dean, describing that job as "a mouse in training to become a rat."

No. You've got that twisted around. A dean is a mouse in training to become a rat. The president is supposed to be the rat!

Anyway, you recall that Numa Adams brought me here as chairman of the Department of Physiology, and I worked to improve this department. One summer Adams was about to go on his vacation, and before he left, he submitted my name for appointment as "vice-dean" to act in his absence. It was during August and he left. He was having some gastrointestinal problems and went to see Lester R. Dragstedt[b] in Chicago. Dragstedt decided to do surgery, and Adams developed pneumonia postoperatively and died from this. I was acting dean for a year, and then they brought in John Lawlah from Chicago as dean, but he and the president soon came to the parting of the ways, and they had to find a new permanent dean.

It was then that President Johnson, for the first time in the history of the institution, called together all the heads of the departments and asked them to name someone as dean. They chose me. At that time I was not in very good favor with Mordecai Johnson, so he threw the decision back to the faculty as a whole; and again, with secret balloting, I was chosen to be the dean. So he was stuck with me.

■   What was your problem with the president?

He had not been giving fair consideration to the members of the faculty, principally in the advancement in salaries, and the faculties of the several colleges of Howard University decided to organize and form a union. They chose me to head the union.

■ I can see how that could make you unpopular with the president. What made you so popular with the faculty?

I think the main reason was the leadership I gave the faculty. I combined all the faculties at Howard University, as well as the nonteaching force of the university. We were the only institution in the country who had teachers, janitors, carpenters, plumbers, everybody in the same union. It was because of my work with the union that I believe the faculty chose me.

■ I'd like to get on to another subject. In the past, schools like Howard had very few white students. Today, with increasing numbers of blacks being accepted elsewhere, the complexion of Howard—pun intended—has begun to change. Does this bother you in terms of something being lost in terms of its past traditions?

No. I don't think so, and probably better stated—I hope not. It would be my hope and my fond wish that all medical schools will accept individuals as students, without regard to color or sex.

■ I seem to detect on the part of some older black physicians some resentment that, perhaps, it has become too easy for some black students to be accepted into medicine. Some older black physicians have the attitude "We made it in our time without any special treatment"; and perhaps some feel that too many special provisions for the current generation may reflect adversely upon themselves. Am I making myself clear on this?

Let me recite an experience which might indicate whether or not you are making yourself clear. As dean of the medical school, I proposed to the faculty that, among the then existing requirements for admission, we include calculus as one of the mathematics requirements. Some faculty members jumped all over me on the basis that they didn't have calculus and were doing all right. So, at various times when we attempted to build up the requirements for admission, we got that kind of reaction. Therefore, I'm not surprised when you tell me of a similar reaction when we talk about preparing Negroes for admission to formerly all-white medical schools.

As dean, and hence a member of the Association of Deans of American Medical Colleges, I fought against the policy of discrimination against Negro applicants for admission to medical schools. Along with some other people, principally Monty Cobb,[b] we carried the fight on up to the federal government, and all the white schools were forced to admit Negroes or risk loss of financial aid from the federal government. My criticism is that these schools accepted Negroes who were not really qualified, and they knew at the time they accepted them that they were going to flunk these students.

■ That's a very good point you are making, and it's one that I, as a former chairman of an admissions committee, can comment on directly. (May I add parenthetically that it took me five years to get accepted to medical school, so I have been through all this, personally.) When I was chairman of the committee at the New Jersey Medical School I can tell you, categorically, that we made a sincere and earnest effort to accept as many qualified black students into our school as we could. This was about ten years ago, and we actually had to comb the country to come up with some candidates whom we thought might be able to do the work. Black students were certainly not beating down the doors to get in at that time. We found that Yale, Harvard, Cornell, and other prestigious schools "skimmed off the cream," and we were left with considering people from little colleges in the South where the "Biochemistry Department," for example, consisted of a single biochemistry professor dropping by once a week to give a lecture. Now, we did accept students who were poorly qualified: I admit that. But we got to a point where we were so desperate to find students, that if we happened upon some who, we felt, had any chance at all we decided to give it a try, knowing that an appreciable number of these students might not succeed.

At the end of the first year there were a number who did not make it. They didn't receive any special treatment or programs other than those provided the rest of the students, although they were less well prepared than the white students. As a result, about half of them were considered unable to continue in school. This almost caused a riot. The medical school is in the middle of the central ward where almost all the Newark blacks live. They poured into the faculty council meeting on promotions, barred the doors, called us racists, said that we intended to flunk all these students out right from the beginning, and then they threatened to close the whole school.

Now, I'm not denying that we probably had some white racists on the faculty; there may have been some people who felt like that. But we, on the committee, and most of the faculty teaching these students did not. We lowered the qualifications in an attempt to bring in more black students, and then wound up in a "no win" situation.

Don't misunderstand me. I don't say that all of the medical schools took these students in, knowing that they were not qualified and with the intent to flunk them. But there were some schools that really did.

■ Well, we didn't, but we were accused of doing that, and it was a "bum rap." Let me toss another "hot one" at you. What do you think of the *Bakke* case?*

I have never favored a quota system, either in the school where I was dean or in other schools. In the *Bakke* case, Davis decided on a policy of admission that would give preference to black and other minority students because, over previous years, they had been denied this opportunity. They adopted a policy of trying to bring these minority students up to the level of qualification for admission and admit them in preference to some whites who, although not the most qualified in their group, were better qualified than the Negroes, for instance. I agree with that.

■ I think the University of California really lost on a technicality. If they had used race as a consideration, but not the *only* consideration for those places in the medical school class at Davis, the opinion of the Supreme Court might have been different. But you raise an interesting point. During one afternoon I interviewed two applicants. The first was a young white man whose father was a banker or wealthy businessman or something of the

*Allan Bakke, a white student, was refused admission to the medical school at the University of California at Davis in 1972. After he was rejected despite excellent grades, he challenged the University of California on this decision inasmuch as Davis had set aside a number of places for minority students, places for which others could not compete. The case ultimately went to the Supreme Court of the United States, which found that the exclusion on the basis of race violated his rights and ordered the University of California to admit him. The Supreme Court decision in effect stated that taking race into account because of past injustices was permissible, but not to the extent of absolutely excluding all other races from consideration for a specified number of places in a professional school. Bakke was later admitted to the medical school at Davis and graduated.

sort, and this fellow had a B average. Right after him, I interviewed a black girl who was the first of *twenty* children in her fatherless household ever to complete college. She went to a much less distinguished college than the young man and only had a C average. I asked myself who was the more accomplished of the two, and it was obvious to me that it was the young woman. She was obviously a much more outstanding person than the young man, and I think anyone should be able to appreciate this.

As I said, I have always been opposed to setting quotas. I had to face that as dean of Howard Medical School. There were always a large number of women applicants; always a large number of white applicants.

■ Were there quotas ever at Howard?

No. I refused to permit it. I just considered all the cases on their merit. I insisted upon a minimum standard of academic requirement for admission no matter who the applicants were. Then I had requirements as to individual character that they had to meet.

■ I think that nobody can deny the quality of the physicians that Howard has produced, and I think it is a tribute to you and your faculty that they have been so good over the years. The maintenance of such quality is important because there is a tendency on the part of many whites, nowadays, to think that if a black gets ahead it is because of the color of his skin and nothing else. I know of a black car salesman who was made sales manager of the outfit where he worked not long ago, and all his white coworkers, who considered themselves friends, kidded him about the "advantages" of being black and getting these promotions. The truth of the matter was that the sales record of this black fellow was better than that of all his white coworkers and he fully deserved the promotion, although it wasn't recognized by the others. That bothers me.

I have my own feelings with reference to that. I think that, in many instances, Negroes do get opportunities and considerations now because they are Negroes. At the same time, there are many, many more instances where they are denied consideration because they are Negroes.

■ Maybe it's balancing out a bit, then . . .

No, I don't think it is balancing out; I think it is still one-sided. I think in my own case some opportunities were given to me because I was a Negro. If not opportunities, at least estimates in people's minds. When I was working at Billings Hospital, for instance, I'm convinced that patients, in their own minds, gave me credit for being a better doctor than I was because they had made up their minds that I must have been that good or else I never would have gotten into the place. That doesn't necessarily follow.

■ As an educator you might be pleased to hear that we don't have the problems in recruiting able black students that we did ten years ago. We generally get a very high-quality black student in now. Of course, there are always a few "losers," but we have those among the white students as well. But now we have a different problem. The message has been out now for over ten years that there are opportunities for blacks in medicine, but the total number still remains underrepresentative. There are still only six percent black students in our medical schools, with an overall black American population of about twelve percent. Do you have any theories about why there are not more blacks in medicine?

One of the considerations is the same that faced me when I began college: Where is the money coming from? With tuition costs continually mounting, it's becoming more and more of a problem, not just for black students, but for any student who wants to study medicine.

■ Are there any other considerations? Is there anything about medicine—to use a current expression—"turning off" the black students?

Yes, I do. I think another reason is that many of the students who have the qualifications and probably could handle the financial end of it look the situation over and decide that the course of study is too long. There are opportunities arising in other fields where they don't have to spend so much time in school before they can get out on their own and start a family.

There was a time, for example, when there were very few opportunities for Negroes in the various phases of engineering. They couldn't get a job. It may surprise you to learn—and it isn't generally known—that Abraham Flexner, who at the time was chairman of the board of trustees at Howard, proposed closing the School of Engineering on the basis that their were no jobs awaiting the students that we graduated in this field. To Mordecai Johnson's credit, he fought against that proposal, and the majority of the board upheld him. Today General Electric, Ford Motors, and a number of other big industrial concerns send their representatives to Howard every year, attempting to recruit our engineering students.

■ That brings us pretty much up to date. Tell me, looking back on it all now, you spent forty years of your life at Howard. Which aspect of it did you find the most rewarding—the work in physiology or as a dean?

What gave me the most satisfaction was working with the young men and women. Both in a teaching capacity and as the dean.

■ Do you, by any chance, have any regrets about anything?

No, I have no regrets at all.

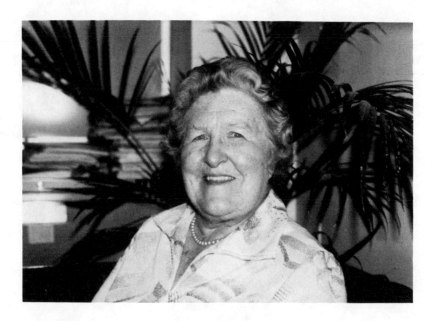

Marian Ropes, M.D.

CHAPTER 13

Marian Ropes, M.D.
(1903–   )

THE FIRST American woman physician is believed to have been Dr. Elizabeth Blackwell (1821–1910), who graduated from Geneva Medical School (now Hobart College) in upstate New York. It was a rather bizarre entry into medicine. When the young woman applied to the school in 1847, the faculty dodged the responsibility for taking any stand, leaving the decision to the members of the entering first-year class. This all-male student body met on the issue, and, as a huge practical joke, voted unanimously to accept Miss Blackwell. In a way, this episode established a pattern: until only quite recently, women in American medicine have remained the butt of a continuing series of cruel and irrational hoaxes promoted by the male-dominated medical establishment.

As for Dr. Blackwell, although she graduated first in her class, it was many years before Geneva Medical School accepted another woman, and Dr. Blackwell was forced to go to Paris to study in her chosen field of obstetrics and gynecology.

For the last half of the nineteenth century and the beginning of the twentieth, it seemed that only through creation of medical schools expressly formed for the training of women could there be any chance for any significant numbers of them to become doctors in the United States. The first of these schools, the Boston Female Medical College, was established in 1848 by Dr. Samuel Gregory, a lecturer on midwifery who

was concerned about the embarrassment and immorality involved with male physicians attending women during childbirth. Shortly thereafter, in Philadelphia, the Women's Medical
College of Pennsylvania was begun, and in 1865 Dr. Blackwell,
with her sister Emily and a German physician, Maria Zakrew-
ska, set up the Women's Medical College of the New York
Infirmary.

Admission of women to predominantly male schools followed, but progress was slow, uncertain, and severely restricted. In the 1890s, as has been pointed out previously
(p. 5), Johns Hopkins Medical School in Baltimore opened its
doors to women thanks to Mary Garrett, as did Cornell Medical School in New York City. But most medical schools continued to shun them. Even the innovative atmosphere of a
Harvard did not permit the presence of women medical students until quite late in its history. A riot attended Dr. Oliver
Wendell Holmes's attempt to liberalize the admission policies
for women and blacks in 1850, and it was not until 1945 that
women were finally permitted to earn a degree there.

The persistent exclusionary policies of the main-line medical colleges of the country fostered the establishment of a
number of schools catering exclusively to women, and by
1895 nineteen such institutions had come into existence. But,
as with the black medical schools of the period, these were
often considerably less well funded and equipped than the
white male institutions. In the aftermath of the 1910 Flexner
Report, which deprecated the then current low academic standards of many American medical schools, as with the black
colleges then extant, most of the women's medical schools
were forced to close. After 1910 only two survived, and by 1969
only the Women's Medical College of Pennsylvania remained
as an exclusive enclave for the training of women physicians.
In that year "Women's" was dropped from the title, and the
school became coeducational.

Except for a short period at the time of World War II when

the percentage of women medical graduates in the United States reached 12 percent of the total, up until the late 1960s women continued to be underrepresented, constituting only 5 to 10 percent of the nation's physicians. Three developments then gave a great impetus to increasing opportunities for women in American medicine. The first of these was the enactment of federal antidiscrimination legislation as contained in the Civil Rights Act of 1964 and then Title IX of the Education Amendment of 1972. The second factor was the commitment on the part of the Association of American Medical Colleges in 1970 to provide more opportunities in medicine for women, blacks, and other disadvantaged groups. Finally, there was the rise of activism with the feminist movement.

The changes these have effected are indeed striking. Until the 1970s, only 5 to 10 percent of medical school applicants and first-year enrollees were women. By 1980 this has risen to approximately 30 percent. In the forty years between 1930 and 1970 American medical schools graduated only 14,000 women; in the decade 1970–80 they have produced 20,000 new women physicians. Among the nation's doctors, in 1870 less than 1 percent were women; in 1970 this figure was 7.6 percent; by 1978 it had increased to 10.4 percent; and the trend continues.

If we are in the process of creating more women physicians, it is of interest to know just what types of doctors they are tending to become. If one looks at the percentages of males and females in different hospital residency training programs, certain patterns can be discerned. In recent years there has been a nationwide emphasis on producing proportionately more primary care physicians; that is, those trained to deal with the daily general medical needs of the population as opposed to specialists who concentrate on the rare and/or more complicated aspects of medical care. Both male and female graduates are tending to gravitate into such primary care fields. In 1978 this was demonstrated by the number of resident trainees in internal medicine (24 and 28 percent, respectively, for men and women) and family medicine (9 and 11 percent, respectively). As has been the trend for a number of years in pediatrics, there has been a greater proportion of women (20 percent) as compared with men (7 percent). Ironically, and probably much to the chagrin of Boston's Dr. Gregory were he alive today, only a small number of women (9 percent) were electing obstetrics and gynecology in 1978, although the figures for men (7 percent) were also quite low. Surgery and its subspecialties have always been particularly inhospitable to women, and this continues to be the case. In 1978, 29 percent of male graduates were entering such programs, while only 9 percent of women fell into this category.

The attitudes of American male physicians toward women in the profession have improved, but it is doubtful that all remnants of previous prejudice have disappeared. The Victorian portrayal of women as frail and delicate creatures, unsuited for the rigors of the medical life, have given way to other, equally debatable male objections. Some diehards have continued to insist that the time required for the birth and rearing of children by women physicians represents a "poor investment" for society as a whole; that months or years of physician services are lost to the public, and therefore that the funds expended in training women are less efficiently spent than those for men. Contrary to this belief, a number of studies have shown that, despite the special demands of motherhood, women are indeed proving to be "cost-effective." They live longer than their male counterparts, are more likely to go into primary care medical types of practice where the need for new physicians is greatest, and—shame on us—are often paid considerably less than male physicians with equivalent training and experience.

It will be interesting to see what future roles and attitudes American women physicians will develop in the future and contrast them with patterns observed in the past. It seems that those women who formerly went into medicine in this country fell into one of two behavioral modes. Some women, those like Elizabeth Blackwell, did not openly challenge the male establishment. In a self-effacing manner they worked hard and uncomplainingly at their profession and accepted whatever rewards, personal and professional, thereby accrued. Others, perhaps anticipating the feminist movement of the 1970s, were more militant in their demands for equal opportunity and recognition. The two women contributing to this collection of interviews represent examples of these extremes.

Dr. Marian Ropes spent almost the entirety of her medical life at the renowned Massachusetts General Hospital in Boston. A few words first on Massachusetts General Hospital, itself, will place her into better perspective.

Opened in 1821, Massachusetts General Hospital has been the scene of many memorable medical advances, the most dramatic of these being the first clinical demonstration of the feasibility of ether anesthesia in surgery. This was performed by Frederick Morton under the famed "ether dome" in 1846. This historical site, the Bulfinch Building, like many other prime examples of this noted architect, still stands in Boston, much as it was almost 150 years ago. Massachusetts General Hospital also became the first of a number of hospitals in the Boston area that provided clinical training for Harvard medical students.

By the early 1920s the hospital, already noted for its high standards, was the focus of a different type of intellectual ferment. Dr. David L. Edsall,[b] soon to become the first full-time chief of medicine at Massachusetts General Hospital, was in the process of sending a number of bright young physicians to prominent research centers in order to prepare them in research techniques. Many of these would later become world famous, men like Paul Dudley White,[b] who went to London to study cardiology under Sir Thomas Lewis, and George Minot, who went to Johns Hopkins in Baltimore to study blood disease with Drs. William S. Thayer[b] and W. H.

Howell[b], and who would later be the codiscoverer of liver therapy in pernicious anemia.

Also among these promising new physicians was James H. Means.[b] He first studied at the Carnegie Nutrition Laboratory in Boston and then traveled to Copenhagen to work under the famous August Krogh,[b] learning hemodynamics and respiratory physiology. He would later become a world authority on thyroid disease and succeed Edsall as chief of medicine at Massachusetts General Hospital in 1923, when the latter went to Harvard as dean of medicine.

One of Edsall's last accomplishments at Massachusetts General Hospital was the establishment of a small research ward (Ward 4) where patients could be admitted for in-depth studies of particular diseases. It became one of Dr. Means's responsibilities to oversee this unit, and the first of a long line of outstanding investigators to work there was Dr. Joseph C. Aub.[b] In 1925 Aub was commissioned by the National Lead Institute to study the effects of lead poisoning, which was becoming a recognized industrial hazard at the time.

Dr. Ropes, after completing her undergraduate studies in chemistry at Smith in 1924, obtained a master's degree at the Massachusetts Institute of Technology in 1926. She was then hired to work as a laboratory technician at Massachusetts General Hospital, assisting Dr. Aub in his lead work but becoming well known to others in the closely knit research group, including Dr. Means. This experience convinced her that medicine rather than chemistry was to be her life's work, and she applied and was accepted to the Johns Hopkins School of Medicine. Finishing her medical school training and a year's internship at Hopkins, she was accepted, through Dr. Means's intercession on her behalf, as the first woman resident in medicine at Massachusetts General Hospital in its one hundred-year history.

She now continued in her work, assisting Aub but also interacting with a number of other investigators. Among them was the legendary Fuller Albright,[b] who pioneered in the studies of parathyroid disease among many other noteworthy accomplishments in endocrinology and metabolism. Another member of the group was Dr. Walter Bauer,[b] who formed the Arthritis Unit in 1928 and succeeded Means as chief of medicine upon the latter's retirement in 1951. Dr. Ropes continued a close association with Dr. Bauer throughout all these years.

A notable achievement of this collaboration was the publication of *Synovial Fluid Changes in Joint Disease,* published in 1953 by Drs. Ropes and Bauer. This summarized their groundbreaking work in 1,500 patients over the previous twenty-nine years in describing normal joint fluid and the changes that were brought about in its chemical and cellular constituents by various arthritic diseases. Dr. Ropes, during her years at Massachusetts General Hospital, also developed a special interest in a relatively rare but devastating connective tissue disease, also with joint manifestations, lupus erythematosis. She became an acknowledged authority on this disorder and finally in 1976 published her experience with 142 patients who had been followed by her at Massachusetts General Hospital over a thirty-four-year period. Her active clinical practice came to an end in 1976, and at present she lives in retirement with her husband, although she continues to maintain some contacts with the institution at which she spent her professional years.

Dr. Ropes obviously fits into the Elizabeth Blackwell mold. She met the male members of her profession on their own terms and, in her irrepressibly cheerful way, managed to carry on a very successful career despite any obstacles that might have existed in the milieu in which she operated. Although one might question how much sacrifice in personal terms she may have been forced to make to achieve her professional goals, there is no question that the role of wife and mother was also amply fulfilled when, in middle life, she married a widower who had two small children.

When I was looking for the right kind of woman to interview for this book—for obvious reasons those of Dr. Ropes's
generation were few and far between—Dr. Phoebe Krey, an
associate of mine at the New Jersey Medical School, suggested
Dr. Ropes. Krey had been one of the many trainees in rheumatology who had studied under Dr. Ropes at Massachusetts
General Hospital. She cautioned me, though, not to expect to
find a woman burning with the cause and message of equal
rights. Dr. Ropes's sanguinity was one of her hallmarks, and I
was, therefore, not surprised at her cheerful mien and positive
view of life.

Times change and, with them, the sorts of people who arise
to meet their challenge. Dr. Krey, who came to New Jersey at
the time her husband, Vincent Lanzoni, assumed the deanship
at our school, has a view of women in medicine that is a far
cry from that expressed by Dr. Ropes. No doubt Dr. Krey's
daughter will have an even different story to tell *her* children.

Passing the rheumatology office not too long ago, I saw a
young girl of about eleven or twelve awaiting her mother's
arrival. I recognized the features at once, and, in a jocularly
accusing manner, I pointed a forefinger at her, saying, "You are
a Lanzoni!"

Without a moment's hesitation the little girl shot back, "I
am a Krey!"

■ Among other aspects of your professional life, I was wondering what particular problems you might have had as a woman. But apparently this goes even further back. You were born in Salem, Massachusetts, where so many women were burned as witches.

Yes, but they hanged them, actually.

■ How did you become interested in medicine? Anyone in the family in the profession?

No. My father and his brothers owned a store and dealt mostly in grain. I had two brothers and a sister, but I was the only one who went in for medicine. I had always been fairly interested in medicine. Perhaps it began when I was about ten years old. There was a very big fire in Salem in 1913, and many homes were destroyed. There were about twenty-five tents erected for the care of the homeless infants rescued from the fire—well, babies, actually—and I helped the nurses care for them. That intrigued me quite a bit, but I wasn't firmly set on medicine until I finished college.

■ You went to Smith. Were you premed there?

No, I majored in chemistry at Smith and graduated from there in 1924. Then I went to MIT [Massachusetts Institute of Technology] and got a master's degree, which consisted of work mainly in chemistry.

■ Chemistry was also an unusual field for a woman at that time, was it not?

Yes. At Smith there were two thousand women without any men, and at MIT there were only thirty women among three thousand men, and most of the women were studying architecture, so it was quite a change. From MIT I came here to the Massachusetts General Hospital to work as a technician in the biochemistry laboratory, and it was this experience that convinced me. After a year of working in the hospital I knew I wanted medicine more than chemistry. I then decided definitely to go to medical school.

■ How was this decision received by others?

My family liked the idea, but people in general thought it wasn't a very womanly thing to do. It was quite amazing to hear people say, "Why do you want to do that as a woman?"

■ To what schools did you apply?

Only [Johns] Hopkins. As you probably know, when they got started Mary Garrett gave them a lot of money with the proviso that they would accept women on equal terms with men. In my class, which totalled seventy-five, there were about twelve women.

■ A number of prominent women came out of Johns Hopkins Medical School, not all of them remaining in medicine. I'm thinking of Gertrude Stein in particular. Helen Taussig[b] had to go there to complete her training because she was only allowed to take a few medical courses at Harvard and couldn't get a degree in Boston.

They wouldn't admit any women to Harvard Medical School at that time, and it was years before they did. Helen was about three or four years ahead of me at Hopkins, and I don't think Harvard accepted women for another fifteen, until the mid-forties.

■ Who were your most influential teachers at Hopkins?

I was quite influenced by Longcope,[b] who was chairman of the Department of Medicine. He was very precise, somewhat dogmatic, very knowledgeable, and very interested in students, although in a sort of distant way. Most of the students liked Louis Hamman[b] because he was really for them. But I was much more impressed by Longcope as a medical man. There were others—Williams in obstetrics, Adolph Meyer[b] in psychiatry, Park[b] in pediatrics, MacCallum[b] in pathology, Marion Hines in anatomy. I'm sure there are a number of other good ones that were there at the time.

■ Were your experiences as a woman student totally unclouded in Baltimore? One shudders to think of them now, but even in my time there were always those pranks on women that seemed to be a tradition at most medical schools. At times it was pretty brutal at our place in Brooklyn, and the psychiatrists were just as bad as anyone else. At the state mental hospital adjacent to Kings County they would routinely put the most innocent girl on stage with some poor old fellow with progressive brain disease which on questioning somehow provoked him into a continuous flow of the most vile diatribe of a sexual nature that I ever heard. The poor unsuspecting girl student selected to interview him would be on show to the class for the whole performance, and the more sheltered her previous background—a Catholic women's college, for example—the better.

There was very little of that at Hopkins and, really, I have no bad reactions of any kind. The only thing I can recall is that the urology professor always made the women sit down front and have them discuss the male GU [genitourinary] cases, but that was his interest, apparently. He wasn't bad at all.

■ You were an intern at Johns Hopkins during 1931–32 and then came back to Massachusetts General Hospital as an assistant resident in medicine. How did your return to Boston come about?

Prior to entering medical school I had worked for over a year as a technician in the laboratory of Dr. Aub[b] at Massachusetts General Hospital. He was one of the first to study the effects of lead poisoning and measure its biological characteristics and lead concentrations in tissue. He also did a lot of work with calcium. Dr. Means[b] was chairman of the Department of Medicine at Massachusetts General Hospital and also knew me and wanted me back. But Massachusetts General Hospital was a Harvard-affiliated hospital, and they had never taken a woman intern in internal medicine. Dr. Means had asked me to apply nevertheless and told me, "Put your name in because we want to get good women to apply." I applied for an internship and was turned down. But the following year Dr. Means wrote me and said: "We now have a new assistant resident position which Harvard Medical cannot tell me we can't fill with a woman because it's a brand new position. Apply and we'll give it to you." I did and became the first woman assistant resident in medicine at Massachusetts General Hospital. They had had a few women in pediatrics before, but not medicine.

■ I thought the chairmen were pretty autocratic in those days. Couldn't Means have taken you earlier as an intern?

I don't know whether it was hospital or medical school policy, but they were not for having women here at the time. Henry Christian,[b] violent as he was, even said at an open faculty meeting one time, "All these people who want women to go into medicine! It's all right if they go someplace else and get their training, but we don't want them at Harvard." Of course, at the time he was referring to women medical students rather than house staff.

■ What was your experience as the only woman medical resident like?

It wasn't bad except that the Harvard fellows just couldn't believe I had taken all the courses they had. Every once and awhile something would come up and they'd say, "Did you study that?" The Harvard graduates were very different from the men at Hopkins; they weren't used to having women doing exactly the same things they were and who had had all the same courses they had studied. But they soon discovered that I had, and they treated me better after the beginning.

■ Were those two years as resident happy ones?

Yes, very. I enjoyed them.

■ After your residency you became a research fellow at Harvard.

Yes, and a clinical fellow at Massachusetts General Hospital. But it was much the same as it is today as a fellow. You do research and clinical work together.

■ Who were the prominent people in medicine then at Massachusetts General Hospital?

There were Dr. Means, the head of the department, Dr. Aub, Chester Jones,[b]"Fully" Albright,[b] and about that time the Arthritis Unit was really going under Walter Bauer[b] and I worked under him.

■ Fuller Albright has become a legend in our lifetime. Do you remember much about him?

Very much. I worked with him closely for a couple of years. He was a charming person. He loved entertaining and was almost childish in his enjoyment of things despite the difficulty he was beginning to have with Parkinson's disease. I worked with him even before this began, however. He was a very interesting person and very original. Every morning he would come into the laboratory and say, "Well, Ropesy, I got another idea last night." He'd do that every day. He was the envy of all of us. It was a tragedy when they tried surgery on him for his Parkinsonism, but "Fully" finally decided to try it when his disease got to the point when he had so much trouble he couldn't even talk. I don't think that Cooper[b] ever had so bad a result, and it was many years later that "Fully" finally died.

■ It must have been terrible, lingering on that way, totally useless as a human being, for all those years. There seems to be a perverse twist of fate that so often strikes down some of the most brilliant young people in medicine. I'm thinking of Soma Weiss[b] and his brain tumor as another tragic example. You also had a long and close association with Dr. Bauer. After all, your monograph on joint fluid is "Ropes and Bauer," and he later became chief of medicine as

well as head of the Arthritis Unit at Massachusetts General Hospital. What was
he like?

You can hear all sorts of differing reports about him. Just the
other day one person who knew him pretty well said, "I was
always afraid of him," because he was pretty "down" on
things he didn't like and very harsh on the people involved
whether they were in the army with him down in Texas during World War II or around here at Massachusetts General
Hospital. But he was a very quick thinker. He had good ideas
but didn't know anything about fundamental research or the
ways of pursuing these ideas. He was very, very good, not only
at getting ideas, but picking out the flaw in anyone else's idea.
This was a great advantage: when anyone started to do some
investigative work, he could pick out the flaw with very simple questions. ("Well, what does that really prove?") He was
also very stimulating, if not irritating. He stimulated some
and irritated others, but his attitude frequently pressured people to get things done. But he wasn't "pushy" in other ways.

He was often in at the very beginning of things with the
idea to do something. When "Charlie" Short was chief resident, Bauer had the idea for him to write up a monograph on
rheumatoid arthritis. All Charlie did was write up what was
the state of our knowledge at the time, and it's still an excellent referral source, although, being twenty years old, it is a
little out of date.

Bauer could get people to do things, get things accomplished.
He was not a research person in any way but had many good
ideas and got others to act on them.

■ You worked with him a great many years.

Yes. Although I started with Aub and did some work for
Albright, I really spent the bulk of my time at Massachusetts
General Hospital with Dr. Bauer. He headed the Arthritis Unit
until he died in 1963.

■ Did you take over the Arthritis Unit after that?

No. The only time I was ever in charge of the unit was during World War II when he was away. And that was as long as I wanted to have anything to do with the administrative end.

■ I must be frank. Was this your decision, or was the post denied to you? These are things people are interested in knowing.

I have no recollection of really wanting the post. I really don't like that approach to people. I'd much rather work on problems, see patients, teach, and things of that sort. I started seeing patients privately here in 1935. This is one of the hospitals that would let you have an office and practice here as all of us did—geographic full-time you would call it.

■ Are you still in practice?

No. I retired three years ago.

■ Do you miss it?

Yes, and yet you find a lot of other things to do. I come in to attend rounds, and if I have anything to say about them I say it, but I don't see patients anymore. A good many call me up, but I stay out of the problems. Sure, it's a different life, but that's all right.

■ At the time you went into medicine it was unusual for a woman to do this. A number of women who did surrendered to a certain extent—at least outwardly—some aspects of their womanhood in order to become doctors. Correct me if I am wrong, but one of the reasons I wished to talk with you was that I had been told that you did not fit into this mold: you were a person who remained a woman and a physician throughout your life and, I must say, I detect no trace of bitterness as I talk to you. If one speaks to many of your contemporaries who went through at the same time or shortly before, a good deal of resentment can be perceived.

That's true. Even Helen Taussig,[b] who has accomplished so much and surely shouldn't have resentment after all she has done, has some of this.

■ Helen Taussig wouldn't even talk to me!

That's too bad, but I guess she is that sort of person. Others were quite different. Miriam Bradley was very different, for example. Much more outward going, like her brother, Allan. A fair number of people told me that it wasn't feminine to go into medicine; that is, people in general, probably some teachers as well. My family liked the idea, however, and most of my close friends did. But I'm sure it didn't change me. I have always been interested in helping people, ever since I helped with those babies as a young girl. When people ask me what it is that I want most, it is to help. I never went into psychiatry, but I like this approach to patients. There isn't a patient who doesn't say to me, "My, you talk a lot—and you ask different questions!" To me the most interesting and important thing is to combine this aspect with the rest, and I have attempted to do this ever since the beginning. One of the things people don't like about my little book on lupus erythematosus is that I have put in too many of the "emotional factors" and not enough of the "steroid factors." But I never changed from my original approach.

I didn't get married during my early period as a physician. In fact, I thought I wasn't ever going to get married. I wasn't one of those determined souls who was never going to get married, but I just didn't think it was going to happen. Still, I enjoyed life very much. I did a lot of camping; I went to lots of parties and enjoyed social activities with all sorts of people. I did get married, to a widower in 1948, and so I have stepchildren and grandchildren now, and that turned out to be a very good solution. But I never changed from being a woman, although I was never a domineering woman. Some of the fellows used to say, "You're the worst argument for trying to help women in medicine because you never do anything about it or talk about it." I would simply answer, "I just did it."

■ If some women physicians, especially of your generation, have chips on their shoulders, there's every reason for them being there. It's amazing that someone like Helen Taussig, who has done such a tremendous amount for medicine . . .

Yes, she's one of the outstanding doctors in the country.

■ . . . male or female. And I suspect she must harbor a great deal of bitterness within her. I have never managed to get her consent for an interview. I've tried twice and struck out twice, but I'm going to try again.*

She's sort of a strange person, and I didn't know she was quite as bitter as that, but I'm not surprised. I know a number of bitter women in medicine who talk so much about lack of opportunities. But I always felt that you had to try what you wanted and do it.

■ A "victim" kind of attitude can be self-defeating. Some people will blame their lack of success on the fact that they are women or black or Jewish or whatever and say that this was the reason for their failure. To a certain extent this might be true, but that is not necessarily the whole story.

I guess I was lucky because Hopkins was a very good place for women; it really was. I doubt that many of the women left there with this attitude. Ann Kuttner,[b] for example, did a lot of excellent work in rheumatic fever and headed Irvington House up on the Hudson, where all these cases once went. She never had any bad experiences at Hopkins or in medicine, I'm sure. She's dead now.

■ I must say your attitude seems so rosy! You're making me feel like I am from some sort of scandal-mongering magazine looking for "dirt," but didn't you have *any* unhappy experiences in medicine?

Of course, everybody says that I have rose-colored spectacles, and I think I do. In college I smiled all the time, and most people didn't think college was as wonderful as all that. It's something people always challenge me about, but, in all truth, I have always been able to enjoy myself in my medical work

*Strike three.

and get whatever I wanted out of it. Sure, I thought about the process of getting married in the early days, but there wasn't anyone that really "took me over" then, and I therefore felt I wasn't missing anything.

On the other hand, I felt very different at the time I got going into matrimony in 1948. I don't think medicine interfered—well, possibly a little, because people occasionally said, "You're too much of a 'medical man,' too much of a 'doctor.' " But that was rare, and it didn't bother me because I usually wasn't too keen about the people who said it.

■ Are there any mistakes you have made?

As for individual patients, this comes to my mind fairly often: the things that I did that might have been bad for particular patients. From my point of view that is one of the worst things that happens to you, but you just have to take it. As for my research activities, I think that if I had gone into synovial fluid culture a little earlier, right after the other analyses I reported, it would have been better, but I didn't. That's just something I missed.

■ To go back for a moment, you were interested in specializing in internal medicine right from the start. Weren't many women of your time sort of pushed into pediatrics?

I guess so. At the Massachusetts General Hospital, at the time I became an assistant resident in medicine, they had never had a woman as either an intern or resident in medicine, while there had been some women accepted as interns in pediatrics. Surgery was hopeless, practically. I think only one of the twelve women in my class went into surgery. She did all right for the first few years, but I haven't kept up with her. Most of them went into medicine or pediatrics and did quite well as far as I know. I've already mentioned Ann Kuttner and her work with rheumatic fever.

■ You, yourself, must have seen an awful lot of rheumatic fever in your time.

Oh, yes; it was a very common disease, and I was interested in it because of the joint manifestations. I used to visit at Children's Hospital and Chelsea Naval Hospital because they always had so many cases there.

■ And yet we see very little of it today, at least in this country.

Because that is one of the diseases that was changing its character even before antibiotics came in to prevent it. Diphtheria also was changing before antibiotics. My disease, the one I've done the most work on, lupus, was changing in its nature even before we got anything to treat it, steroids or anything else. Of course, the difference in prognosis has dramatically altered: whereas forty years ago eighty percent of patients used to die within a couple of years, today only ten percent die within five years. That's amazing.

■ Do you think this is due to therapy or to the natural history of these diseases?

I don't know. I suspect a little bit of both. At the Good Samaritan where Drs. Jones[b] and Bland[b] were so active, they noted that the diseases were getting less severe in patients well before sulfonamides became available to prevent strep infections and the ensuing rheumatic fever attacks. The same was true of diphtheria. And yet when I suggest that lupus, too, has been changing in its manifestations, people are surprised despite the obvious past history of these other two diseases.

■ It's interesting. Louis Weinstein has also commented on the changing nature of many diseases even without specific treatment. Syphilis certainly changed, and even bubonic plague tended to pretty much burn itself out in the fourteenth century. What do you think of the future of rheumatology?

I think it is an excellent field to go into, still. It's a big, broad field with all kinds of patients ranging from the very severe acute illnesses to the chronic ones which are difficult to handle and go on forever. I remember when cortisone first appeared. We were one of the first centers to test it on arthritis, and the initial results were really very dramatic. That was before we were aware of all the side effects of steroids and their eventual shortcomings in treating various diseases. Our three research fellows came into my office one day and told me, "Well, we certainly made a mistake, all right. We never should have gone into this field. It's all over." I told them that they were perhaps rushing things a bit and that they better stay in. I still think it's a good field to go into.

We have seen that rheumatic fever has become very much less of a problem than it once was, and even lupus, although still a dreaded disease, is getting better to treat. But I don't see where much has happened in rheumatoid arthritis despite all we have learned about it. We have expended a tremendous amount of work and money on learning many interesting facts about the disease, but none of them seems to be helpful in treating it. Perhaps we are treating it somewhat more effectively now with a combination of a little help from environmental factors, a little from the emotional approach, and a little help from strictly medical means.

■ Gold therapy seems to be a recurring vogue for the treatment of rheumatoid arthritis. Do you have any comments on this?

It depends upon which doctor is reporting the results. I think it is one of the many modalities of treatment that causes a lessening of the inflammation in some patients, a fair percentage in some series; but I think that there is no evidence that it really alters the course of the disease. We still don't even know what causes it. I have always believed that there was some inciting agent, perhaps a very small virus which is either the main cause or plays a precipitant role, but there's no very good evidence for this, and many people have looked for something along these lines without any success.

■ If you had a daughter or granddaughter today with thoughts of going into medicine, what would you advise her?

I think the most important thing to know is what it is that

they really are interested in, and this is hard to know. I have interviewed a fair number of girls applying to Harvard or wanting to apply somewhere else, and a lot of them have a very superficial interest in medicine.

Just by talking with them, I get the feeling that they are intrigued with certain aspects of medicine but really haven't thought about it in depth, about the difficulties involved and what they really should get out of it. *That's* the most important thing. Somewhat less important, but along the same line, is that they don't seem to realize that their lives are going to be different if they do get married as physicians. We're obviously different from other women as wives and homemakers. This was even true for me when I married in my forties and found myself with two children, the youngest of whom was eleven.

Your life as a married woman physician is very different from that of other women, and without any question you must be sure that this is what you want. I emphasize that as much as I can to these young women, pointing out that the two roles are surely compatible but that you won't be doing medicine quite as you would if you were unmarried. Similarly, you won't be taking care of your home and children in the same way as a woman who does this as a full-time occupation.

■ Being married to a physician, I am well aware of that. I advise all my women students, "Whatever you do, when you get married, try to marry a doctor: he's the only kind of a husband who will understand the 'craziness' of your career." What about your own spouse?

He was a certified public accountant before he retired, a partner in an international firm, Haskins and Sells.

■ Was there any resentment on his part about the demands of your profession?

I guess not. He never showed it in any event, and, of course, he knew what he was getting into. But he was a professional man, himself, and accounting, at least in those days, was very demanding and he was a very hard worker. He was worse than I was, practically, and therefore expected as much from me. We worked our careers in quite well together in two very busy lives.

■ **Did you ever feel that the children suffered because of the demands of your profession?**

Not from my career, I think. The girl graduated from Wellesley. She was interested in chemistry and got a master's in chemistry from Radcliffe-Harvard. She taught organic chemistry at Wheaton for a few years, and then worked in a research group in biochemistry at Harvard Medical School. The boy graduated from Cornell and got a master's in physics at Rochester. He did research in physics at Rochester for a few years and subsequently around Boston with different companies. Both of the children are married. She has two children and he has three. All of the grandchildren have done very well.

■ **You started your college education at Smith, a women's college, and then went to a coeducational medical school. There are no more exclusively women's medical colleges, but a young woman still has a choice at the undergraduate level. Do you think that there is still a place for the women's college?**

Very strongly. For certain people I have always felt it was right. At Hopkins, I remember, we had a total of about forty women when I was a medical student there, and we always would argue about the pros and cons of going to an all-women's college. There are those women who enjoy their associations with other women and learn better in that environment; there are those women who somewhat suppress themselves among a mixed group of men and women; and there are those a little less interested in the social side of college involving men and women together. For these women I think very strongly that a women's college is the place for them. I surely hope that Smith doesn't take men, because I don't think any good man would want to go to a women's college. I wouldn't if I were a man.

■ Why do you say that? Let's say some young man wanted to study astronomy and that there was a very good astronomy program at a particular school that was, essentially, a school for women. Why shouldn't he go there?

It would be a very unusual situation, I think, in which there would be such an outstanding department in a women's college that couldn't be matched in another school, and I still don't believe an outstanding young man would choose a straight women's college. But perhaps the question is academic because there is so much sharing of classes between the previously all-women's and all-men's schools. Smith, for example, has classes with the University of Massachusetts and Amherst, and anybody can now study anything they want practically along the whole Connecticut River Valley.

■ Well, then, what kind of a woman *should* go to a coeducational college?

The kind that is the other way around, one who enjoys social activities more with both men and women involved, and who is brought out more by a mixed academic environment. I think that there are some women who would fare better in one academic setting and some who would do better in the other. What I object to is that there is too much of an attempt to persuade people to go one way. I think that girls of a college age know what they want in this respect. At least a lot of them know.

■ I think your views on this are interesting. Perhaps you really are a truly liberated woman.

Someone asked me about the equal rights amendment and I said, "Well, I think I just use it. I don't think you really need another amendment to the Constitution."

■ My wife, another woman physician, feels the same way.

The only thing we really need are pockets in women's clothes. Everybody laughs when I say that, but it's the only thing I wish they would have done that they haven't. It's a crime [*laughing*].

■ You really have come a long way, and I think you have managed to do it without scars. So many women of accomplishment do have scars.

I really don't and I don't think I'm hiding them, even to myself. There's no question that I have rose-colored spectacles, and I always tend to see the better side of something. That has always been true.

■ Well, it makes for a happier life.

It surely does. I'm glad I had them.

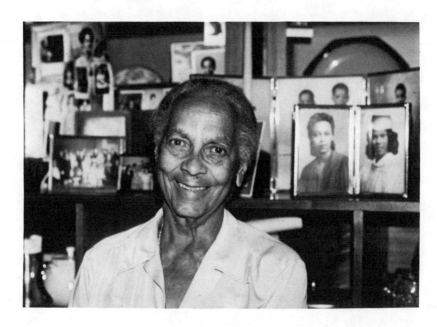

Lena F. Edwards, M.D.

CHAPTER 14

Lena F. Edwards, M.D.
(1901–   )

THE CAREER of Lena Edwards, another woman physician, represents a far cry from that of Marian Ropes. Beyond the fact of her gender, Dr. Edwards had elements of race and religion that determined the course of her life. A black woman with a deep lifelong committment to her Catholic faith, Dr. Edwards had divided her life in such a way that it might be described as a tale of three cities: Washington, D.C.; Jersey City, New Jersey; and Hereford, Texas.

Born to a prominent black family in the nation's capital, Dr. Edwards distinguished herself as a scholar and an aggressive competitor at an early age, earning honors first in high school and then as an undergraduate and medical student at Howard University. Following graduation from Howard and her marriage to Dr. Keith Madison, Dr. Edwards moved to Jersey City and soon established a successful private practice with increasing emphasis in obstetrics and gynecology. She became one of the first black women in the country to receive board certification when this specialty achieved recognition as such in the 1930s.

Recognition of her abilities did not come easily to Dr. Edwards in Jersey City, and she soon became a thorn in the side of the local medical establishment, which refused to grant this black woman the recognition her accomplishments de-

manded. Not content merely with her own personal advancement, Dr. Edwards, over a thirty-year period in Jersey City,
became involved in a number of socioeconomic and political
endeavors within and beyond the strict confines of medicine.

This segment came to an end in 1954 when, stimulated by
the desire to teach and urged toward this goal by the many
young physicians in training she had supervised during her
years at the Margaret Hague Maternity Hospital, Dr. Edwards
left for Washington to assume an academic post at her alma
mater, the Howard University College of Medicine.

But there was an even greater need to be met by this deeply
religious woman, a lifelong desire to serve some portion of her
years as a medical missionary. At the age of sixty-five, despite
a heart ailment and at a time when most of her contemporaries might have been thinking of retirement rather than the
assumption of some new burdensome responsibility, Dr. Edwards left Washington for Hereford, Texas, to assume charge
of the medical clinic that had been set up at the San Jose
Mission for the Mexican-American migrant workers in the
area.

After arriving in Texas in 1961, Dr. Edwards recognized the
great need for a maternity and infant care facility and soon
bent every effort toward the construction of what would become a year later Our Lady of Guadeloupe Maternity Clinic.
As significant as the construction of this maternity hospital,
itself, was Dr. Edwards's recognition that personal involvement in the creation of the facility by the migrant workers,
themselves, was critical to the success of the effort. This pattern of community involvement led to this project being recognized as a model for subsequent similar programs throughout the nation. In recognition of this achievement, in 1964 Dr.
Edwards received from Lyndon B. Johnson the Medal of Freedom, the highest civilian honor that a president can bestow
upon a civilian.

The demands of family required Dr. Edwards to return to

the Northeast, and after a few more years in central New Jersey, not far from her activities in Jersey City, Dr. Edwards settled in Lakewood, Ocean County. "Settled," not "retired."

In her eighth decade, still ardently devoted to a career of humanitarian service, she continues to be active in such endeavors as the Ocean County Cancer Society, Alcoholics Anonymous, the Council on Aging, the Board of Regents of St. Peter's College, Head Start, the New Jersey Task Force for the Early Diagnosis of Genital and Breast Cancer, and a number of senior citizen groups, to list only some of her wide-ranging activities.

Incredibly, despite a life of outstanding personal accomplishment and social service, Dr. Edwards has also found time to give birth to, love, and oversee the growth and education of her own six devoted children: a priest, a medical social worker, a teacher of business administration, an aeronautical engineer, and two physicians. Throughout her professional life as a physician, educator, and social activist, Dr. Edwards has maintained a zest for living and openly espoused the often controversial, if not dangerous, causes to which she has felt committed. These have been the hallmarks of her character. In receiving one of her many awards for public service, the Bronze Medal of the American Cancer Society, Dr. Edwards was introduced by one of the officials, who said, "I am glad to be here to help present this award to Dr. Edwards because she 'tells it like it is . . .' "

And so she does.

■ Tell me about the early years, your parents, your upbringing.

I was brought up in Washington, D.C., and greatly influenced by that city, which was a "rascal of a city"—and still is. My father and mother were opposites. My mother was a "princess," a descendant of the aristocracy of Washington through what I plainly like to call the rape of her ancestors. My father's background was more humble. He graduated with a teaching degree from Howard in 1897, but, being married to my mother, he had to do more than that. So he went to dental school at Howard during the day, while he worked at the post office at night. He got his degree in dentistry and then began teaching oral surgery at Howard in 1911. He continued on the faculty there for the rest of his life, until just before he died in 1936.

He was a philanthropist if there ever was one. He loved people. He hated no one, and he taught us how to love even the "bum" on the street because you didn't know how he got there or who put him there.

Washington is a city of castes, and back at the turn of the century the castes among the blacks were very pronounced. You first had the professionals; below them were the teachers; then you had the government employees; then the houseworkers; and then the laborers. I belonged in the top caste because my dad was a professional. The children in our household, my brother, sister, and I were little devils and grew up tending to think we were better than anybody else. My mother would say to me "Who are you associating with?" But my father invariably brought us down off our high horse. He would say, "Everybody's good and everybody's bad. So just don't follow what other people tell you. Think for yourself; that's why you have a mind."

There was a race problem in Washington, there was quite a problem, but we ignored it. My father would say, "People who are that way are stupid and ignorant, so ignore them." My mother would say, "Hold your head high and walk straight because there's no difference in God's eyes."

We were expected to be the best children in Washington. Our parents taught us: "good, better, best; never let it rest until your good is better and your better's best." If you do that no one can keep you down. I went through school with high honors. I wouldn't cry if someone beat me up, but I did if I wasn't tops in the class.

I decided to be a doctor when I was twelve. Because of my admiration for my father, I first wanted to be a dentist. But he was a great student of people and their personalities. He knew I was fidgety, so he told me, "You'll never be able to stand by a chair all day long. You've got to be on the move." So I told him "All right. But I like the way you treat patients, and I want patients too, so I'm going to be a doctor." And nothing stopped me.

I graduated from Dunbar High School at the top of my class. Because of segregated schools in Washington in those days, in order to place someone in a prestigious place of learning, they would take the top boy and top girl graduating from Dunbar and send them to an Ivy League school up north. But even at the age of seventeen I knew who I was and was proud of it. I knew that as long as I could be good at whatever I wanted to do, I would make it. So I didn't want to go to one of those schools and come back brainwashed. I decided to go to Howard instead. This was a great disappointment to my high school teachers, and in the autograph book they signed for me there were all these expressions of sadness about the opportunity I was passing up. You see, most of these people were mulattoes like me—I was quite fair when I was younger—and they had a way of looking down on those poor little black people they were going to teach. I didn't want that; there was too much of my daddy in me for that. So I went to Howard. I told these teachers that I wasn't missing *anything*. I've always had the philosophy that no one can *teach* you anything. They can expose you to knowledge, but you dig it out and learn it for yourself.

■ Did you have any trouble as a woman going to Howard as an undergraduate and then as a medical student?

No, there wasn't any difficulty for me going through Howard except the same kind of heckling that all women get. The men would really go after you if you were a woman and sort of sharp. I always used to say I had to "chase the wolves," but other than that, intellectually, I had no difficulties. Howard has always been mixed. One tenth of our class was white and chiefly Jewish fellows. We respected one another, but there again I had to be at the top to win prizes.

■ Was your husband in the same class with you at medical school?

He started out one year ahead, but we graduated together inasmuch as I accelerated my program. I wanted to relieve my father of some of the economic burden of educating the three of us, so I wanted to hurry up and get out of school. I always had to crowd my program. I finished four years of undergraduate work in two years and three summers by taking extra hours of credit, and I then finished medical school in four years.

■ After Howard there was a very large segment of your life that took place in Jersey City, about thirty years, from 1924 to 1953. What made you decide to come to New Jersey?

We learned that a Negro doctor had died in Jersey City. As a matter of fact, he had been killed in a political battle. His wife was a former resident of Washington, D.C., and we knew her.

It occurred to me that we might take over his practice. The advantage of working in Jersey City was its proximity to New York City. I wanted to further my medical education, but knew that I couldn't do that at the other medical colleges in Washington and would be limited there to only what Howard had to offer. I figured that if I came to Jersey City I would be able to go across the river and continue my studies.

■ What was Jersey City like in those days?

Jersey City has always been a middle- to lower-middle-class town, and at that time was full of European immigrants, especially in the Lafayette section to which we moved. There were people from Czechoslovakia and Poland; there were Irish and Italians who had been there longer than the others. I fitted in beautifully with those people because they were used to a woman taking care of the family, whether it was a midwife or just some kind of healer. I built up a practice very rapidly and also picked up a little Polish and Czech to go along with the French, German, and Spanish I learned in college.

■ Did you start right out in obstetrics and gynecology?

There was no defined specialty in that at the time. There were two men who did obstetrics in town, and at the Jersey City Medical Center they had some kind of a residency in it. Then in 1931 they decided to build the Margaret Hague Maternity Hospital, which turned out to be one of the greatest institutions of its kind, and people came from all over the world to study there. In order to drum up public support for the Margaret Hague they put representatives from all groups on the staff. They had a black, a Jew, Catholics, and Protestants—representatives from all cultural backgrounds. They picked me because at the time I was doing a lot of home deliveries and didn't hesitate to call someone in on consultation if I had a problem. These consultants were the influential medical people who were "going places" in town, and although I had been interested in pediatrics and had hoped to go to New York to study it, I decided to take the opportunity that came in Jersey City when it presented itself.

■ You had some problems with the people at the Hague.

It was the same sort of thing I described to you back in my childhood. There are people who are Ivy League and others who are not. The Ivy Leaguers may recognize your ability, but they let you know just how far you can go.

When I came to Jersey City there was no such thing as a specialty board in obstetrics and gynecology. When these were established in about 1936, if you had been an established practitioner of the specialty you could get your boards by simple endorsement (a grandfather clause type of thing), or else you could do a residency and then take an examination. I was determined to take the residency and the exam rather than be beholden to any of the senior staff at the Hague who could have obtained an endorsement for me. The thing that made me so adamant about this was an experience I had had with a poor patient who had also been seen by a consultant. I thought the patient should have had one kind of treatment, and he recommended another. I interpreted this decision as simply a matter of poor man's treatment versus rich man's treatment. I went home that night and actually cried, thinking about the "crap" I had to take from that so-and-so when I knew what I had recommended was the proper treatment. I said to myself, "Darn it. I'm going to become assistant to the chief in that hospital if it kills me."

Well, when I applied for residency training "the man" decided to let me know who I was, and I was sent to Harlem Hospital in New York for an interview. The director there said, "Why are you coming here? The Margaret Hague Hospital is a wonderful place to train." I said, "I guess they think that I should be where blacks are." He told me that he would take me if I wanted to come, but asked me what was the matter with those people in Jersey City.

After this episode they got off my tail a little in Jersey City and let me do a little more than I had done in the past, but they still wouldn't give me the residency and kept trying to talk me out of it. They would say, "Look, you have a wonderful practice and you treat your patients well. Why do you want to go through all the trouble of being a resident? What about your six children? What will you do about them?" Well, my children were right at home with me in Jersey City, and it was obvious that I could do the residency there much better than in Harlem Hospital. So I wouldn't go to Harlem, and they kept turning me down in Jersey City.

Finally the thing came to a head in 1945. Dr. Cosgrove was then chief at the Margaret Hague. He was a great guy and recognized my ability, but that black-white thing still existed, as it does today, and there were pressures exerted not to give me my due. At that time Dr. Cosgrove had just received the brotherhood award from the YMCA of Jersey City, and the day following this I went to his office. I told him, "You give that award back to the man." (I've always been kind of fresh.) I said, "Give that award back because you don't believe in *sisterhood.* I've been coming here now for six years trying to get a residency, and I know you don't like women because you've only had three of them here at the Hague."

As I was talking to him in this way, his secretary finally said to him, "Dr. Cosgrove, you know Dr. Edwards is one of the best doctors here; she has wonderful success with her patients. Why don't you give her a break?" And he said, "Okay, when do we have an opening?" So the following spring I started my residency. It only required eighteen months at the time. I completed these, took my examination, and was certified in 1952. As far as I have been able to find out, I was probably the second black woman in the country to become board-certified in obstetrics and gynecology.

■ At the time you practiced in Jersey City, were most of your patients black
or were they European immigrants?

Most of my patients were white throughout my time in
Jersey City. This is because we blacks have an inborn lack of
confidence in one another, and this is a great impediment to
our becoming full citizens of this country. The fact is that
many times they don't trust you.

■ Black patients don't trust black doctors?

That's nothing new. It kind of still exists.

■ You practiced in Jersey City during the reign of Mayor Frank ("I am the
law") Hague. Did you know him?

Not intimately, but I met him.

■ What was he like?

I called him "The Good Thief." Did you ever read the book
of that title? It is the story of a priest who was in a prison
camp during the war, and he used to sneak out and steal things
from the commissary to take care of the prisoners. That's how
I thought of Frank Hague. He had a heart as good as gold. He
grew up during a very depressed period in that city, but he had
ambition to help the poor. He probably did some things he
shouldn't have done in order to get money for the poor, but he
really helped.

■ The story goes that he believed his mother to have died for lack of good
medical treatment and that's why he was always concerned about good medical care.

That's why he built the Jersey City Medical Center and
named the Hague Maternity Hospital for her. He grew up in a
tenement in downtown Jersey City. People who knew the family and where they lived used to say they could hear the old
lady in the middle of the night beating the rats out of the
house. The medical care then available for the poor, black or

white, was not good. That's why he was dedicated to doing something for them in this way.

■ I worked in Jersey City during the sixties when the medical facilities were really falling apart, and the old-timers would tell me if Hague were still alive he would never have let that happen. They told about him coming around to the hospital in the middle of the night to see that everyone was doing his job properly. If not, there would be hell to pay.

That's right. But after he went out of power the real politicians took over, and then you began to have all those no-show jobs. To this day the disciplinary situation is terrible in Jersey City. None of the city workers are supervised, and as a result it has become a slum town. I remember when even the tenements were beautifully cleaned, and you didn't mind climbing three or four flights to get to an apartment. But then the real estate brokers came in, bought up the tenement houses, and divided each apartment into two or three units. The people in the front often had no fire escapes because the fire escapes were in the back. How they got away with it, I'll never know. Naturally, the place went down.

■ Was your husband in general practice or some specialty?

He practiced general medicine, but he was a sick man and not too active.

■ You spent an awfully large part of your life in Jersey City. What made you leave and go to Howard?

I've always been a teacher like my dad, who was a born teacher, and I formed many ideas about obstetrics during my years of practice. I became a strong believer in natural childbirth, and emphasized the importance of a very close relationship between the doctor and the mother. You learn a great deal from your patients when you take the time to spend with them. The house staff at the Hague used to hang around me asking my opinion on all sorts of problems they had with their patients. It was they who asked me, "Why don't you go to a medical school and teach the things you are teaching us here?"

I resisted this at first. I would say, "As soon as my children are grown I'm going into missionary work." What finally changed my mind was a conversation I had with a son of a friend of mine with whom I had grown up in Washington. He told me, "Doc, if you go on a mission you will help only that group of people, but if you go to medical school and teach a number of doctors your philosophy and skills, through them you will be helping many, many more people in the end." That convinced me I should teach. I had an opportunity to join the new medical college in Jersey City, Seton Hall; I could have gone to Meharry in Nashville; but, because of my dad, and his association with Howard, I chose to go there.

■   Your physician son, Edward, told me that it was his impression that you were a pretty tough taskmaster at Howard.

I was. We would have about one hundred students in a class, and sometimes only sixty would show up for a lecture. I started passing out an attendance sheet, because in medical school you're not there to play around, you're there to get an education. One day I caught a fellow signing in twice, once for himself and once for his "buddy." I called him to account and told him, "You're not going to play games with me. If you're dishonest as a student, God forbid, you'll kill somebody when you become a doctor!" But they loved me. Don't your children love you and doesn't anybody love you when you show real concern? Otherwise, they'll say you just don't care.

■   What made you leave Howard after your six years there?

It was that yen for missionary work. I have been a Franciscan for years. I was born on the feast of St. Francis, and my middle name is Frances. Those Irish fathers had a great devotion to things such as the saint you were supposed to be born under, and I loved St. Francis's life because he was headstrong in his youth just as I was. So when I went on a pilgrimage to Rome during the Holy Year of 1950, I spoke to one of the priests that accompanied us and told him that I had always wanted to be a Franciscan but did not think I was good enough. He said, "That's ridiculous. If you want to become a Franciscan then you *are* good enough, because God will see it that way." So when I returned from Rome I joined the order as what you would now call a lay Franciscan. We had the rules of poverty and obedience, as did the priests and nuns, but poverty was the main thing.

Well, there I was at Howard approaching sixty, and I was afraid that if I didn't get out to do missionary work then, I wouldn't be able to do so much longer. You see, I've had a heart lesion since I was eighteen. I nearly died during the "flu" epidemic at the time, and it left me with a leaking mitral valve.

■ How did you pick out Texas for your mission?

Tommy, my priest son, was a member of the Graymoor Friars, a Franciscan order in Graymoor, New York. Whenever I could, I would go up to visit him, and one day we were having dinner with some of the other seminarians. My children always spoke frankly about me because I encouraged it, and during the course of our conversation he turns to one of the other fellows at the table and says, "You know, this crazy mother of mine thinks that she wants to do missionary work." And one of the young men in my son's class said, "Well, then, she should see the clinic they have down at St. Joe's. It's terrible. Why doesn't your mother come and take care of it so they can have a doctor? All they have now is a nurse." He was referring to this little clinic they had set up for migrant workers down in Hereford, Texas. I said, "I'll think about it."

I then made arrangements to visit the place. I'll never forget my first visit there, because it was another time I cried when I saw human beings treated worse than animals. Even though it was a mission, the patients just stood out in the doorway while a nurse would see them and *just maybe* call a doctor to see what could be done for them. I went home and told everyone that this was where I was going.

By that time all my children were out of high school and into college and getting along pretty much on their own, so this didn't hold me back. But they didn't want me to go because they knew I was so outspoken. "Mother," they said, "if you go south they're going to lynch you!" I said, "With the grace of God, if you're doing his work and you're friendly with people, nobody is going to touch you." And that's exactly the way things turned out.

The townspeople—the "Anglos"—lived in the center of Hereford; St. Joseph's Mission was on the outskirts and had about fifty or sixty of these old converted army barracks from World War II. Each was broken up into several apartments and were the living quarters for the migrant workers, who were about eighty-five percent Mexican—Chicanos. About one hundred of them were permanent residents and had jobs in town or on the farms; the rest came and went, and numbered as many as eight or nine thousand at times, depending upon the season.

■ Just where is Hereford, and what was the medical setup at the time you arrived in 1961?

Hereford is up on the Panhandle part of Texas about halfway between Amarillo and Albuquerque, New Mexico. It's situated in Deaf Smith County—named after an early politician named Smith who was apparently deaf—and the local hospital was called Deaf Smith County Hospital. They would take the migrant workers there, but they would have to pay, and they had so little money that their last penny might go for medical care. Frequently they could not afford any at all.

At the Mission there was a clinic that had about ten to fifteen beds for all the migrant workers. What was really needed was a maternity hospital, because the Chicanos lived in very close quarters, had many communicable diseases, and more often then not had no immunizations. It was important to keep the pregnant mothers and especially the newborn babies separated from the rest, so the maternity hospital became our goal.

■ Did you have any trouble with the townspeople?

No. I simply told them what I wanted to do. I said, "I don't want to take any practice away from your doctors, but they have so much to do they haven't got much time to bother with these migrant workers. I just want to help because people are dying." One woman had just died from hemorrhaging at home during childbirth with a midwife. I said, "Any time I go too far, let me know, but I just want to help them."

So there was no opposition from the town. Interestingly enough, at the time I arrived in Hereford, at Deaf Smith County Hospital they were getting ready for a review of their accreditation by the Joint Hospital Commission, and they knew I was the only board-certified obstetrician-gynecologist within sixty miles. So they added me to their staff in time for the inspection. I was therefore able to admit patients to their hospital while awaiting the completion of our own.

■ Were you able to communicate as well with the Chicanos?

I had studied Spanish in college, and this came in handy, although it was very different from the local Tex-Mex dialect, which I gradually picked up. But we had to build for the people, and the one thing we did there which is not customary for people doing missionary work was to go there and *be* one of them. These people were farm laborers, and it was real hard farm labor. I wondered how they did it. After we got going I would go into the fields with them to pick up whatever was left after the crop gathering. This was good exercise for me, and I liked the soil anyway.

When we got ready to build the hospital and needed a hospital board, I insisted that it be composed of the Chicanos themselves. They said, "But Doctor, we have no education." I said,
"You may not have schooling, but you have education. Schooling is one thing, but you have been educated by life, and when
you apply that, it's the most wonderful thing in the world."

■ How did the maternity hospital get built?

It was built by the Chicanos themselves, with some super-
vision from the kind people of the community. For example,
one fellow could lay cinder blocks (it was all block building in
those days); another worked for a town plumber as a common
laborer, and the plumber very kindly supervised his work.
Another knew a little carpentry. I taught them how to lay tile
and supervised the painting. Labor was free, and the only
thing we paid for to any extent was building materials, and
these we got at a discount.

After things got going in building the hospital the Anglos
offered to give me some furniture they didn't need, but I told
them, "With all due respect for your kindness, this is one time
in their lives that these people are going to have everything
brand new, even if it takes the last thing I have."

■ How was the hospital financed?

There was my own money* and contributions from friends
mostly. The Margaret Hague Hospital in Jersey City took up a
collection from the janitors and elevator operators on up to
the chiefs and donated twenty-five hundred dollars. I like to
tell about the contribution of my son, the priest. It was customary in our church for newly ordained priests to bless people and receive contributions from them. When Tommy was
ordained, he kept blessing people at All Saints Church in
Jersey City from four in the afternoon on into the evening. A

---

*Dr. Edwards contributed over $10,000 of her own funds to the project.

doctor friend of mine had given him a briefcase into which he had all these parishioners drop their money. When he came home that night there was $1,650 in that bag, and he gave it all to me for the hospital.

At that time they had just come out with those special transparent covered cribs, each with a shelf for the baby's things underneath. These were each $150, and I was able to buy ten of them with the money Tommy sent. That was one of the biggest donations we received, and when the Anglos in town saw we really meant business, little by little some of them also made donations.

When we finished building in 1962 it was a lovely place, with ten beds and ten cribs. Upstairs, over the maternity hospital, we built five rooms on one side to train the Chicanos in nursing, and on the other side a little apartment where I hoped to live with my mother when she came down. After we finished that, we revamped the preexisting clinic in the other building, which was badly in need of repair and updating for the other patients.

■ Your work in Hereford between 1961 and 1965 was obviously a high point in your life, and you received the presidential Medal of Freedom in recognition of it. Do you know how this came about?

After we began to work on building the new hospital, *Ebony* magazine got wind of it, and an editor and photographer came down to do a story. They spent several days running around with me gathering material and taking pictures, all of which resulted in a six-page spread. In the same issue (February 1962) there was a story on the coming-out party of Nat ("King") Cole's daughter. President Kennedy was very friendly with Nat Cole and came across my story as he was reading about Cole's daughter. He had somebody investigate who I was and what I was doing and recommended me for the Freedom Medal. Because of the assassination I actually received the medal from President Johnson.

■   What led to your leaving Texas?

I had wanted my mother to come down and stay with me, but her health was failing and there was other illness in the family. They did not want to send my mother down to Texas and therefore put her in a nursing home in Washington. When I learned of this, I went to the father and told him, "I have put five years of life into this Mission and now my mother is in a nursing home. If she died there and I was not taking care of her I would want to die myself. So I have to go."

My son Tommy had been ordained by then, and was ill with hepatitis in a small town in Brazil. I was afraid he might have a serious type of hepatitis related to an amoebic infection and that he might not be receiving proper medical care in South America. I was prepared to go down there to bring him back. Fortunately, he was sent back, so I did not have to make this trip.

Finally, I had had a very severe heart attack while I was in Hereford, and this also contributed to my decision to leave.

■   Was it a bona fide "coronary," then?

Oh boy, was it! I'll never forget that night. I had just finished delivering a baby. Someone was supposed to have come to help me but had not shown up. Then this attack came on, and I thought I was dying. I got the baby into a nice little crib and, with a whole lot of praying, managed to get the mother into bed. I told her I wasn't feeling too well and gave her a bell to ring for me right in the next room if she needed me. I had this terrible chest pain with vomiting and diarrhea all coming on me at once. I lay there and prayed like a son of a gun for hours until I was able to breathe. I slowed down after that, and it was about three weeks before I dared to travel. I came back to Jersey City where my daughter took me to a cardiologist who examined me and took an electrocardiogram. She then turned to my daughter and said, "How in the name of God did your mother have a blowout like that on the posterior part of her heart and not die?" My daughter said, "My mother prayed." The cardiologist said, "Well, don't push God too far!"

■ What did you do after leaving Texas?

I had to get things lined up for my mother in Jersey City. I had given the two houses I had owned there to my two daughters for their families and didn't want to bother them, so I rented a little apartment for my mother and myself. I took her out of the nursing home and brought her to Jersey City where she died ten months later. That was in December 1966.

After leaving Texas I had originally planned to move with my mother to a house I owned in Gillette, New Jersey, out in Morris County. I had informed the tenants that I intended to occupy the house at the end of their lease in January 1967, but the day after they left the house was burned down.

■ Are you implying that this was intentional?

Definitely, very definitely. I knew exactly what happened. When I bought that place in 1937 it was farmland, and it was one of the smallest pieces of farmland I could find, not more than two or three acres. I was "a fly in a pail of white milk," but over the years, as the area became more settled, the suburbanites didn't know me because I wasn't around much—I had been in Washington and Texas for eleven years. When they found out that I was going to move in with my mother and I had the real estate agent arrange for this, the tenants moved out on a Saturday and the next day, Sunday, the house was burned down. When I went to get a building permit to rebuild, they told me, "You can't rebuild on that lot; it's not the right shape." I said, "You must think I'm stupid, but it's you who are stupid. I can build a house just like the one that burned down." They made out that something was wrong with the original house and that was why it burned down. "If the original was all right, why did it burn down?" they asked me. "I

would have to ask you that question," I told them. Some of
the neighbors had told me just what happened, but I couldn't
be bothered with a person who was that small.

I did build a house, not exactly like the original, but a bilevel
one which was easier for me with my heart trouble. I lived
there for five years, from 1967 to 1972, commuting back and
forth to Jersey City where I had my office and other activities.

■ Your last stop was Lakewood, Ocean County. Why here?

The family felt I was getting older, I was almost seventy-
three, so they wanted me closer to one of the children. My
daughter Genevieve is a social worker down here, and her
husband had died when her baby was only a year and a half.
She had never remarried, so I thought I would come down here
and help her out. So I found my own place here and moved in.
I don't ever want to live with any of my children. I love them
and they love me, but I don't want to live with them. As long
as I have a breath in my body I'll do things on my own.

■ Was there anything else for you to do when you came here in 1972?

I first thought of practicing in a poor neighborhood, but this
was not realistic. I think that I was the first black woman
doctor ever in Ocean County, and the prejudice here was worse
than I've seen anywhere in the South. Even the black people
coming from Jersey City complained about it. Another factor
was my age; I was already going on seventy-three, and I knew I
wouldn't get on the staff of any hospital. Without hospital
privileges a doctor cannot really practice adequately, so I decided that I wouldn't practice medicine here.

I nosed around to see what they did have here that I could
volunteer for, because I had been doing volunteer work all my
life; homes for unwed mothers, well-baby clinics, cancer society, and so forth. I couldn't find any of these in Ocean County.
I went to the chief of the health department and told him
"This is the damndest place I've ever lived. You folks think

you're a bunch of millionaires here, and you're not. There are plenty of poor people here, and I want to volunteer my services to help. You have not one single well-baby clinic; you have no medical screening services for the aged. How about starting up something like that?" Finally I said, "I'm going down on Fourth Street and start a well-baby clinic." They felt threatened by this, and I think some of it got into the paper, but anyway the well-baby clinic got started.

Then I got on them real heavy about the senior citizen business. Ocean County is one of the greatest retirement areas in the country. One day I was talking to a nurse, a friend of my social worker daughter here, and she told me that if I could only take blood pressures on the people living over in the low-income senior housing projects, it would mean so much to them. I told her that I would take blood pressures and nothing else, but I would talk to these elderly people. "Wonderful," she said, "what they need more than anything else is a sympathetic ear." So I finally got active on the advisory board of the office on aging for Ocean County, and have been busy with a number of groups.

■ There are many things you have done that are well known, but one of the things that may not be widely known, and that I can especially appreciate, is your helping send young people through college.

I saw to it that my six children went through professional school, and I would also help outstanding young people that I thought could be helped. There were two in Texas—one at the state college and one in nursing—then three, four—gosh, five students in graduate school for whom I paid tuition. They wanted to improve themselves but came from families that just couldn't afford it, so I paid the tuition. I'm still paying money out like that, but the students themselves have to do their share. They have to get a little job, live at home if possible, and not worry about room and board. I supply the tuition. I have now established an endowment at Howard University for the education of a black woman who will be a family doctor. I've gotten the principal up to a point where the interest is one thousand dollars per year, but I'd like to double that.

■   **You have sent all these youngsters to college, you've given away houses, you've helped build a hospital with your own funds. Where do you get the money for all these things?**

I never spend money; I have always saved money. My father used to tell us, "You can have your needs, but not your wants." So I grew up as a very disciplined person as to time and money. Up to the time I had my last baby I had to spend money to buy homes in which my children could live, but after that it was different.

■   **I have always wondered where you ever got the time and energy to have those six children, what with all your other activities.**

Well, I was in very severe heart failure with my fifth child and was told that I couldn't have any more: that if I got pregnant again I would have to have a therapeutic abortion. I knew that was good medicine and was well aware of the risks of childbirth, having seen two women die during it just about that time. That hit me real hard. But I have this old Franciscan belief that God is going to help me because I like to help people. I have felt and acted this way since I was a kid. So when I became pregnant the sixth time I said, "I'll tell you what I'll do; I'm going to go through with it. I will slow down a bit and I promise God that if He helps me to have this sixth child (I had wanted a dozen and I was thirty-nine then)—if He lets me have this one, I promise Him that I will go to church every day of my life to thank Him." And, believe me, that child is forty-two years old this year, and except on very odd occasions, I have kept this promise. So, you see, I have this compulsion to do the things I believe in.

■   **You talk of the joy of having children, but now there is such great controversy on the abortion issue. I know your position on this as a Catholic, but you are also a black woman. The other side of the argument is that the people who** will suffer most from repeal of abortion rights are young poor black women. They will be the ones without access to good medical care; they will be the ones being butchered on kitchen tables. Do you have any conflicts with yourself on this issue?

I have no conflicts at all. As far as blacks are concerned, as I have said, we are the products of rape, of illegitimacy. But even when we were forced to have babies, even in those days the parents and grandparents loved those babies. Up until very recently you never heard of a black woman having an abortion. There's a well-known expression among them: "That's my flesh and blood," they'd say. "God will punish me if I get rid of it." And I'm not talking about Catholics now; I'm talking about blacks.

■   Then you believe it is a cultural thing, that blacks are more willing to have children out of wedlock than whites . . .

Why sure, and I am certain that all the problems of the "abortion racket" are being underplayed: sterility, complications from inducing the abortion, and so on.

Sterility problems were my "hobby" in gynecology. They came to me from Florida to Boston because I had the reputation of being able to help women get pregnant. I used to tease them and say, "I don't have the 'basic ingredient', but I'll look you over and see what's wrong with you and your husband so that you might be able to have children." I've always had a love of helping women to have babies.

There's another thing about abortion: guilt. Not long after I went to Jersey City to practice, one of the good Catholic foreign-born women came to me and asked to see me because her nerves were bad. She said to me, "Mrs. Doctor" (that's what thay all used to call me), "I come to you because I can talk to you and 'cause you won't tell nobody. I killed the baby; I had an abortion." That had been years before, but she was still having nightmares, seeing babies in her dreams. The psychic trauma of abortion is more than people think it is.

But now the morals of the world are so low, especially in this country, that abortion is no longer a cultural no-no, even for the black man. And abortion is encouraged to eliminate the black man for fear they'll overpopulate and become predominant in this country if they continue to have many children while whites have only one or two.

■   I won't deny that among some whites such a view is held, but you certainly cannot say that this is true of all of them or that this is the primary consideration of the whole issue.

No, no. There's nothing that you can say or nothing that can happen in life that's going to be the same for everybody. If some woman asked me to perform an abortion I could not do it, but I would not condemn her. That is between her and God, what she does. I tell them how I feel about it, and they have a right to feel about it as they wish.

■   If you'll pardon me using the expression in your presence, I would like for a moment to play the devil's advocate. I want to put something else to you. In Newark we have these girls—fourteen, thirteen, twelve years of age—coming in with babies. Now, in the nineteenth century that might be something that was routine, but what this is doing now is forcing these kids into a lifetime of poverty, of dependence on welfare. You would be the first to admit that you, individually, came from a very good background. At the time you grew up there weren't many blacks with parents like yours: there weren't many white people around with your kind of family credentials! You had a good start in life. I see these kids coming into the clinic having babies at twelve or thirteen and trailing three or four kids after them at the age of seventeen. Some of them might have a lot of potential, and yet they are never going to have the opportunity to go to college, to better themselves, to make something of their lives. They're going to live on welfare for the duration.

I do not believe in Welfare. It has been the condemnation of the black person. There may have been a reason for it at the beginning when times were so terrible, but by the time it got around to the second generation, you could see that it was being encouraged by the bureaucracy. I used to say to patients, "What in the name of God are you doing on welfare? Why don't you get up and go out and work?" Time and time again I would get the same answers: "My welfare worker says I don't need to work. If I get a job I'll have to buy clothes. I'll have to pay income tax. So I might as well stay on welfare because it's better."

This is the curse of the country: demeaning poor people in order to preserve the jobs of bureaucrats. They get jobs paying ten to twenty-five thousand a year in order to keep poor people poor. And the poor people are saps, as I've told them in speeches all over the country. We're not going to go anywhere unless they get rid of Welfare. It's a form of genocide.

■ We've talked so long and covered so much ground and there are still so many things we haven't discussed. But let me ask you one last thing. You have had such a rich and full life. Is there anything about it you regretted?

I guess I haven't sense enough to regret anything. But I know there is no such thing as perfection, and I know I've made mistakes, but there's a song called "I Did It My Way." That's my song.

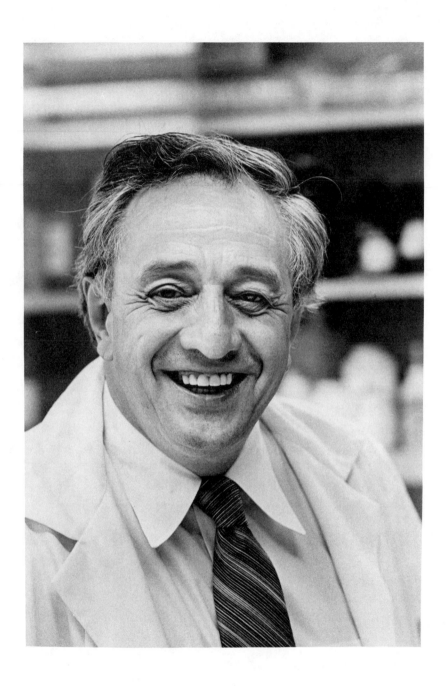

CHAPTER 15

Robert A. Good, Ph.D., M.D.
(1922–   )

IMMUNOLOGY IS at once one of the oldest branches of medicine and, as Sir Peter Medawar, a 1960 Nobelist in the field, has termed it, "the most brightly lit domain of the medical sciences." We recall the story of Edward Jenner, the English physician who, in 1796, began vaccinating patients with fluid from the cowpox lesions he found on milkmaids in order to protect them from smallpox. But, as colonial Americans such as Cotton Mather had learned from their black slaves, the practice of inoculation had been carried on in Africa since antiquity as, indeed, it had also been practiced in the Orient. (Some aspects of this have already been discussed in Chapter 1 and with Dr. Francis Moore's comments on Zabdiel Boylston.)

Vaccination has had a noble history in the prevention of bacterial diseases such as diphtheria, whooping cough, and tetanus. The use of the immunological approach to viral disease has been even more important, since these infections are almost invariably unresponsive to antibiotic therapy. Such work was given an enormous boost by virologist John Enders and his associates, who developed tissue culture methods for mumps, measles, and especially poliomyelitis virus. The latter enabled the development of the Salk and later the Sabin vaccines for polio with profound effects on public health.

In 1954 there were 18,000 cases of paralytic polio in the United States. In 1955, one year before the use of the Salk vaccine, there was an epidemic of 55,000 cases. Three years later this had fallen to under 200 annually. Between 1973 and 1980, at which time the Salk vaccine had been replaced by the attenuated virus in the oral Sabin preparation, the number had fallen to less than a dozen annually.

Perhaps the crowning achievement of vaccination can be attributed to its control of the scourge that led to its development, smallpox. The last naturally occurring case in the world was reported from Merka Town in Somalia in 1977. Current and future application of immunological science extend far beyond the sphere of ordinary infectious diseases and the problems recognized as common allergies seen in the offices of physicians every day. A variety of immunodeficiency disorders have been defined and treated with considerable success. And they are much more common than once appreciated: the most frequent pure form is an isolated immunoglobulin A deficiency estimated to be present in about 1 in every 600 of the general population.

The recent outbreak of AIDS (acquired immunodeficiency syndrome) in homosexual and Haitian men, intravenous drug abusers, hemophiliacs, and other susceptible groups, with its alarmingly high mortality of over 40 percent, would be even more frightening if immunologists were not able to characterize it by an imbalance between those lymphocytes that assist and those that interfere with the immune functions of the body. Given these findings as a possible indication of the disease, physicians at least have the opportunity to follow its course and obtain clues as to cause and cure.

In a variety of other illnesses—cancer, alcoholism, and other chronic states—the immune system has been found to be compromised. In other conditions, the autoimmune diseases such as that involving the thyroid, lupus erythematosus, multiple sclerosis, and a wide range of other disorders, a deranged response of the immune system has been uncovered and studied extensively in a search for cures.

The twentieth century opened with Karl Landsteiner's discovery of the ABO blood groups of man in 1901. The problem of self-identification has continued to absorb the interest and efforts of medical investigators. The future success of organ transplantation depends almost entirely upon our ability to find ways to prevent the body's rejection of implanted tissue from others and, conversely, to prevent its antithesis, the graft versus host reaction in which implanted cells begin to attack the recipient.

The discovery of the major histocompatibility complex in mice and later its counterpart the HLA (human lymphocyte antigen) system in man have provided vital information about the immune response and introduced a new basis for better tissue typing to insure improved future success of transplantation.

Finally, with the development of hybridomas and the production of monoclonal antibodies, new ways are being found for the production of cancer-cell-specific antibodies to help identify subclinical cancer and, in the future, may lead to new methods for its eradication.

It is difficult now, with the wealth of data available to us regarding the immune system, to appreciate how ignorant we were about it in 1943 when Robert Good, then a medical student working toward a Ph.D.-M.D. degree at the University of Minnesota, began his work in the field. The progress of immunology is, in many respects, simply the story of Robert Good's scientific career.

In the early 1940s it was known that antibodies were contained within the electrophoretically defined gamma globulin fraction of the serum, but little else was known about immunoglobulin structure and function. At that time it was widely held that macrophages were the source of antibodies, and only gradually did the role of the lymphocytes and plasma cells become recognized. Making a perfect combination of bedside observation as a clinical observer and laboratory bench work as a basic investigator, Dr. Good gradually came upon the finding that the lymphocytes themselves evolved in one of two ways after their origin from precursors in the bone marrow. The T lymphocytes are processed through the thymus gland and become responsible for cell-mediated immunity reactions involved in certain types of chronic infection and graft rejection, among other functions. The B lymphocytes (after the chicken's bursa of Fabricius) are responsible for antibody production (immunoglobulins) to combat other infections, primarily following their conversion into plasma cells. Today even these subsets can be subdivided with T helper cells, T suppressor cells, killer cells, natural and otherwise, defined— all adding to the complexity of the immune process as well as our understanding of it.

Such complexity has not prevented Dr. Good and others from treating immune deficiency disorders. A milepost was reached with the first successful bone marrow transplant accomplished by this group in the treatment of severe combined immune deficiency disease, where both T and B lymphocyte subsets are depressed. Other entities in the immunodeficiency sphere have been recognized and treated along the way: the DiGeorge syndrome (failure of thymus development resulting in absence of T lymphocytes); Bruton's disease (X-linked agammaglobulinemia, a B lymphocyte deficiency); common variable immunodeficiency (a variation of combined immunodeficiency); the Wistkott-Aldrich syndrome (cellular deficiency associated with high immunoglobulin levels, low blood platelets, and eczema); and the Good syndrome (combined B and T cell immunodeficiency in the presence of thymoma).

Much of this work was done at the University of Minnesota where, spanning the Departments of Pediatrics, Microbiology, and Pathology, Dr. Good (except for one year at the Rockefeller Institute, 1949–50) worked for twenty-six years following his graduation from medical school.

In 1973 he left Minnesota to become president and director

of the Sloan-Kettering Institute for Cancer Research in New York City. It too was a time for progress but was marred in 1974 by an episode that was to haunt the medical community and Dr. Good for years thereafter. Medical fraud is not an event limited to the twentieth century, but in the period of flourishing medical research in the United States that followed World War II, when public confidence and support had not yet quite begun to waver, what came to be called the Sloan-Kettering affair was looked upon as a disaster. In the light of similar, perhaps even worse scandals that have since been uncovered at Boston University, Massachusetts General Hospital, Mount Sinai Medical School, Yale, and even sacrosanct Harvard, the events at Sloan-Kettering diminish in magnitude. What happened was that Dr. William T. Summerlin, a transplant researcher who had previously reported success in avoiding the rejection problem, was having trouble repeating the work with mouse skin transplants in New York. In desperation, just prior to a visit to Good's office to discuss this with his chief, he took a black felt pen, darkened the fur of two white mice, and carried them to Good's office as examples of his transplant work. The fraud was revealed to Good by an observant laboratory worker; Dr. Good exposed it but suffered a blow to his own reputation and standing as a result, despite his exoneration by a review board.

The Summerlin episode was believed by many to be a major contributing factor leading to Dr. Good's departure from Sloan-Kettering in 1982 to assume his current post as member and head of the Cancer Research Program, Oklahoma Medical Research Foundation, in Oklahoma City. His frank discussion of this shattering experience provides some lessons for the rest of us within the scientific community.

■ If I were one of those "soap box opera" writers and using you as a model, I might start off a program like this: "Can a poor boy from a small town in the hills of Minnesota find happiness and fulfillment in Minneapolis, New York City, and beyond?"

My birthplace, Crosby, was indeed a small town, about eight to ten thousand, and about 150 miles somewhat north of Minneapolis. My father was the principal of the school in Ironton, a smaller city just outside of Crosby up on the Cuyuna Iron Range. My mother was also a schoolteacher. When I was still a boy, we moved to Minneapolis where my father became principal at one of the large elementary schools so that he could complete work on his Ph.D. degree. Just before he did, however, he contracted a highly malignant type of testicular tumor and died.

It was this that first stimulated my interest in medicine. I remember the surgeon who attended my father, a professor at the University of Minnesota, coming to our home. He was very friendly to me and encouraged my interest, explaining my father's disease to me. I was five years old at the time, but, whether I really understood anything about it or not, I maintained from then on that I wanted to be a doctor. My interest in science and mathematics as I went through public school later reinforced this attitude.

It was a difficult time for the family after my father's death, and my mother had to go back to work as a schoolteacher. I was the second of four sons. My oldest brother was six then and my youngest only one. We all ultimately became doctors.

We received a great deal of encouragement from our mother

despite the problems she had raising four little boys by herself during the depression. She was a very intellectual person and very much in favor of advancing our education, so there was never any real question in my mind about my goals. This was further strengthened during my undergraduate years as a pre-med by a paralytic illness with which I was stricken right after the final exams of my second year.

After a short febrile period I found myself paralyzed, essentially from the shoulders down, and was diagnosed as having polio. But there was an aspect of chronicity about the illness that got people talking about "Lou Gehrig's disease" [amyotrophic lateral sclerosis, a progressive and fatal disorder], and this was rather frightening. In retrospect, it was probably Guillain-Barré disease [see page 174], because I finally recovered almost completely from it. I still have a foot drop, however, and have to wear a brace.

I was never really handicapped by this, but it made me determined not only to do medicine but to be a medical scientist and spend my life asking questions. At that time there was really nothing known about the illness I had experienced. My father's illness had also been a complete enigma. Why should he have contracted cancer in the first place? Questions like this were constantly stirring about in my head, so I was determined to spend my life as a medical investigator. When I finally went to the medical school at the University of Minnesota, I therefore worked simultaneously toward a combined M.D. and Ph.D. degree program, the first one to do so there, I believe.

■ What were some of the experiences as a medical student that directed you further along your way?

Well, I really didn't start out as an M.D.-Ph.D. candidate, but when I was a freshman in medical school, thanks to my paralysis, I was able to start doing research and I happened to make a discovery.

This was 1943, and at that time, you may recall, we didn't have the luxury of a relaxed medical curriculum; we were on a three-year program in order to provide physicians for the army. Because of my disability I didn't have to do drilling with the other guys in my class and was able to work in the laboratory of Berry Campbell, a neurophysiologist who had previously been at Rockefeller. In this part-time job I had with him I was using a herpes virus to try and produce an ersatz kind of polio model in rabbits. I was also studying the effect of the two neurone-two axone reflex. I used herpes virus infection as one means of producing chromatolysis of the nerve cells and was helping Campbell time the consequences of this influence on the reflex function. It was at this time I was befriended by Fred Kolouch.

Kolouch was a Czech from Nebraska who, five years earlier, in 1938, had made a discovery from a question raised by a patient he was following who had subacute bacterial endocarditis [a heart valve infection]. As always, in those preantibiotic days, the patient ultimately died, and at the postmortem Kolouch noticed a fantastic accumulation of plasma cells in the spleen and bone marrow. So he asked Hal Downey, a great teacher of hematology, what these plasma cells did. Downey didn't know, but he had often seen them in bacterial infections and thought they might be some sort of secretory cell just on the basis of their appearance under the microscope. It was a pretty good guess, because that's what they eventually proved to be.

Kolouch also asked a pathologist, Ben Clawson, about plasma cells. Clawson had been working with experiments infecting rats with streptococcus viridans, the same one that killed Kolouch's patient. Clawson thought they might be associated with some kind of allergy. So what Kolouch did was make a vaccine by heat killing the strep viridans that he had grown from his patient and injected this repeatedly into rabbits. The repeated injections produced a rapidly developing plasmacytosis of the bone marrow in these rabbits. This was especially true if the rabbits signaled their immunity by developing anaphylactic shock. Kolouch published his experiments and drew from them the conclusion that the plasma cells are responsible for producing the antibodies following antigenic challenge.

■ This was not the accepted view at the time, was it?

No. At that time most of us were thinking that it was the macrophages that were the source of antibodies, as suggested by Florence Sabin.[b] She was in a very prestigious position at the Rockefeller Institute, and her studies sort of indicated that it was the macrophages. Kolouch's observations about the plasma cells as an alternative source was published in a little "Proc.-Soc." [*Proceedings of the Society for Experimental Biology and Medicine*] note. But he had to discontinue this work for six years because his father, a physician from down in Schuyler, Nebraska, had had a "coronary," and Fred had to go down to take over the practice until his father fully recovered.

Four years later he was back at the University of Minnesota, but his father, a great admirer of Wangensteen, insisted that Fred go into surgery under the great man of the time. He was working in the surgical dog labs when I met him, but he was still thinking about hematology.

One day he came over to me and said, "Why don't you cut this crap you're doing with the two-neurone two-axone reflex and help me with my experiments?" I said, "Well, if you've got something that's exciting and important to you, tell me about it." He then recounted his experiences with the strep viridans and the plasma cells five years earlier.

Because of my work with virus infection I had been studying some immunology and knew a little about it, about the different types of reactions and responses involved, and I said, "Well, if we compared passive with active anaphylaxis we could sort out whether the physiological events associated with anaphylaxis are responsible for plasma cell development, or if it is rather the antibody production initiated by secondary exposure to the bacterial antigen that is responsible."

Thus I designed this experiment to test in a new way whether it was, as Kolouch thought, that plasma cells made antibody. The experiment came out beautifully and Kolouch let me publish a paper on this by myself in "Proc. Soc." in 1945. From then on I was an immunologist, absolutely committed.

But that was really Kolouch's discovery. However it was a second discovery, one I really made myself, that made me leave medical school temporarily for graduate school to get some more "tools" for my laboratory efforts. This came a little later and was largely due to lack of funds and the need to reuse some of my old rabbits who had survived my neurophysiology experiments with the herpes virus. You see, being short of funds, in order to carry on some new anaphylactic shock experiments, I had to take some of these survivors for my studies. However, when I put them into anaphylactic shock, I got something I wasn't looking for; I activated the virus that had simply been lying dormant within them. I remember it was the day when my uncle Mark was visiting from Montana and I was just taking him around to show him what I was doing in the laboratory and the little place where I did my work. We then went into the animal quarters and there was old number 370 paralyzed again. Seven days before I had put him into anaphylactic shock, and this had reproduced the paralytic viral disease. I showed that I could do this repeatedly, reactivating the virus. Thus I discovered that a virus infection could be reactivated from a latent state by an unrelated immunological event. This was my own discovery, a function very largely of chance and my own bumbling experiments, but it captured me forever for scientific research. For the first time I was seeing something new that was a consequence of my own scientific effort.

Years later Lew Thomas[b] was interested in this and asked

me to reproduce the experiment for him, and I did. He later said that was the first time he had ever seen someone coming into the laboratory waving a rabbit, but that was an exciting discovery and, as I've indicated, made me go for the combined Ph.D.-M.D. degree.

Kolouch, who got me started on all this, had a very interesting career after this, because after becoming an associate professor in surgery, he left academia. He was very smart and had a sort of cyclothymic personality. He lost an eye in a skiing accident which wasn't the best thing to happen to a surgeon. But he then got interested in hypnosis as a means of preparing patients for postoperative early ambulation and better management. This was written up in *Time* magazine. He further developed this kind of interest and finally became professor of psychiatry at the University of Utah in Salt Lake City. A brilliant guy, and I enjoyed working with him.

Because of Kolouch I was really quite interested in surgery when I was still a medical student. As a junior clerk I would sometimes be brought up by Kolouch as first assistant in operations ahead of the surgical residents. This didn't make me too popular with them, but it was great for my education as I went back and forth between the laboratory and clinical medicine. I was very fortunate as a young man in school, same as now, in that I really didn't require much sleep. Four hours a night are plenty for me.

■ I understand that you frequently used to come into work at four or five in the morning.

I still do, and it isn't anything I've motivated myself to do. When I was a little kid, the worst punishment they could give me was to make me stay in bed until seven.

■ You're lucky to be on that edge of the curve.

That's right and it enabled me to do a lot. I worked very hard but was highly motivated and had a lot of fun at my work. I always had my research going along with my schoolwork in medical school, and when I was house officer I always had laboratory experiments going. Sometimes, however, I got into a little trouble with that. In lieu of the usual medical clerkships I had a sort of rotating internship, and so I served on various department services. Once when I was working as junior intern on the Medical Service, I admitted a patient of the great Dr. Cecil Watson, the head of the Department of Medicine then. After working up his patient, among some others, I ran back to my laboratory where I was engaged in some experiments, leaving word with the ward nurses regarding my whereabouts.

Dr. Watson called me to discuss his patient who had a very interesting metabolic problem involved with his diabetes, but I got this patient confused with another who had been admitted with a trivial complaint, probably on a psychosomatic basis, and began presenting the wrong patient to him. After I informed Dr. Watson of all I had done with "his patient," he said, "Dr. Good, your description of my patient is very inaccurate. I understand you are in your laboratory. I think you should spend your time on the wards when you're an intern."

■   Who else influenced you during your time as a medical student? The name of Richard Varco keeps popping up when people talk about the Department of Surgery at Minnesota then.

Richard Varco was an assistant professor of surgery about the same time Kolouch was training there and they were sort of friendly competitors. All the students were afraid of Varco because he was so tough, so critical, and so smart. I remember when he first came into surgical clinic where I was working and called out to me, "Hey, Skeezix, will you bring me the dressing tray?" He called me Skeezix after the old comic-strip character because my hair was always standing up on end like his—which it still does. That was my first meeting with Varco and I sort of feared him in the beginning, although later I really came to admire him and he became one of my closest friends and scientific colleagues. Varco was a great teacher of surgeons and, with Wangensteen, trained some of the great men in surgery like Lillehei[b] and Norman Shumway.[b]

Irvine McQuarrie,[b] the chairman of pediatrics, had a great influence on me. He taught me to pay attention to the experiments of nature and the scientific questions that were being asked by the patient in the clinical setting. He helped me to learn to think at the bedside in a physiological, microbiological, immunological way so that I could carry these questions into the laboratory with me.

■ To backtrack just a little, it must have been difficult for your mother to send you and three other sons through medical school, often concurrently.

It was incredible. We all worked to pay our own way along with the help of local scholarships. A man by the name of Drew gave needy intelligent youngsters some financial assistance, but most of the time we paid our own way. We did anything to get it together. Once I got into medical school I did a lot of tutoring, and that really paid well for that time. I would promise kids a letter increase in their grade or else would forgo the fee. I was charging fifty cents an hour, and with a class of ten or twenty could clear as much as ten dollars a hour, which was a lot of money then.

■ What happened to your brothers?

The oldest, Charles, is a neurophysiologist, mainly involved in nonacademic work now. Roy is a general practitioner, still active in Minnesota. Tom is a pediatrician. He worked in Utah with Leo Samuels in biochemistry for a while and then in Maryland, finally becoming a professor at the University of Wisconsin. He left there a few years ago and is now practicing pediatrics in Carson City, Nevada.

■ Let's get back to the plasma cell story. When was it finally accepted that they were indeed the source of antibodies?

Kolouch and I were sure that it was the plasma cell that was the source of antibody, but now a new controversy arose because some investigators began to bring forth evidence that it was the lymphocytes that were the antibody-producing cells. The "plasma cell hunters" in our corner—and there weren't very many of us—were convinced they were wrong. Then the Swedish virologist Astrid Fagraeus came out with a beautiful paper in which she showed that little bits of red pulp tissue from the spleens of hyperimmunized animals rich with plasma cells could make antibodies in vitro, whereas the lymphocyte-rich Malpighian corpuscles did not. This fit with all our observations and was further supported and extended by Al Coons at Harvard when he developed his methodology of immunofluorescence microscopy analyzing the distribution of antigenic proteins in tissue sections.

■ Tell me how you came to discover that there were two different lines of lymphocytes: the T lymphocytes and the B lymphocytes.

After I finished my formal pediatric training in 1949, Dr. McQuarrie got me a job at the Rockefeller Institute where I was to spend a year working on a problem. When I first went to the Rockefeller, in 1949, I was assigned to "Mac" [Maclyn] McCarty. He was interested in C-reactive protein, an interesting protein that goes up early in infections, the acute phase, something I had been interested in while doing biochemistry with David Glick and Vincent Kelly back in Minnesota. McCarty had previously crystallized C-reactive protein from effusions in patients with streptococcal infections, but now with the ready availability of penicillin, these effusions were no longer clinical problems and another source of fluid had to be found.

I found a ready source of effusion fluid right across the street from Rockefeller at the Sloan-Kettering Cancer Institute where Hodgkin's disease patients were being followed by Dr. David Karnowsky. Since there was no really effective chemotherapy then available for these patients, they frequently had pleural effusions, and Karnowsky encouraged me to study them. From the chest fluid obtained from these patients I was able to crystallize C-reactive protein for McCarty, but as I observed these individuals with Hodgkin's disease I was struck by a curious selective kind of susceptibility that they had to infection. They were very susceptible to tuberculosis, fungus infections, and certain viral infections but apparently not so susceptible to infection by the pneumococcus, streptococcus, *Hemophilus influenzae,* or pseudomonas.

During this time I was also befriended by Dr. Henry Kunkel, who knew I was a "plasma cell hunter" and who was interested in studying the proteins in the serum of patients with multiple myeloma, a disease in which plasma cell proliferation is the most striking characteristic. He was having trouble getting his hands on serum of such patients who produced myeloma proteins but knew that I, as an expert on plasma cells, was often called to see such patients. What struck me in this group of patients, however, was that compared to the Hodgkins disease patients there was an entirely different spectrum of susceptibility to infectious disease. Here the organisms that were causing the patients the most trouble were pneumococcus, streptococcus, and *Hemophilus influenzae.*

So here we had two groups of patients with hematopoietic malignancies with totally different susceptibilities to infections. It was this that first got me to thinking about the possibility of there being two different types of cell lines separable for immunity and two major bulwarks against infections. I began, through a haze, to see these experiments of nature dissecting the microbial universe.

■ What were some of the developments along these lines that occurred when you returned to Minnesota?

Dr. McQuarrie had bought this impressive machine to do electrophoresis and when I got home to Minnesota his associate Vince Kelly taught me how to use it. Then in 1952 Colonel

Ogden Bruton, who had never seen a case before and has never seen one since, described agammaglobulinemia. Right on my wards I had three patients who turned out to have agamma-globulinemia when I did electrophoresis on their blood: two brothers and a third boy who later had a brother develop this X-linked inherited form of the disease. I ultimately called it Bruton's disease, giving him credit for his beautiful description of it. Like the multiple myeloma patients, these patients were highly susceptible to pneumococcus, streptococcus, and hemophilus but had no trouble with tuberculosis and could resist well many virus and fungus infections. But rather than *defective* plasma cells, as in myeloma, these patients had *absence* of plasma cells, while their lymphocyte counts were perfectly normal.

We soon found that they could develop and express delayed allergy normally. I found they could exhibit the reactions we later called cell-mediated immunity. So already by 1955 we were talking about two kinds of immunity: one based on lymphocytes (cell-mediated) and one on plasma cells (circulating antibodies, gammaglobulins).

There was another experiment of nature that really directed my work, a patient that Richard Varco and I saw together in 1952. This patient had a tumor of the thymus, and Varco thought he was becoming addicted to the antibiotic, Terramycin, which he was taking because it "made him feel better." The fact was that he had a broadly based kind of immunodeficiency, the first I recognized as being related to an abnormality of the thymus. Varco finally removed the thymic tumor, but it didn't correct his immunodeficiency and he died from viral hepatitis. But this did start me thinking about the thymus and the immune system.

We started on some thymus work in the lab but removing them in experimental animals did not seem to influence immunity very much. Then in 1959 my friend Harold Wolf told me about Bruce Glick's work on the bursa of Fabricius which had appeared in *Poultry Science* in 1956.

■ That is certainly a fascinating story.

And I love to tell it.

Bruce Glick is a Ph.D. in biology was was a graduate student at the time working for Knauf at Ohio State. Knauf had told Glick that he would be famous if he could find out what the bursa of Fabricius did because, ever since Fabricius had described this outpouching in the intestine of chickens in the sixteenth century, the function of that organ had remained unknown. Challenged by this, Glick began taking out the bursa in all ages of chickens and studying the effect on physiology, egg laying, and anything else he could measure. Now, as part of his responsibilities Glick had to teach a course which involved the demonstration of bacterial agglutination reaction of the serum of chickens sensitized to *Salmonella typhimurium* when later challenged by this bacterium. Glick, on this occasion, sloughed off the job of preparing antibodies for the experiment which is accomplished by prior injection of chickens with heat-inactivated *Salmonella.* He got another graduate student, Timothy Chang, to do it for him. Chang, by mistake, selected for immunization some of Glick's chickens that had been bursectomized in the neonatal period. When it came to the class demonstration the experiment didn't work, because the bursectomized chickens that Chang had injected had not produced antibodies. Glick, Chang, and the other fellow, Jaap—who, I think, helped with some of the methodology—realized that this fluke had led to an important discovery. They had found a function for the bursa of Fabricius. They submitted their paper to *Science* which rejected it as being of no general interest. So it wound up in *Poultry Science.*

■ Who in hell reads *Poultry Science?*

Exactly. Not many of us did, but Harold Wolf did. He was a

bacteriologist-immunologist at the University of Wisconsin and a "real professor." His life's work basically involved studies on antibody production in chickens, and there were a series of perhaps twenty-three to twenty-five papers, each with elegant methodologies and different graduate students for which he was responsible. So Harold read *Poultry Science,* and when he caught the paper by Glick et al he told me about it.

I was particularly prepared to accept Glick's work and interpret it appropriately because of Hal Downey. Downey was a comparative hematologist who had taught us that once Jolly had called the bursa of Fabricius a "cloacal* thymus." This stuck in my mind, so that when I learned that Glick's removal of the bursa in the newly hatched period interfered with antibody development, I was stimulated to do similar experiments with thymectomies in the newly born mouse, rat, and rabbit. We just hadn't been doing it early enough before. This, as you know, led to the demonstration that the thymus is a crucial site for immunological development.

■ Have we found the human counterpart to the bursa of Fabricius? If we have B cells, then we should have a bursa or at least some anatomical counterpart to it.

That's a very important and interesting question. It may be more relevant than anyone thinks right now, but we haven't truly answered it. We thought for a while that it was the Peyer's patches in the intestine, but that is probably wrong. Basically, the Peyer's patches are a site for major expansion of the B cell system and for developing the cells that become the local immunity system, the cells of the lining of the gastrointestinal tract, and the salivary glands and all of that.

A few years ago Max Cooper went off to work a year with

*In the chicken, contents from the urogenital and gastrointestinal tracts pass through a final common chamber, the cloaca. This, more precisely, is the structure from which the saclike bursa of Fabricius arises before regressing and becoming atrophic by about the tenth month of life.

Raff and Owen in London, and they concluded that probably everything the bursa does in chickens is done in mice and humans in the fetal liver, which is a lymphoepithelial site as well as a hematopoietic site. But later it can even be in the bone marrow, which may even be the case for the chicken at some later stage after the involution of the bursa. In brief, then, we haven't found a gastrointestinal site similar to the chicken's bursa in humans or any other mammals.

■ Getting back to the thymus, it appeared that you and Miller came up with the same idea just about the same time.

[J. F. A. P.] Miller was working at the Chester Beatty Institute in London and came to the same conclusions as we did about the thymus but from a completely different direction. It had been shown back in 1944 that if you took out the thymus of newborn mice, you could prevent the development of leukemia in the AKR strain which had been developed by Jake Furth to study the disease. Using that strain and investigating it immunologically, Miller discovered by taking out the thymus that this organ is essential to immunological development.

Now, the first public presentation of our findings took place in the spring of 1961 at the Federation Meetings before the American Association of Immunologists in the United States. Miller presented his findings for the first time before a CIBA symposium in England that summer. His *Lancet* publication, entitled "A Preliminary Communication," appeared in October of that year, while ours on neonatal thymectomy in mice, although submitted earlier than Miller's to *Lancet*, did not appear in "Proc.-Soc." until January 1962.

■ The battle for priority in science is a recurring one, but I like it best when it's settled amicably. I'm sure you know the story about Irvine Page[b] and Braun-Menendez when they came up with the discovery of the same vasopressor substance in 1939. Page and his associate, Helmer, called it "angiotonin," while Braun-Menendez had named his substance "hypertensin." When they met at a heart association meeting in 1958, they acknowledged to one another that the two substances were one and the same and agreed over a couple of martinis to call it "angiotensin" thereafter.

At the Thymus Conference in 1962 which I had organized, Miller and I had both been very tense. But we were both young, aggressive guys and were fighting for the credit, although there was no way the discovery could have been anything other than simultaneous. It was funny because, in retrospect, the time for the thymus had come, and in two other parts of the world they were just about to make the same findings as those reported by Miller's and my own group. Fortunately, at the conference we had Fichtelius from Uppsala, Sweden, chairing the meeting, and he really took all the heat off. He said, "I yust vant to tank you all for leafing the tymus to me for so long." He had been working on it for a great many years and hadn't come up with a real understanding of what it did. But he was a persistent investigator and scholar.

■ Where did the actual terms "B lymphocytes" and "T lymphocytes" come from?

Ivan Roitt from London was the first to use these terms when it became awkward to talk about "thymus-dependent lymphocytes and bursa-derived or bone marrow-derived lymphocytes."

■ Now I'd like to get to another story, and one of great human as well as scientific interest. Tell me about David Camp.

There were several important developments that led to our discovery of how to use marrow transplantation to cure disease. We now recognized that there were two immunity systems: we knew the thymus was the source of one of these, and if the bursa of Fabricius was the source of the other in the chicken (and other birds), then there had to be some counterpart to this in humans. Starting with this knowledge, we wanted to see if we could now correct any of these immunodeficiencies as they existed either experimentally or in man. We started with neonatally thymectomized mice and found ultimately that we could correct the induced immunodeficiency, first by the transplantation of a neonatal thymus, and ultimately even with a transplant of a little wet membrane of embryonic thymus, the precurser of the thymus. Edmund Yunis,[b] now professor of pathology at Harvard, was then one of my students and associates working with Carlos Martinez and me on these experiments. Now, Ed Yunis wanted to reconstitute the neonatally thymectomized mice with lymph node or spleen cells but found if you gave a mismatched transplantation of lymphoid cells to a neonatally thymectomized mouse you got a graft versus host reaction and the mouse died.

Martinez was originally an endocrinologist, and a buddy of mine who had been working for years with me developing what we called the Minnesota System for studying tissue and organ transplantation. Our studies were based on Gorer's[b] work in the mouse (the major histocompatibility system). The HLA (human lymphocyte antigen) system would later prove to be the counterpart in man. By use of the Minnesota System, Yunis, Martinez, and I were able to match the mice to a degree and succeed in these transplants: no graft versus host reaction. So we wrote in the last sentence of an important paper in the *Journal of Experimental Medicine*, "This will have clinical application" because we were sure that matching would ultimately be possible in humans.

Meanwhile, Max Cooper and Ray Peterson in our labs were taking the bursas or thymuses or both out of irradiated chickens and demonstrating the differences between T and B subsets of lymphocytes. Finally, one day Max was presenting his findings at a pediatrics meeting in Philadelphia in 1965, explaining that chickens without bursas were just like patients with agammaglobulinemia—they couldn't make antibodies and had no plasma cells or germinal centers—while chickens without thymuses were like Hodgkin's disease patients who lacked normal cellular immunity. And I'll never forget Max Cooper coming back from the meeting and telling me how this guy ran to the microphone, shaking it and shouting, "That's it! That's it! That explains what we've been seeing in Philadelphia."

This was Angelo DiGeorge, an endocrinologist who had these patients born without a thymus and who had plasma cells which could make antibodies but lacked cellular immunity to defend against tuberculosis, virus infections or fungus infections.

We then had this Conference on Immunodeficiency in 1967, and several of us agreed there that we knew how to correct the DiGeorge syndrome. We felt that we could do it either with fully matched peripheral lymphoid cells or a thymus transplant. After the conference a guy from Miami, Bill Cleveland, found a patient with the DiGeorge syndrome. The child had repeated infections and an absent thymus and parathyroid gland (DiGeorge's patients had already died). Meanwhile Humphrey Kay in London had been developing an organ bank collecting and freezing organs from aborted fetuses. He provided a thymus from this source for Cleveland, and a successful transplant was performed, curing the patient.

Now, at that same 1967 conference we had proposed that in severe combined deficiency disease (both T and B cells deficient), a genetic disorder with which we were more familiar because it was more common, treatment was also possible. We figured that the basic defect there had to be in the bone marrow because both T and B cells originated from stem cells there or fetal liver before going their separate ways. I thought the best source of stem cells would be bone marrow or fetal liver, and we used the latter on a little boy, N. F., who was brought to us with the disease.

However, the house officers who were with us made the mistake of giving the child a blood transfusion to help him, and the kiddy developed a fulminant graft versus host reaction and died. Afterwards we were not sure, though, whether it was this blood transfusion or something about the fetal liver cells that caused his death.

For the next patient that came our way I wondered whether it might be wiser to use a bone marrow transplant, but I felt sure that a mismatch at the major histocompatibility complex with this would also result in a graft versus host reaction and probably be lethal. I kept thinking about the genetics of it, and then one night after coming home from a party and when I was a little in my cups and just falling asleep, I realized exactly how it could be done. I got up immediately and called Dick Hong and then Ed Yunis on the phone and told them that we had to use marrow from an HLA-matched sibling. Then the whole major histocompatibility locus would be matched. It kept Hong up all night he was so excited about it. "You're absolutely right," he said. "Why didn't we think of it before?"

■ It all seems so straightforward now, in retrospect.

Today you wouldn't even hesitate to think about it, but then it was an exciting new idea. We wrote a theoretical paper on this, saying that to correct severe combined immunodeficiency disease and avoid graft versus host reaction you had to get a matched sibling donor. David Camp's physician in Connecticut heard about our work, and the family made a pilgrimage to Minnesota.

David certainly had the disease, with multiple male deaths in his family before from it, but he also had four healthy sisters. It was theoretically possible, on the basis of the genetics involved, that one in the four would be a perfect match. This was not to be the case. The best partial match among the sisters was Doreen. She was matched at what we would now call the C, B, D, and DR loci, but not at the A locus. She was also mismatched for the ABO blood grouping, being a type O while David was type A.

We considered about whether or not we should proceed, lacking a perfect match, and finally decided that we had to go ahead. The disease had already been lethal in twelve male members of David's family; it was clearly an X-linked recessive severe combined immunodeficiency, and without the bone marrow transplant the end result was likely to be the same for David. So we went ahead. He got a take that corrected his immunodeficiency but he also got a severe graft versus host reaction. Doreen's transplanted lymphoid cells began destroying all of David's blood elements: red cells, granulocytes, platelets, the whole "ball of wax." He progressed to an aplastic anemia.

I remember the discussion as to whether or not the graft ought to be terminated to save the kid's life from the graft versus host reaction. But I said, "If this child were a mouse he would not die from this graft versus host reaction; he would survive. David may get over the reaction and survive. We must leave the graft in place."

And we still had Doreen. So we gave another bone marrow transplant from Doreen to David to treat the aplastic anemia. This second marrow transplant took hold and switched his blood type completely. Now, fifteen years later, all of his cells function absolutely normally hematologically and immunologically in every way. Our theoretical formulation was correct. But if you test his cells, they have the female karyotype, thanks to his sister.

■   How many of these bone marrow transplants for severe combined immunodeficiency disease have you now done?

There have been about one hundred performed, of which we have done about forty. And it's absolutely like creating life. Let me just show you some pictures [*removing several from file*]. Here's a little kid the way they usually come to us with fungus infections, pneumocystis infections of every body orifice . . .

■ It looks like a child from a death camp . . .

At death's door, exactly. First we treat his infections with antibiotics and then we give him a bone marrow transplant from a matched sibling. Now, look at this chubby little baby. It's like creating life all over again, and it works with all seven different forms of the severe combined immune deficiency disease.

■ Are all children with this in the United States now getting proper treatment for it—bone marrow transplants?

No, they're not. First of all, some cases are still not recognized by their doctors. Then in the beginning we felt it necessary to have a matched sibling, and that occurs only twenty-five percent of the time. With American families becoming smaller and smaller, perfect matches become more difficult to find. Then we found that the match did not have to be so perfect and not necessarily from a sibling. This discovery came about when I was asked to go to Copenhagen to see the child of a pathologist there with severe combined immune deficiency disease. They wanted to know if there was anything we could do. We found an uncle in the family who was matched at the D locus but mismatched at the A and B loci. Because of our experience with David and Doreen Camp I said, "Let's do it." That kid was also cured, and then another in the family was transplanted with his father's marrow. So we then found that even without perfect matches we could treat another eight to ten percent of patients who came to us. But that was still under fifty percent of the total.

We returned to the laboratory and, with others, began exploring ways of avoiding graft versus host reactions to increase our level of success. We figured that if we could only get rid of the "bad guys" in the transplanted marrow, the T lymphocytes that attacked the cells of the host, we could be more successful and avoid graft versus host disease. There have now been several ways developed to approach the problem with increasing success.

Another development has been the use of bone marrow transplantations in acute leukemias resistant to chemotherapy. There, after radiating the bone to destroy the malignant cells, the bone marrow transplants can be performed. So it's still exciting as it ever was, and we can now treat more than twenty-two otherwise fatal diseases by this revolutionary technique of bone marrow transplantation. And this is only the beginning.

■ Let's get back to Robert Good, subjectively, again. You had such a wonderful setup in Minnesota and did such great work there. Why did you leave it?

In other words: Why the hell did I ever go to New York? That's an interesting question, and the answer is very complicated. I really loved Minnesota. That was my home; I had always been there; and I was very comfortable there. I had a lovely life in Minnesota. I think I went to New York because my work had taken me to a point where I really wanted to bring immunology to bear on cancer. I had always worked with cancer patients, and I felt, and still do, that the immunological approach to cancer is going to be the most powerful to understand the nature of cancer, the definition of cancer cells, and finding cancer cells in the body when they are occult, hidden from other ordinary methods of diagnosis, and even eventually to treat and prevent cancer.

To do this I felt that I should to to New York where I could do this at Memorial Hospital and the Sloan-Kettering Cancer Center right across from the Rockefeller Institute. I went there originally as a visiting professor, but there was an element of timing: I had just been named to the President's Cancer Panel and the opportunity at Memorial seemed a real challenge to me to get on with the conquest of cancer.

I don't regret it at all, going to New York. I had a tremendous experience there, but the time was not ripe for the application of immunology to cancer the way, as you saw, things fell into place with the thymus discovery. I'm absolutely certain that the immunological approach to cancer will be the right one, and the seventies were a time for beginning to learn about this. The only regret I have was that I took on so much administrative responsibility that it was distractive to my scientific work. However, I always worked hard and was able to develop some exciting new ideas while I was there.

■ This is, after all, a historical book, and I would like to broach another subject. Baseball stories provide paradigms for much else that we experience in American life, and I am reminded of the National League pennant race in 1951. It came down to the bottom of the ninth inning in the last game of the season, between the Giants and the Dodgers. I'm sure even nonbaseball fans recall how the Giants were behind with two out when Bobby Thompson came to bat with men on base and hit a home run to win the game and the pennant. For years after that memorable game the pitcher for the Dodgers, Ralph Branca, would recall that no one ever remembered him as one of the best pitchers year in and year out for the old Brooklyn team. They would remember him only as the Dodger pitcher who served up that home run ball to Thompson. Ralph Branca reminds me of you and your own bizarre experience with Summerlin. It is now almost ten years since it all happened. Are you able to philosophize about it?

I don't mind discussing it because the Summerlin phenomenon hurt me a great deal. I got criticized because people said I was not on top of things. That was not true. I was right there, and I was making observations right along with Summerlin. Regarding the whole affair, there are three things that have to be considered: the event, the science, and the men.

The event. There was no question that Summerlin behaved erratically. He faked data, and there is no doubt about this—he painted the mice. He admitted that. The reason he did this was that he was trying to make skin grafts take by culturing them in vitro first, as he had done before coming to New York, but which he was then having trouble reproducing. It is likely the conditions of the experiment had been changed some way in New York.

The day the incident occurred, I had called him up to my office to discuss with me his working with John Ninnemann, a research fellow who had come with me from Minnesota and who had been unable to produce Summerlin's earlier results. Summerlin maintained, "You can't do it, but I can." Then he showed me these "salt-and-pepper mice," as he called them. I really didn't inspect them very closely and said, "Bill, don't give me salt and pepper. I want to see real black grafts of skin growing on white mice in a proper genetic context." Like what we had seen back in Minnesota. Later the animal boy who saw him paint the mice reported this to John Raff and the whole story came out. So Summerlin faked the data, an inexcusable behavior in science. My worry initially was that he might be manic. I had previously had a manic scientist in my laboratory, and this bizarre act was in keeping with such behavior.

The science. In Minnesota, Summerlin had observed something that turned out to be absolutely true and reproducible. I am convinced of this. I think that even at that time in New York I had reasoned that the cause of his failure might be related to his culturing the skin under adverse conditions. In the skin epithelium are these Langerhans cells that carry the major histocompatibility determinants. If you can make these cells disappear, then you can achieve dramatic long-term survivability of these grafts with later transplantation, just as Summerlin was doing sometimes. The problem was that these cells were probably still intact at the time he was attempting these transplantations. Since then, it has been shown that in skin as well as endocrine organs such transplants can now be successfully achieved. So it is clear that the basic science of what Summerlin was attempting was correct.

The men. In retrospect, there were signals along the way about Summerlin that I failed to recognize. Summerlin was criticized by one of his associates, Douglas Bigger, who came to me and said, "I don't want to work with Summerlin. I don't trust him." I should have picked up on this and said, "Now, wait a minute. Why don't you trust him?" and didn't. I attributed the dispute to internecine strife which is very common between young scientists.

What people don't realize, however, is that Summerlin and I never published a paper on this. Summerlin did present a paper at a California transplantation meeting and one in Atlantic City. And he was really good at presenting! It really brought the house down especially in Atlantic City where everybody was just overwhelmed. I had a very high scientific profile at that time and was clearly identified with the work, for it had come out of my laboratory. In a sense I really set myself up for what was to follow. I had to give this big address to the Federated Society [of Experimental Biology] and, discussing Summerlin's work, which I called the "Summerlin phenomenon," I ended with, "And there will be big surprises," looking forward to all the transplantation and other implications of the work.

When the disclosure of his faking results came out, I came in for a lot of hostility and personally suffered greatly from it. It took me several years to really once again become confident enough in myself to have the guts to make discoveries. You know, it takes guts to do that. What you have to do in making a real discovery is to show that all of your friends and the people you admire most are wrong. But I'm completely recovered from that aspect of uncertainty now.

■ I'm glad you feel free to talk about it now. Do you feel that the Summerlin episode led to your leaving Sloan-Kettering?

I don't think so. I think my leaving Sloan-Kettering was mainly a consequence of my having been there long enough. I had been there just about ten years. Then Lew Thomas retired from his post as president of Memorial Hospital and Sloan-Kettering Institute and became chancellor. Although he was nominally my boss as head of both institutions, I had pretty much of a free hand at Sloan-Kettering under him. The replacement they finally hired, Paul Marks, and I were completely incompatible. He was a hard-nosed administrator and sometimes hard on scientists, and I don't believe in that. I don't believe in pressing people.

In retrospect, Paul Marks was the best friend in the world to me because his appointment helped me to decide to come to Oklahoma City. I'm having the time of my life here. I have a great laboratory setup; good people to work with; and, if you look on the map, you'll see that Oklahoma is really the guts of the country.

■ Do you have anything to say to future generations of scientists about what you have learned from the Summerlin case, because it will surely come up again in some form or another?

I've thought so much about this. It has been present throughout all of scientific history. It is present now and, unfortunately, more than people think. It happened once before in my own career. I found a young fellow who was faking data, and I just sat down with him and said, "You know, you don't belong in science, so just don't try. Just get out of this game." I didn't make a big thing out of it. He was a young medical student doing research, and he was just too anxious to please. The rules of the game require that scientific data be impeccable.

I think this thing occurs, but I think there isn't a lot I would like to change either in the way I work personally, by myself, or with my fellows. A mentor has very few things he can do for a fellow. One, he can set a tone; he can work his butt off and show that it is really worthwhile to try to push aside the mundane part of science, the rituals, false beliefs, misinterpretations and really make observations. It's a matter of setting a pattern. Secondly, he can understand what his fellows are doing, analyzing and appreciating the work. Third, he can be critical, and I was highly critical. It was my critical approach with another fellow that led to the discovery that things were not going well with Summerlin. To avoid this sort of thing in the future I would also advise those in charge to listen very carefully. It's like making discoveries: you don't pay attention to the things that fit. You'll never make a discovery if you do that. You pay attention to the things that don't fit, and the same thing is true of people. If I had to teach people how to avoid events like the Summerlin affair, I would tell them to listen for signals, the often subtle signals that people are willing to give you, because there were people who were trying to tell me something was wrong and I didn't hear them until I began to see for myself.

Finally, you can encourage, encourage, encourage and wait, wait, wait. You cannot hurry discovery.

■ Let me try to close this discussion of fraud with a smile if I can. We had an example of this in our own backyard not long ago, and the fellow involved obviously had something wrong with him. He was constantly saying and doing outrageous things. When he finally tried to publish a paper in which most of the data were the product of his imagination, he was quietly made to leave. When his supervisor was later asked by one of my friends why he had kept such a person on his staff, the answer was, "Well, I like to have controversial people around. It livens things up." To this my friend suggested, "If you want somebody controversial, then why don't you just go out and hire the Ayatollah Khomeini?"

It's hard to draw superficial conclusions about a thing like that, and I would hate to go through it again. I'm a little gun-shy now. One of the wise things that I have done here and I didn't do before was to require that when anything really new is observed in the laboratory it must be confirmed before we publish it. This slows things down a bit and is probably a little unfair to the younger people who are trying to build up their bibliographies, but there is really no need to rush into publication. You can present the material at a meeting and have an abstract to establish priority, et cetera, but there is no real harm in delaying the final publication until confirmation is at hand.

■ I know there are many new things cooking in your field that I'd love to discuss, but I have to mention something that struck me about your early life concerning the death of your father. As a medical student like your father, I, too, had a highly malignant testicular tumor and spent about two months in the hospital undergoing some radical surgery. That was over twenty years go, and thanks to my doctors, I survived. I've always maintained that that experience made me a much better doctor than I would have been. I see so much callousness among physicians, especially younger ones. If I had my way, I would make every medical student deathly ill for one month of his life as part of his education and then effect a cure. Their future patients would surely benefit from it. I am wondering if your own serious illness has affected your own outlook in a similar way.

I am absolutely certain that my skill as a physician, my attention to detail with patients, and concern for them was very much influenced by my own experience with disease. After all, for a while there I thought I had a lethal disease (amyotrophic lateral sclerosis). I was scared and I know how it feels. When I have a patient or the parent of a patient with me, I can sense that fear, and I am at least reactive to it, and try to be supportive.

■ While we are still in the past, is there anything about it that you regret? I'm not talking about the Summerlin thing now, because something like that could happen anywhere, anytime, to anyone.

To be really honest, if I had it to do over again, I think I would be a lot more encouraging and a little less pressing on my oldest child. I really wanted a boy to follow me, as a scientist and scholar. Michael wasn't anything like me, although he's a great guy. He always said, "Well, the first one is just for the trial and error and you just have to let that one go by." He's a successful businessman in Minneapolis with a lovely family now. He learned from his father's mistakes. With my other kids I was pretty good, I think, which means, among other things, that I have tried to understand what *they* want to do.

There's something else that I sometimes think about. I

should have done a sabbatical. I always figured that I didn't
know anybody that I'd rather take a sabbatical with than myself, but that was a conceit. I would have done well to take
some sabbatical time on vacations to learn a new wrinkle. I
was always good at picking up new ideas and developing them,
but there are some things that take a little more time and
effort, and a sabbatical or two would have afforded such opportunities.

■ Looking to the future, it seems that immunology will be involved with so
many things: allergy, joint disease, infections, endocrine disorders, blood problems, organ transplants. But more than anything else it seems to hold the clue
to cancer. Why can't we attack the cancer cells immunologically? Why do they
keep outsmarting us?

Because we haven't learned enough yet. When we look back
on our knowledge of immunology today and compare it to
that when I started in 1943 it's incredible. It was thought then
that it was the macrophages that made antibodies. Ridiculous!
The immunological system is an amazing system in itself as
well as with its interaction with two other major networks,
the brain and the endocrine system. There are extraordinary
controls that we are just beginning to fathom. It's remarkable
that we have been able to do the cellular engineering we have
with the fragmentary information at our disposal. But when
we get our act together, and really understand immunology
we'll be able to turn off tumors; we'll really be able to do
cellular engineering to control cancer.

■ Well, you certainly have approached it with a lot of different hats. I look
back on your titles, and they're all over the place—pediatrics, pathology,
medicine . . .

Basically, that's because I really am kind of undifferentiated.

■ I'll leave it at that.

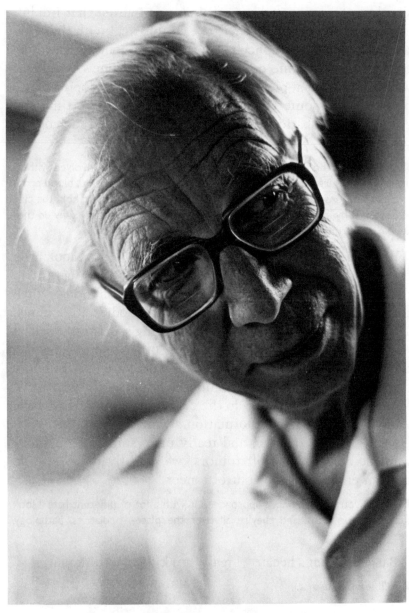

Willem J. Kolff, M.D., Ph.D.
(Courtesy of the University of Utah Public Relations Office)

CHAPTER 16

Willem J. Kolff, M.D., Ph.D.
(1911–)

B Y THE TIME this is being read hundreds of thousands of patients with acute or chronic renal failure will have owed some part of their lives to Willem Kolff, developer in 1943 of the first practical and widely used artificial kidney, and responsible in 1945 for the first long-term survivor of acute renal failure through renal dialysis.

The term "dialysis" (the technique of diffusing solute molecules from an area of high concentration to one of lower concentration across a semipermeable membrane) was originated by a Scottish chemist, Thomas Graham, in an 1854 paper entitled "On Osmotic Force." In this he described experiments with different solutes using a membrane fashioned from an ox bladder. The German physiologist Adolph Fick, best remembered today for his principle in determining cardiac output (see p. 113), one year later found that the syrupy liquid, collodion, when dry became a porous membrane. This became the basic material used for many subsequent diffusion experiments that began to appear in the scientific literature.

The first application of the dialysis principle for the treatment of renal failure occurred at Johns Hopkins University in 1913. There John Jacob Abel, a pharmacologist working with L. G. Rowntree and B. B. Turner, built a prototype for, and gave the name to, the "artificial kidney." Conducting experiments in animals, they utilized a collodion membrane (celloidin) formed into tubes through which blood could flow and all mounted within a glass cylinder containing dialysis fluid. Heparin not yet being discovered, to keep blood from clotting within the system they used as an anticoagulant, hirudin, extracted from the heads of thousands of leeches.

Two other notable contributions to the development of renal dialysis were made by Heinrich Necheles of Hamburg and by another German investigator, George Haas, of the University Clinic at Giessen. Necheles, greatly moved by his experiences as a drafted medical student in the German army during World War I where he saw many young soldiers dying in renal failure, later attempted to use sheep peritoneum as a dialyzing membrane, sandwiching multiple layers of the material in a dialyzing solution. This introduced critical elements that were incorporated into subsequent dialyzers: the ability to use only a small amount of blood and exposing it to a wide surface area of dialyzing membrane.

Haas, using a collodion membrane in a device more similar to that of Abel, Rowntree, and Turner, performed the first human dialysis in 1924 after working on the problem since 1915. At first using hirudin, he later produced his own heparin for anticoagulation. Despite some promising results, he discontinued his work when it was not received with any enthusiasm by the surrounding medical community.

By the late 1930s the basic requirements of an acceptable artificial kidney had become clear:

- the availability of a practical and efficient dialyzing membrane
- the ability to distribute blood in the device in a thin enough film so that its waste products could be efficiently transported across the membrane and into the dialysate
- the need for only a small amount of blood to prime the dialyzer so that the patient would not become hypovolemic when attached to it
- the availability of a safe and efficient anticoagulant

In 1937 a German chemist, Wilhelm Thalheimer, found that cellophane (cellulose acetate) could be employed in removing solutes from the blood; and R. Brinkman, Kolff's professor of biochemistry at Groningen in the Netherlands, had begun to conduct experiments with this membrane by the time Kolff came under his influence. This inexpensive, efficient membrane was already being produced on an industrial scale in the form of casings for sausages and other meat products.

Kolff, after leaving Groningen and working in the small town of Kampen during World War II, combined the cellophane, heparin, and his own innate mechanical ingenuity in designing the rotating drum artificial kidney. This would become the worldwide standard for this purpose, especially after an improved model was developed with Kolff's assistance by the Peter Bent Brigham Hospital group in Boston.

As the Kolff kidney achieved general acceptance and its inventor's abilities became known, the way was prepared for Kolff to assume a research position at the Cleveland Clinic in 1950. He remained there until 1967, working on a variety of artificial devices, including a heart-lung machine, a membrane oxygenator, and early models of the artificial heart. He also worked on improvements in the artificial kidney, finally evolving the disposable double-coil model that, for a time, was also a leader in the field.

To bring the artificial kidney story up to date, it was soon recognized that, to achieve long-term survival, the kidney would be most useful in those patients with acute reversible renal failure such as that due to trauma or certain poisons. The artificial kidney could then take over the function of the natural organ and prevent patients from dying from uremia while awaiting resumption of function by their own kidneys. Such, in fact, was the case with Kolff's first long-term survivor. The use of the Kolff-Brigham kidney spread and was of immense importance during the Korean War when used by Paul Teschan at the Eleventh Evacuation Hospital to treat

American soldiers who had gone into acute reversible renal failure as a result of battle wounds.

A major obstacle to effective long-term dialysis in patients with end-stage renal disease and permanent kidney failure was the need to isolate blood vessels surgically each time the patient required dialysis, perhaps two or three times weekly. This was initially overcome by the construction of an external Teflon shunt between an artery and vein in the forearm, as developed in the late 1950s by Belding Scribner and Wayne Quinton at the University of Washington in Seattle. This external shunt provided easy, rapid access to the bloodstreams of patients requiring repeated long-term dialysis, although shunt disconnection and infection were hazards of this external communication. The external Scribner shunt was superseded by the preferable internal arteriovenous shunt introduced by Dr. James Cimino and his associates at Bellevue Hospital in New York in 1966. New types of dialysis units have continued to proliferate until at present a compact capillary type containing thousands of small hollow tubes constructed of an improved cellulose product and thus reminiscent of Abel's original device is currently the most favored.

With the feasibility of chronic dialysis established, the next problem to address was the cost, which was well beyond the means of most patients requiring this treatment. In the early years of dialysis, committees were set up that determined the life and death of patients by selecting which patients would be allowed to gain access to the limited dialysis facilities available to the public. In 1972 this treatment was guaranteed to all Americans by the United States government through medicare funding, although increasing cost-effectiveness continues to be sought through the training of patients in home hemodialysis. There has also been a revival of interest in a simpler form of dialysis more adaptable to home use and also investigated by Kolff and his associates in the early days in Kampen. This is peritoneal dialysis, where fluid is introduced to the abdominal cavity through a permanent access tube and allowed to remain there for periods of time to allow the waste products of the blood to diffuse into it before removal.

Returning to the Kolff story, in 1967 he left Cleveland for the University of Utah in Salt Lake City where he has remained ever since as professor of surgery, heading the Division of Artificial Organs, and as Distinguished Professor of Medicine at the medical school while also serving as Research Professor of Bioengineering in the College of Engineering. His efforts in directing a number of investigations in artificial organs have continued undiminished, although the operation involving Barney Clark as a result of the artificial heart program has received the most publicity.

The features of the Kolff character that have been commented upon by most of those who have known and worked with him have included a single-mindedness of purpose, inexhaustible energy, superb organizational ability, and an unfettered eclecticism in the selection of men or materials, with the sole criterion of having them best serve his purposes. He has been quoted as saying, "I'll take a good technician over a mediocre doctor any day," and he has not hesitated to use such items as a Ford water pump coupling, orange juice cans, and clothes washing machines in the construction of machines to meet his needs.

His reputation for efficient use of time and punctuality is legendary. It therefore came as no surprise to me when he suggested that, in order for me to conduct an interview with him, I should pick him up in Washington, D.C., where he had business at the Food and Drug Administration and drive him to his surgeon son's home in a suburb of Philadelphia where he was to spend the weekend. I made a point of arriving well ahead of time at the FDA to await the appearance of this medical pioneer, whom I had never before seen in person.

As I sat in the car I recalled the words of a close associate of his in Cleveland, heart surgeon Donald B. Effler, who referred to the "pioneer" label as applied to himself with some distaste. ("I always think of pioneers as being unshaved, dusty, and scruffy looking, much like Hopalong Cassidy's sidekick Gabby Hays.") When Dr. Kolff appeared I was somewhat surprised to see that, like Effler, he was very erect and distinguished looking. He squeezed his over six-foot lanky frame into the back of my tiny Japanese compact and was introduced to our chauffeur, my charming Dutch wife, whom I counted on to smooth the way with what one writer described as a "dour Dutchman." This label really did not fit well. Dr. Kolff's pungent remarks and devastating judgments were frequently punctuated with wry humor throughout the trip.

We stopped for refreshments halfway to Philadelphia, and as we walked from the parking lot to the dining room, a shiny rebuilt American motorcycle and its Hell's Angels-type owner was in our path. Unselfconsciously, Dr. Kolff stopped to inquire enthusiastically about its performance and about how it compared with similar Japanese models. After probing several minutes as to the bike's qualities, he seemed on the verge of asking to go off on a test spin. We later resumed our trip, which was certainly enhanced by the presence of the youthful, friendly Dutch woman in the driver's seat. The paternalistic Kolff repeatedly referred to her as "little van Raalte" (her maiden name) and provided instructions to her as to how best to ventilate the vehicle along the way.

Our rendezvous with Dr. Kolff's daughter-in-law was a McDonald's hamburger stand in Villanova. When she arrived, I placed his bags in the rear of her station wagon and then shook hands in farewell. I was not the least surprised, however, when, like a Dutch uncle, he offered his cheek to "little van Raalte," who dutifully bussed it before he drove off into the night.

En route from Washington, D.C., to Philadelphia
May 19, 1983

■ Wherever one reads about the development of the artificial kidney, there is usually an early note that the first practical one for human use was developed by Willem Kolff in "war-torn Holland." I would like to know more about how you became interested in medicine, and especially renal failure.

Although my father was a doctor, when I was very young I didn't want to follow in his footsteps because I could not bear the thought of seeing patients die. As I grew older, I revised that opinion and never changed. My father ran a tuberculosis sanatorium, and his attitude toward patients impressed me. He would agonize over his frustrations in treating them, and I recall seeing him weep on several occasions.

My interest in kidney failure was aroused soon after I graduated from medical school in Leiden and took an unpaid teaching assistant's position at the University of Groningen in 1938. I was married during my last year of medical school, and thanks to a little income that my wife had, we were able to live on this while I furthered my training. I had responsibility over four beds on the Medical Service at the University of Groningen, and in one of these was a young man who was slowly and miserably dying from renal failure. I felt helpless, having to tell his poor mother that there was nothing we could do for him. I began to reason at this time that, if only we could remove the amount of urea and other excretory products that he produced each day, we could keep him alive.

I was fortunate in coming under the influence of two outstanding people who were at Groningen. These were Professor R. Brinkman in biochemistry and Professor Polak Daniels, head of the Medical Department. Brinkman had shown that cellophane was a good dialyzing membrane and had used it to concentrate blood plasma and determine osmotic pressures of fluids.

He had thought about using it in an artificial kidney, but nothing came of it. My first attempts along these lines was to take some cellophane membranes (the same kind used for sausage skins), fill them with a little blood, expelling the air, and adding some urea to see if, by agitating this in a bath of physiologic saline, the urea would be removed. To my surprise, I found that in five minutes nearly all the urea I had added to the blood sample, four hundred milligrams, had disappeared from the blood and entered the saline bath.

This initial experience led me to proceed with the development of an artificial kidney, with which I later succeeded in Kampen. Polak Daniels was important to me because, instead of ridiculing this idea as some other senior people might have done, he encouraged me to pursue it.

The initial work in Groningen was interrupted by the German invasion on May 19th, 1940. On that day I happened to be in the Hague to attend the funeral of my wife's grandfather. When the German planes appeared overhead dropping bombs and pamphlets, instead of attending the funeral I went to the main hospital in town, the Ziekenhuis aan de Zuidwall, and asked the director if I could help. Anticipating the need for blood transfusions, I asked if they had a blood bank. The director told me no. I then offered to set one up, and he agreed.

I got an automobile, requisitions, a soldier to sit next to the driver, because there were snipers on the roofs, and went from one shop to another picking up what I needed: bottles, rubber tubes, needles. In four days the blood bank was set up. It was the first of its kind on the European Continent and is still in existence.

The planned Dutch defense in the east and through the middle of Holland was to flood the area, but this didn't work. As soon as Professor Daniels realized that the Germans were overrunning the country, he and his wife, who were Jewish, committed suicide. Instead of accepting the candidate recommended by the Groningen faculty to fill the vacancy, the Germans decided to appoint a Dutch Nazi with a German name, Kreuz Wendedich von dem Borne, to the professorship of medicine. I had resolved never to serve under him, and this led to my going to Kampen.

After the initial German attack, which found my wife and me in the Hague, we had to make our way back to Groningen. Since the Dutch had destroyed all the bridges, the only place where we could cross the Ijsel River to get to Groningen was at Kampen. I stopped to talk to the mayor of Kampen on my way, and while we were commiserating with each other about the Germans, he told me that they were thinking of getting an internist to work in the ninety-bed municipal hospital at Kampen where he happened to be chairman of the board of directors. I told him I might be interested.

Back in Groningen the Lord was with us in that he gave this Nazi, Professor von dem Borne, tuberculosis with pleurisy, so his arrival was postponed at least six months. In the interim, the secretary of curators of the University of Groningen had papers for my resignation conveniently all drawn up and ready with the exception of the dates, pending his arrival.

While awaiting this eventuality, I noticed an ad in the newspaper for the internal medicine post in Kampen and formally applied. I was the youngest and last of the applicants, but since the facilities were outdated, I was insistent about what I expected: an up-to-date laboratory for which I provided the plans, and a modern X-ray room for which I gave them specifications I had acquired from Phillips. Without these, I told them, they could not compete with the neighboring hospital in Zwolle. Despite all my demands, they finally decided to choose me, although there was a time I was unemployed between Groningen and Kampen, and we had to live with my father and mother.

I recall leaving Groningen the evening before the National Socialist von dem Borne was to take his post, thinking that his tuberculosis was over. It was a year and a half later that I saw him again. This was towards the middle of the war one day on the way to Groningen when my little car was forced off the road to make way for a cannon carriage drawn by two black-draped horses. On the carriage was the body of von dem Borne, who had died from miliary tuberculosis and meningitis. I have to say I could not have been more content.

■ Was it at Kampen, then, that you built your first successful artificial kidney?

There was one unsuccessful model built by a manufacturer for me when I was at Groningen, but it wasn't until I got to Kampen and received the cooperation of Mr. H. Berk that we finally got a workable model. He was a director of the enamel factory at Kampen, the town's main industry.

After my initial experience with the sausage casings in Groningen, simple arithmetic dictated that I would have to use tubing at least ten to twenty meters long with one half to a liter of blood in order to dialyze a patient adequately. This was finally accomplished by wrapping twenty meters of cellophane tubing around a horizontally placed drum, which in turn was placed in a trough containing dialysis solution. Any blood within the tubing sinks by gravity to the lowest point in the drum, and as the drum is rotated with its lower half in dialysate, the blood is constantly coming in contact with the solution through the tubing, of course. Now, the blood has to get into one end of the cellophane tubing wrapped around the drum and then out the other end. This was best done by leading it through the hollow axle of the drum. We first tried rubber rotating couplings for connecting the tubes to and from the patient to the rotating drum but had some trouble with them. They kept getting twisted as the drum rotated. I then went to see the local Ford dealer and took over the idea that Henry Ford had used in constructing the seal of the water pump of his engine. I copied it, having only to drill a hole in it for my purposes. The first artificial kidneys had drums made of aluminum around which the cellophane tubing was wrapped. When aluminum could no longer be obtained due to wartime shortages, we used wooden laths. They worked fine, except that often the wood was not aged properly and warped.

■ Your first patient was a twenty-nine-year-old woman, Jenny Schrijer.

Yes. We began with her on March 17, 1943, and she received a total of twelve treatments with the artificial kidney. She had malignant hypertension and advanced kidney disease with renal failure. We observed no ill effects from the dialysis and were able to keep her alive for twenty-six days before she succumbed to her disease. This encouraged us to attempt additional dialyses on other patients, constantly learning how to improve the technique.

We started off with intermittent dialysis, removing fifty milliliters of blood from the patient's vein and dialyzing it before returning it. We then found it possible to dialyze more effectively by letting blood continuously run through the artificial kidney from the patient, entering in one end, then exiting out the other as it rotated.

At first we used two veins from the patient to remove and return blood. We then learned that cannulating the radial artery in the wrist provided much better access for the removal of blood. We knew very little about using heparin in the beginning under these circumstances. Although this was a necessary ingredient to add to the dialysis machine to prevent clotting, it also had the risk of causing bleeding when returned to the patient, and a good form of antidote for excessive bleeding, such as protamine, had not yet been developed. Gradually we learned how to use it safely and effectively. And, of course, we became very aware that complete cures could be obtained in acute reversible renal failure as opposed to chronic failure.

Between March 17, 1943, and July 27, 1944, we treated a total of fifteen patients, among whom there was one survivor, although I do not credit the artificial kidney for this. He had been given a sulfa drug which had crystallized in his kidneys and blocked the ureters. He went into acute renal failure, which was relieved when the mechanical blockage of the ureters was relieved, and I credit this rather than the artificial kidney with having saved his life. That man is still alive. I was back in the Netherlands thirty years later, and he called me to speak with me. After all, our aggressive approach to his problem, with or without the artificial kidney, was what saved him. He would have died in many other hospitals in Holland at the time.

■   Tell me about Sophia Schafstadt, your first real success, in September 1945.

Sophia was the wife of Mr. Schafstadt and was sixty-seven years old when she came to us in uremic coma. Following her treatment, when she opened her eyes the first words out of her mouth were, "I'm going to divorce my husband." And she did! And lived another seven years. She was a Dutch National Socialist [Nazi], and although I don't have any proof of this, everybody believed that she had betrayed her countrymen to the Germans. It is a beautiful example of a saved life to start philosophizing about.

■   You think of all those good people who died, and then you have your first success in a woman like this . . .

That's just the point. If a patient needs help to save his life, you give that help and don't ask whether or not he is a National Socialist or anything else. In regard to the selection of patients for the dialysis program, they originally set up these life-and-death committees, which I always fought tooth and nail and will continue to fight. They asked such questions as: "Are you married?" "Do you have children?" "Are you employed?" "Do you go to church?" And when you happen to be divorced, without children, unemployed, and the member of no church, you are deemed unqualified to be dialyzed. This is true. These were the selection criteria developed by the life-and-death committee in Seattle; and the more they talk about "cost containment" and whether we can "afford" to take care of people who need treatment, the greater likelihood there is of return to this. This is something we must guard against. If we do not change our production-oriented community to a service-oriented one, we will have nothing but trouble.

■ After Sophia Schafstadt you began to have more consistent results. Was it clear sailing after this?

The technique began to be accepted, of course, after our initial successes, although there were some strange developments. I'll tell you about one of them, since it is now so many years later.

There was this young man, a law student, who was engaged to this beautiful blonde girl, the daughter of a physician. He was very nervous even after he had passed an examination, and the girl, in order to calm him down, offered him a pill from her father's case. The bottle was labeled "Luminal," which is a sedative, but what the pill really contained was bichloride of mercury, a poison. As a result, the boy's kidneys went into acute shutdown, and he was brought to me. The prospective father-in-law felt very guilty, naturally, and said he would willingly pay all the costs of treatment with the artificial kidney. That is until he saw the bill, although he finally did pay for the treatment, which was successful.

The dilemma I faced with this boy, however, was that I gave him a very thorough physical examination, as I did with all my patients in order to present a proper report to the referring physician. On examining his genitals, I found that the testicles were no larger than the nail on my little finger. And here the referring physician was the father of his fiancée. Should I include this finding in my report? That marriage never took place. The boy was later wed to another girl, but they divorced and never had children.

The upshot of all this was that, years later when a reporter was interviewing all the survivors of the early dialysis treatment, the family was very bitter about it because they blamed the artificial kidney for the small size of the man's testicles.

■ Holland was occupied by the Germans then. Did you have to conceal your work on the kidney from them?

Not really, although I did not want to publish my work in a German journal and be claimed as a "good German." I did send manuscripts to *Acta Medica Scandinavia* in Sweden, to a Swiss journal, and to the French *Presse Medicale* in order to make the work known.

I still had to get along with the local Germans, however, since they had a garrison in the city of Kampen and would send patients over to the hospital for me to treat.

A German medical officer came over to see the artificial kidney one time and remarked, "Das ist der Apparat den ich es aus die Literature kenne." (This is the apparatus as I recognize it from the literature.) In point of fact, it had not been published yet. Typical.

■ I gather that you built something like ten artificial rotating drum kidneys while you were in Holland and, at the end of the war, sent one each to Hammersmith in England, Royal Victoria Hospital in Montreal, and Mt. Sinai in New York. Are any of these original models still in existence?

I think there must be two. One that was left in Kampen is now in the Medical History Museum in Leiden. The one that was sent to Hammersmith, I believe, was acquired by Travenol Laboratories, which uses it in a traveling exhibition. The very first one I kept but later allowed an associate of mine to cannibalize it when he needed one of its parts for a heart-lung machine model we were working on.

■ It seems that when in Holland you were fortunate in having the right people to work with, but were short on supplies.

The cooperation of Berk was very important, and I had very good nurses. Nanny DeLeeuw, a Dutch physician, worked with me during the war, and she later went to Montreal to teach the people how to work the kidney. Bob van Noordwijk was a medical student who was a Socialist and put in a concentration camp by the Germans early during the occupation. When released, he came to us, and we gave him room and board in Kampen where he was very helpful with the work we carried on. He later completed his medical studies, went to London, Ontario, and became professor of pharmacology in Utrecht. Dr. Piet Kop also worked with us, but he concentrated on peritoneal dialysis and wrote the first extensive book on it. And there were others.

We were not as fortunate in terms of supplies. Although I had the foresight to buy up adequate amounts of sausage casings to use for our studies, as the war progressed we ran short of just about everything else. Needles were in short supply; rubber tubing was so scarce that we only used it to make flexible joints, substituting glass tubing for greater lengths of the material.

Toward the end of the war we had to temporarily stop all work on the kidney. The Germans considered every able-bodied Dutchman to be a potential terrorist after their experiences during the retreats from Brussels and Paris. To prevent a similar thing from happening in Holland, they decided to round up all the men and ship them to Germany to work on fortifications. They started with Rotterdam, surrounding the city with eighty thousand troops, herding thousands of men and boys into a giant stadium there, and then shipping them out on these large coal barges they use on the Rhine. Each of these ships carried about eight hundred prisoners, and they were towed across the Zuider Zee to Kampen. From Kampen they were to be transported by train to Germany. One morning ten of these ships were docked in Kampen with eight thousand prisoners, among them blind people, some paralyzed, others deaf, others severely retarded, diabetics that had not had insulin for days.

That whole mess was at the riverside, and a doctor who lived there came to me at the hospital and said, "Kolff, could you please come over. Something should be done about it. People are dying on my doorstep."

I went to see the German commander, Oberleutnant Baatz, a "Sonder Commando der Wehrmacht" who really wielded authority over the regular Wehrmacht [army]. I told him that there were some very sick people in the boats and that I would be willing to take them out. He said, "Who will be responsible? All these people are terrorists." I said, "I will be responsible." "Very well," he told me, "and if they run away, you will be shot."

We finally managed to get twelve hundred patients off these convoys, and I became the head of eight emergency hospitals. Among the people we took off were many Jews and members of the underground, and we wanted to get them away from the Germans. We had much of the male population of Rotterdam going through, with accountants, managers, even doctors. I told them that we would set up a very efficient administration to impress the Germans, using a system of cards, et cetera. This we did, and then forged identity cards to help people get away. The Germans never found out what we were up to, but I was responsible for all the dealings with them. I wasn't very fat when I started, but during that last winter I lost twenty pounds.

■   After the war you came to the United States. How did this come about?

My first contact was with Isidore Snapper,[b] who was also Dutch but whom I had not met either before or during the war. He had worked in Amsterdam and I in Leiden. Being a

Jew, he had gone to China and later came to the United States in a prisoner-of-war exchange. He was at Mt. Sinai Hospital in New York at the end of the war, and in 1947 I wrote him, sending reprints of my work and offering to donate an artificial kidney to Mt. Sinai Hospital. I also offered to come over to the United States to show them how it worked.

I had no money at the time, and he offered me three hundred dollars to support myself and my wife during the three months we were to live in New York. I found out that it would not be enough only after we arrived, and the situation was impossible. No doubt about it; we lived in deep poverty in New York.

At Mt. Sinai I was to use a microphone, and I planned simply to speak from brief notes, as was my custom. I had seen in London that when a non-English-speaking foreigner reads from a paper his accent is all the worse, and it just doesn't work. Snapper insisted I write out the speech and showed it to an editor, who added things like "your great country the United States"—and all that sort of garbage. As I gave the speech, Snapper was constantly at my elbow whispering, "In the microphone! In the microphone!" which I learned right away. The speech went over very well, and Snapper was delighted. He arranged for me then to speak at a number of hospitals, including Harvard and other major teaching institutions such as those in Montreal and Minneapolis.

George Thorn[b] at Harvard soon after was very helpful in winning for me the Francis Amory Award from the American Academy of Arts and Sciences in Boston. This was for thirty-six-hundred dollars, a lot of money for me then, and this later was used as a down payment for my house in Cleveland.

The year 1947 was the centennial of the American Medical Association, and I was also invited to give a talk there. After four months of travel in the United States, it was time to go home, although our four children were doing quite well without us. The two youngest, Albert and Kees, I recall, were going through a stage of wanting to be dogs and were eating from their plates on the floor at the home of my secretary's parents. They had a wonderful time.

I came back to the States in 1949, this time actively looking for a position. This was quite difficult, because all the returning GIs could take positions without pay while getting support through the GI Bill. I found that the only place available to me was the Cleveland Clinic where I was hired by Irvine Page[b] to work in the Research Division. He had just gotten an old building assigned to him and had adequate space.

In my earlier communications with him, I had pointed out that, with him working on hypertension and me on the artificial kidney, we could form a very strong team. After I arrived in 1950, however, I found that he wanted me, too, to work on hypertension rather than the artificial kidney, to which he became very unfriendly. It was only after five years, in 1955, that I finally felt strong enough in my relationship with Page to tell him that I saw very little use in taking out the kidneys of dogs and making them miserable when we had patients in which kidneys had been removed anticipating transplantation.

■ Do you mean to say that during the first five years you were in Cleveland you couldn't do any work on the artificial kidney?

When I arrived there was an Allis Chalmers artificial kidney waiting for me. It was a six thousand-dollar version of the old two hundred dollar model but worked just as well. The first years, however, I didn't even have a dialysis room. If I wanted to dialyze a patient, I had to clean out a dog laboratory and bring in a bed to assemble. We had to carry the patient down four steps in our arms. The patients were miserable and would die. The dogs that we had removed from treatment for two or three days would also be miserable and also die. It was awful.

Finally they gave me an artificial kidney room, and then the clinical service for the kidney began to flourish, but it took seven years at the Cleveland Clinic to build up the same staff I had at that small hospital in the Netherlands. After being very productive in Kampen, where I had five technicians, an instrument maker, two secretaries, specially trained nurses, all working together, I met only frustration in Cleveland. It was three months before I got my first technician, and he promptly stole my wallet!

■ If things were going so well in Holland, why did you leave?

In the first place, I thought the Russians would be coming in. Second, I thought Holland was overcrowded; it had lost its colonies, and there would not be enough space for our four children—five by the time we immigrated. Last, I had been working on a heart-lung machine in Kampen at a hospital with only one surgeon and one internist. A ninety-bed city hospital was too small to start an open-heart program. So I felt I had to give up my independence and join a large team where they could use and develop both the artificial kidney and an improved model of the heart-lung machine.

When I came to the United States, though, none of the surgeons were immediately interested in using the heart-lung machine, because Charles Bailey had just started doing his mitral valve commissurotomies. This was a blind procedure done without bypass, which the surgeons loved because they hated complicated apparatuses anyway. It was only four or five years later, when the limitations of closed-heart surgery became evident for valve problems other than mitral stenosis and also for complicated congenital heart disease, that interest in open-heart surgery with bypass was revived. In 1955, five years after arriving in Cleveland, I took out of the closet all my heart-lung equipment that I had brought with me from the Netherlands and began to work with it again.

■ Were you aware of Gibbon's[b] work on the heart-lung machine?

Yes. Gibbon was professor of cardiac and thoracic surgery at Jefferson, and I stayed at his home in Philadelphia during my first visit. We became very good friends and he invited me to join him at Jefferson, but I felt it would be unwise to be working in his institution on exactly the same project. I also sensed that his relations with the chief of surgery were not the best, so I decided in favor of the Cleveland Clinic, where there was more space and at least some guarantee of a salary on which I could support my wife and five children.

■ Despite all your problems in Cleveland, you certainly accomplished a great deal while you were with them. There were further developments with the artificial kidney and development of the twin-coil disposable kidney. Then, although people generally credit Kantrowitz[b] for the intraaortic balloon pump because he popularized it, the device was developed by Moulopoulos, Topaz, and you at the Cleveland Clinic. You've already touched on the membrane oxygenator and heart-lung machine. I would now like you to tell me about how you and Effler[b] introduced elective cardiac arrest in open-heart surgery.

Experimental elective cardiac arrest in dogs using potassium citrate was introduced by Melrose and his group at Hammersmith Hospital in London. They showed that reperfusing the heart with normal blood could then easily restart it. This was desirable in correcting cardiac defects in open-heart surgery, since the surgeons were not used to suturing moving targets. Donald Effler and Laurence Groves, the cardiac surgeons at the Cleveland Clinic, came into my laboratory and worked together with me, doing this in dogs. We did many of these, but the last ten consecutive puppies went without a hitch.

Then in the operating room this was tried on three children with congenital heart defects. Yet the first baby died, although the second and third lived. You see, no matter how many successful animal experiments you have, you can still lose your first patient when you attempt something new clinically. You must have some leeway for some failures when you are beginning something new and worthwhile.

■ Did you experience the same pressures in the Netherlands when you lost fourteen of your first fifteen patients?

No. There was never any pressure on me there to stop, and if there had been I wouldn't have paid any attention. But if I had been doing that work at the Cleveland Clinic, they would have stopped me.

You have to find ways of evading that sort of obstruction. For example, at the Cleveland Clinic the urologist, Dr. Eugene Poutasse, and I decided to attempt some renal transplants, maintaining the patients on the artificial kidney until they were ready. We reasoned, however, that if their natural kidneys remained in place this might, in some way, affect the survival of the transplants adversely. We planned bilateral nephrectomies in these patients prior to the transplants.

Knowing, however, that there was little room for trial and error, we elected to do a number of these cases at once before any prohibitions could be set up against this should there be an initial failure or two. Six bilateral nephrectomies were scheduled by the surgeon in just a few days, and the transplants rapidly followed before any potential opposition to this could develop at the Clinic. Fortunately, they all turned out well, and at the Saturday morning Clinic conference we were able to present six patients with transplants, all in excellent health. Page, who was very negative about the work we were doing, was called upon to make a comment. He had no choice but to congratulate us.

I knew Charlie Bailey, and he had to do the same thing in regard to the mitral commissurotomy operation.* Now it's

---

*After Dr. Bailey's first three attempts at closed mitral commissurotomy had not succeeded, he realized that any further failures might result in his being barred from any future attempts in Philadelphia. With this in mind, in 1948 he scheduled on the same day one case at the Philadelphia General Hospital where he had morning operating privileges, and another case at Episcopal Hospital where he had afternoon operating privileges. He calculated that if one attempt failed the other would already be underway before he could be stopped from doing it. On the original day of the scheduled surgery, Bailey, at the ripe old age of thirty-eight, developed measles and had to postpone both operations. One month later, the first patient, an older man with far advanced disease and pulmonary complications, died; but the second case, a woman who was a much better candidate for the procedure, survived with marked improvement. The acceptance of the closed mitral commissurotomy for mitral stenosis was therefore assured.

worse than ever with the IRB [Institutional Review Board for Research on Human Subjects] and the FDA breathing down your neck. It took our surgeon William DeVries twenty-two months to get permission to implant the first artificial heart. Twenty-two months!

■ I would like to start at the beginning of the artificial heart and follow through on its history. You actually began work on this in Cleveland . . .

In 1957 Peter Salisbury gave his presidential address to the American Society for Artificial Internal Organs [ASAIO]. He spoke about the possibility of an artificial heart inside of the chest, and when I came home to Cleveland I said to Dr. Tetsuzo Akutsu, "Let's do it." We had also heard about a genius from New Zealand, Selwin McCabe, who was working on artificial hearts at the NIH. He made them by cavity molding of plastisol, a polyvinyl chloride. He could make valves, too. Although we had different ideas about shape, we basically copied his technique and gave him credit for it.

McCabe got into some political trouble and had to leave the NIH. I wanted to get him for the Cleveland Clinic, but when they heard about the kind of difficulty he was in this didn't get approved. So Tet Akutsu and I began this work. He presented it at the ASAIO meeting in the spring of 1958. That was the beginning. I was then put in touch with S. Harry Norton, a retired engineer from Thompson Products, and he made for us the first electrohydraulic heart using solenoids which, when activated, compressed hydraulic fluid in which the right and left "ventricles" were suspended. We took a dog with this electrohydraulic heart to the X-ray laboratory and made angiograms where you could see beautifully how the contrast material was pumped from the right side of the artificial heart into the lungs of the dog and then back to the left side. When my associates and I were presenting this at a later ASAIO meeting, although we had planned our time carefully, it seemed I might run overtime due to the showing of a movie.

As it was running, I asked the chairman of the meeting, "Do you want me to stop now?" He said no, and according to what some people in the audience later told me, they would have killed him if he had answered yes.

This was a beautiful presentation of the feasibility of the artificial heart, and Harry Norton continued to work with us for some time. Later, another engineer, Kirby Hiller, from NASA Lewis Research Center, helped our group and asked, "Why do you use all this mechanical hardware and electrohydraulic systems? Why not just use air, which is light and easily controllable?" I agreed to this, and we built what we called NASA Towers. This was a very beautiful kind of machine where you could program the air pressure wave you wished to use and the amount of pressure you wished to employ and experiment with various combinations to give the best results. And it was easy to get grant money for this kind of machine because, when something is complicated and looks like very clever engineering, people respect it. When you come in with a simple device, you can never get any money to support it.

The problem with NASA Towers was that you needed a pilot's license to drive the damn thing. It was always broken down when we needed it the most. Then and there I decided that, if we were going to build an artificial heart, it would have to be very simple, and this is what has guided us ever since. We have also come to concentrate on air-driven hearts as the most practical.

■ You were at the Cleveland Clinic for seventeen years, from 1950 to 1967. Why did you leave?

The Cleveland Clinic had broken its promises to me so often that it became quite clear that I could never accomplish there what I had set out to do. I was very friendly with the people there, but they just thought differently from the way I did. I managed to circumvent a lot of the obstruction by having appointments in two departments: surgery and research. Then the day came when I was told that I could only be a member of one. I realized then that I would be losing whatever leverage I had and decided to leave.

The same evening when I learned that I would be given the choice of either one department or the other by the Clinic I called up C. William Hall in San Antonio. He had been an associate of DeBakey in Houston and had been running the artificial heart program for him. I figured the best place for me would be one with a strong regional medical program because that was where an artificial organs program would have the best chance of succeeding. I asked Hall who had the best regional medical program, and without hesitation he said, "Salt Lake City." Keith Reemtsma was head of surgery there at the time. I knew him and had a good relationship with him. Although there were other opportunities offered me, I decided to go to Utah to set up a biomedical engineering institute. What especially impressed me was the promise of the associate dean at the medical school, Dr. Tom King, that at the University of Utah there would be a very short chain of command. No red tape would be allowed to stand in my way, and I would report directly to the vice-president of research for action on my grant and contract applications.

I have been in Utah for sixteen years now, and it has worked out very well.

■ One of your major accomplishments, if not the major accomplishment, in Utah has been the artificial heart program. Although you actually began this work in Cleveland and a number of people are involved "behind the scenes," I think most people are interested in how you brought DeVries and Jarvik into the picture.

Robert Jarvik came to me as a premedical student after having been unable to get into any American medical school. He had been going to the medical school in Bologna for two years, but there were Socialist strikes at the time and he did not wish to go back. A Ph.D. from Ethicon first told me about him in 1971 and described him to me as a very ingenious fellow. He assured me that if I took Jarvik on as an assistant he could probably get funds from Ethicon to pay for him. I spoke to Jarvik, who was on the East Coast, over the telephone, and asked him to come out to Salt Lake City. While awaiting word from Ethicon, he needed something to live on, and I asked him how little he needed to manage. This was not because I begrudged him the money but only because I didn't have it in my budget. He asked for two hundred dollars a month. Three months later Ethicon called and told me that funding for his support by their research committee was turned down. So until he got his own research grants many years later I supported Jarvik and we had a very good relationship. It could be described as a father-son sort of thing, but sometimes the son revolts against the father.

DeVries came to Cleveland while I was still there in 1967, I believe, and was assigned to work with us on the artificial heart. He was still a medical student in Utah at the time but wrote a paper on "Consumption Coagulation Shock and the Heart," a problem we found in animals with artificial hearts. This became a classic after publication in 1970.

He completed medical school in 1970 and went to Duke University for one of those terribly long ten-year residencies in thoracic and cardiovascular surgery. He returned to Utah intending to get involved with the artificial heart program even though another man had just been appointed head of cardiothoracic surgery at the University of Utah and there really wasn't room for two. The other fellow, however, decided to go into private practice, and DeVries was appointed to the position.

■ I don't believe there's anyone alive with his head on straight who does not know about Barney Clark, the first human recipient of an artificial heart. I think you should know, however, that in some quarters the University of Utah has been criticized for the way it was publicized. The sometimes "circus" atmosphere there has been contrasted, for example, with the low profile of the heart transplantation team under Norman Shumway at Stanford.

It is very unfair for others to criticize the Utah people for the way they handled the publicity. To begin with, there is no comparison with Stanford; heart transplantation is no longer "newsworthy," having been around since 1967. As for the situation in Utah, you must understand that all these reporters were not invited. They came, probably about a hundred of them, with TV cameras, radios, photographers, et cetera, and we had to accommodate them. You have no idea of what we had to contend with. Finally, it was a choice between dealing with the press in an organized way, as Chase Peterson [vice president for health sciences] did very well, or letting them write whatever crazy things they might pick up from all sorts of odd and uninformed people who happened to be in the vicinity. The reporting of Dr. Peterson was factual, accurate, honest, and complete. I made a statement to the assembled press conference only on the day before surgery to warn them against overoptimism, and spoke only for a minute on the following day in response to a question.

The only thing we were not prepared for was that the newspapers would put such a monetary value on any extra little thing they could get. Photographs of Barney Clark as a young man were obtained from the family and sold in Europe for hundreds of dollars. I have also seen a letter from a reporter to a medical resident whom he mistook for one of the surgical residents in the intensive care unit where Barney Clark was located. It was an invitation to dinner but also an ill-disguised bribe to get some inside information about the patient. This sort of thing went on for the entire period of his hospitalization. Even at the funeral there were more than twenty reporters about and two helicopters flying overhead.

■ While you're answering these charges you might address another, that the publicity regarding Barney Clark was welcomed by Utah to use as a wedge to

pry more money loose from the federal government in support of your program.

This is a loaded question, and it is incorrect. I just said that
we had no other choice but to give the proper information. Yet
it did have a beneficial effect in that the NHLBI [National
Heart, Lung and Blood Institute], following Barney Clark's
implantation on December 2, 1982, increased their allocation
with many more millions of dollars.

We have not been very lucky in getting money from the
NIH. It's true that we get some. We have support for an electrohydraulic heart and also for an air-driven heart. On the
other hand, I have submitted the same proposal in four different versions for left and right ventricular assist devices. So far,
it has not been approved. For a feasibility study we were
awarded fifty thousand dollars, an amount with which we
could do very little. Then one reviewer said that our projected
study of blood coagulation was unnecessary. In the last study
section another reviewer said that the coagulation study was
not sophisticated enough; and so I got nowhere. We have not
had much luck with the NHLBI either. Another manufacturer,
using Jarvik's motor and Jarvik's pump, got funded for the
electrohydraulic heart. We did not.

The NIH was against our putting a total heart in any patient. Fortunately, Schweiker, the secretary of health at the
time, ruled that the FDA, and not the NIH, was the agency to
rule on the use of new drugs and new medical devices. If we
had had to go through the NIH human experimentation committee, do you know with whom we would have had to deal?
It is said, but probably half in jest: two priests, a cleaning
woman, a banker, and a union leader. This is the kind of committee that frustrated all the studies of Jack Norman, who was
trying to develop a left ventricular assist device for Denton
Cooley. The protocol they had to adopt was so impossible that
every patient was three-quarters dead before he could be ad-

mitted to the study. All twenty-three of the patients they tried it on died—not a single one left the hospital alive. That's even worse than the first fifteen patients I treated with my artificial kidney. So you can see why I wanted to avoid the NIH review committee. We got funded from independent sources for Barney Clark's surgery, and they couldn't stop DeVries from operating because, not being subsidized by the government, he was free to act.

■ The public is just not aware of all these things, and often those who contribute a great deal to a project are forgotten by posterity. In August 1980, more than two years before the Barney Clark experience, you sent a staff memo to this effect, anticipating what lay ahead. I'd like to read a portion of it back to you.

"When the artificial heart will be implanted into a human recipient the principal surgeon in charge is the one who takes the greatest risk to his career, the greatest part of the blame when things go wrong, but also the greatest publicity. It is this last part I want you to ponder long before the time of the actual implantation. It may be very difficult for those of us who have worked so very long on the total artificial heart to accept that the total publicity will be handled by the surgeon. His name will be flashed on the TV screen and over the news media. If some of us are mentioned, it will be due to the surgeon's generosity in thinking of us at that moment. You must also assume that although he will probably think of us during the first, second or third news release, he cannot continue to do so. Also, when the artificial heart's successful transplantation is done in man, and we hope its successful implantation will be described, this will be done by the surgeon, most likely at a surgical meeting of a society to which we do not even belong. . . .

"What I want to warn you about is that you may not like the way the publicity is going to be handled. Some of this may be inevitable, some of this may be unjust, none of it is done with a particular design towards hurting you. Our main reward must be to know that we have done our best and that in time, patients will be saved who are now doomed and that they will be saved through our efforts."

I wanted them to know what was coming and have them be thankful for whatever credit they got and not be bitter because, after all, if anything went wrong it would be the surgeon who went to jail and not them!

■ What do you think of the future of the artificial kidney and the artificial
heart?

I am convinced that, with the introduction of cyclosporin A
and other effective immunosuppressive agents to prevent rejection, kidney transplantation from almost any individual to
another will be possible in the future and eliminate the need
for the artificial kidney. After all, we all have two kidneys, and
need only one to live.

As for the heart, you will never get enough good hearts that
you can use for transplantation. Not by any stretch of the
imagination. And there are perhaps fifty thousand patients
dying each year in the United States who might be good candidates for the artificial heart.

■ How far do you think we are from a totally implantable artificial heart?

With an outside source of power delivered transcutaneously
[through the skin] with the use of coils, at least five years. I
had a contract for years for a better approach, a nuclear-driven
heart where the amount of radiation exposure would be minimal. But the nuclear-driven heart is without prospect with the
current hysteria over nuclear energy, an hysteria quite unrelated to the validity of the concept. Before it dies down you
and I will long be buried.

■ You are mostly known for the kidney and the cardiovascular devices you
have developed. What has happened to the others, such as the artificial eye and
ear?

We haven't done anything about the artificial eye for seven
years since the man in charge of the program left for Columbia University. This is very specialized work that cannot
easily be taken over by another. Still, we have gone further
with it than anyone else. We have definitely proven that if you
have an array of electrodes over the visual cortex of the brain
and stimulate them properly, meaningful images will be perceived by a completely blind person. At present, the system

requires a roomful of computers, and the subject has to hold a television camera. But the principle is sound, and all that is needed is miniaturization of the system.

With the artificial ear, miniaturization has been achieved by Dr. Don Eddington and Jeff Orth. Whereas we once needed a roomful of computers to run it, this has now been reduced to a box no bigger than a pack of cigarettes. A tiny electrode coiled up in the cochlea of the ear is stimulated, and a totally deaf man can hear eighty-five percent of spoken words without seeing the lips of the speaker.

■ With all the projects you have going and all that you have accomplished, you must have been very well organized. Your former associate at Cleveland, Donald Effler, calls you the most ambitious man he has ever known.

I don't think "ambitious" is the right word. It has an unpleasant connotation, meaning ambition for oneself. But I can develop a very strong driving force, and I will persevere. I very rarely give up, and if I have to relent temporarily, I usually come back to the project later.

I have had certain goals I wanted to reach, usually in terms of an artificial organ that could create happiness for people. Not simply through the simple prolongation of life, but only *happy* life.

These are honest and good goals and deserve to be pushed. It is true that I cannot stand it if something blocks me from reaching these goals. I may get a little difficult when people try to block me, and if one way is occluded I'll find another.

Financially I have always "walked on a tightrope," but have managed to keep my balance. Calamities and disasters have turned out to my advantage in the long run. For example, when my wife and I were in the Hague for a funeral, the Germans invaded the Netherlands. For us, that was the beginning of World War II. I went to the largest hospital in the city and was given the opportunity to set up a blood bank. It was a wonderful experience because, through necessity, everybody helped. It was the first blood bank in Europe, and it is still in existence.

In Utah, once a large number of our sheep were stolen. I first thought that it was a disaster. They were stolen in a year that I had grants and enough money; the insurance paid us back in a year when we were nearly broke, and it saved us.

When our laboratory at the university burned out in 1973, it was a disaster. However, twenty days later we moved to the old St. Mark's Hospital. Dr. Don Olsen has remodeled its surgical wing into the most advanced experimental laboratory for artificial organs in the world. We could never have afforded such a facility on the university campus.

■ You're seventy-two years old now and have been going full-blast all your life. Are you thinking of retiring soon?

I'm having a good time. Why should I?

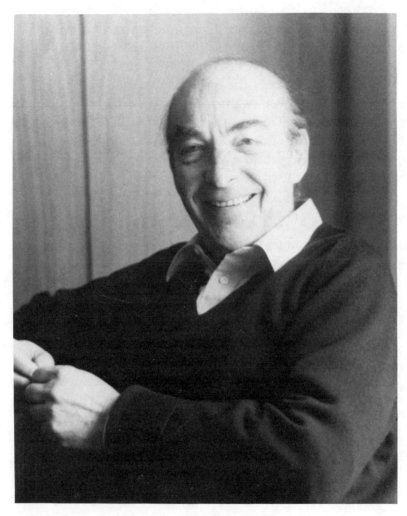

Arthur Kornberg, M.D.

CHAPTER 17

Arthur Kornberg, M.D.
(1918–   )

W HAT IS the medicine of the future, molecular biology, all about? The substance we now call DNA (deoxyribonucleic acid) was recognized as early as 1870 by the Swiss scientist, Johann Friedrich Miescher, who isolated it from the nuclei of salmon sperm cells. It was not until amost the mid-twentieth century, however, that its true significance began to be appreciated.

Begining in 1940 a series of, at first, seemingly unrelated discoveries ineluctably progressed at an ever accelerating rate over the next forty years to lead us into the era of genetic engineering, recombinant DNA, and all the rest. In 1940 at Stanford University, a biochemist, Edward L. Tatum, and a geneticist, George N. Beadle, were working with the red bread mold, *Neurospora.* Inducing mutuations with X rays, much in the way that Herrmann J. Muller in Thomas Hunt Morgan's laboratory had previously done with *Drosophila* (the fruit fly), Beadle and Tatum found that the nutritional requirements of *Neurospora* could be changed by an alteration in its genetic makeup. The dictum "one gene, one enzyme" resulted.

On the other side of the continent, working at the Rockefeller Institute, a physician-microbiologist, Oswald Avery, and his coworkers were trying to develop an antiserum to the pneumococcus, a frequent cause of death in preantibiotic times. In 1944 they reported a hereditable change that might occur when a harmless form of the pneumococcus, one without a capsule, was exposed to a substance obtained from the pathogenic capsular form. The substance was DNA.

In 1946 Joshua Lederberg, a protégé of Tatum, demonstrated sexual reproduction in the bacterium *E. coli*, a ubiquitous resident of our large bowels. That genetic material could be transferred from one generation of *E. coli* to another suggested that this lowly, experimentally accessible form of life might be a suitable model in which future investigations regarding life processes in man might be addressed. A few years later, in 1952, Lederberg and Norton D. Zinder would show that certain viruses that infected bacteria, the bacteriophages, were capable of transmitting chromosomal material from one bacterium to another and thus provide another approach to the study of genetics and cell biology.

Then in 1953 James D. Watson and Francis Crick, using X-ray crystallography, as developed in England under the Braggs at Cambridge University, were able to come up with the correct model for the structure of DNA. Further developments in the United States, Great Britain, France, and elsewhere were soon to be revealed to the scientific community.

All these advances in biochemistry, microbiology, and genetics were catalyzed by the world of physics through one of its eminent practitioners. Erwin Schrödinger, a founder of modern quantum mechanics, was instrumental in this regard through his slim volume published in 1944, *What Is Life?* In it Schrödinger persuasively argued that the very secrets of life itself were now amenable to exploration by the physical and chemical means already at hand in laboratories throughout the world.

It was into this maelstrom of scientific excitement and creativity that Arthur Kornberg plunged in the postwar 1940s as he forsook a career in clinical medicine for one in basic biochemical research.

After receiving his M.D. from the University of Rochester in 1941, and serving a year as medical intern at the Strong Memorial Hospital, Dr. Kornberg had entered the Public Health Service. Following the war he remained in the Health Service at the then fledgling National Institutes of Health (NIH), studying rat nutrition until 1946. He then left the NIH temporarily to study enzymology for a year with Severo Ochoa at New York University and then with Carl and Gerty Cori at Washington University, St. Louis.

In 1947 Dr. Kornberg returned to Bethesda, Maryland, where he organized the first Enzyme Section at the NIH, and carried out fundamental studies on coenzyme biosynthesis, which led to his initial recognition as a leading investigator in this field. In 1953 he left the NIH to become professor and chairman of the Department of Microbiology at Washington University, St. Louis. In 1959 he left St. Louis to head the Department of Biochemistry at Stanford University, where he has remained ever since.

Among many awards for his research accomplishments Dr. Kornberg received the Nobel Prize in medicine in 1959 for his work on DNA replication. This award he shared with his former mentor, Severo Ochoa, who was recognized for parallel work involving the synthesis of RNA (ribonucleic acid).

Because of his unusual background, combining both clinical medicine and basic science, Dr. Kornberg is uniquely equipped to provide a most complete view of his subject and a special insight into the way of an investigator. His gift for lucid and compelling prose, as demonstrated in the ensuing conversation, provides an added advantage. His personal history, with his surmounting of numerous obstacles to the career he ultimately realized, can serve as an inspiration to all in our society, especially to those with humble or disadvantaged origins.

■ Since most of your professional life has been spent in basic science, I suspect that most people think of you as a Ph.D. rather than an M.D. Could you tell me what it was that directed you out of clinical medicine and into basic science?

I grew up in Brooklyn during the depression, and recall that at first I wanted to be a high school teacher because my brother, who was thirteen years my senior, was already teaching elementary school at the time I entered it. By the time I got to City College in 1933, my ambitions had been raised from teaching high school chemistry to college chemistry. But very early at City College I was told by an indulgent and devoted dean (Morton Gottschall) that there would be little future for me in college teaching. There were no openings at City College on the faculty then, nor were there likely to be for many years to come. I had better think of something else.

I was a good and eager student, so during my second year I began to take biology courses in addition to chemistry and became a premed. I originally had no ambition to become a doctor, but going to medical school seemed a natural course to take because it was a refuge from doing something less inspiring, and it would give me several more years of doing what I enjoyed, going to school and learning new things.

You have heard how difficult it was getting into medical school in that period, but I didn't get too apprehensive about it. I had never been farther than twenty miles from New York until then. I drew a perimeter of about four hundred miles around New York City and applied to the schools within it. I was summarily rejected from just about every one: Albany,

Buffalo, Columbia, Harvard, Cornell, and so on. It was a tough time for a Jewish boy from Brooklyn to get accepted to medical school. Columbia, for example, had not accepted a student from City College for ten years even though they had available a full scholarship for a City College graduate, the Jacobi Scholarship. Of my whole class of some two hundred applicants—and it was an excellent group of students—only five or so were accepted to medical school.

I was fortunate to be accepted at two schools. One was the Long Island College of Medicine in Brooklyn, which is now called the Downstate Medical Center of the SUNY system. Then, for some strange reason, the University of Rochester also offered me a place. I would have gone to the Brooklyn school because of my parents' preference, and it would have been more economical, but Joe Bunim, a family friend, and my premed college advisor (Professor A. J. Goldfarb), urged that I go to Rochester. Joe Bunim was a rheumatologist in New York and had a teaching appointment at New York University Medical School. He was a wonderful man. So I went to Rochester. It was an adventure. It was the right choice. Rochester is still a good school, but then it was outstanding, with a dedication to science unusual for the time.

■ Were your parents very influential in directing you during this time of your life?

Oh, no. They had an enormous love and respect for what I was doing and hoped that I would succeed. They were utterly devoted but were in no position to guide me. My father had been a scholarly man but immigrated to the United States when he was twenty-two, as did my mother at sixteen. He was self-taught, never having had any opportunities in Europe for formal education. He had assimilated many languages and was always eager to learn more. In order to earn a living, upon arriving in the United States, he was forced to become a sewing machine operator, "in cloaks" as they called it then. His health was often poor. In the early nineteen-twenties he had an opportunity to open a little hardware store in Bath Beach and barely managed to scrape a living out of it. When I was accepted to medical school, I had some savings from having worked throughout my years in college and some scholarship awards. It would have been sensible for me to have gone to work to help support the family, as most young people did in those days, but my parents skimped in order to help me continue at school. A scholarship of three hundred dollars from Rochester paid my tuition. While I was still a medical student, about twenty years old, my mother died, gas gangrene having set in after a cholecystectomy. By this time my father was blind from a retinal detachment which had been unsuccessfully treated. I had to borrow money from a bank in Rochester to finish my medical education.

■ How did you do as a medical student at Rochester?

Although we were graded at Rochester, we did not learn of our grades until we got home at the end of the year. So when I returned home after the first year, my parents anxiously inquired as to how I had done. You always worried about getting bounced from school, but I said, "If they bounce me, I think they will have to bounce a few more before me." When the letter finally came, I nervously tore it open hoping that I had survived and found that I had been awarded some kind of a prize for my performance during the first year of school.

It was a practice at Rochester to offer fellowships to outstanding students to take a year out of medical school to do research. To be selected for some of these fellowships was to be "anointed" and on the way to an academic career. I didn't get any of the fellowships, some of which I would not have accepted had I been offered them. Many years later, in 1954 I think, as chairman of the Department of Microbiology in Washington University Medical School in St. Louis, I participated in a teaching conference on microbiology and pathology in French Lick Springs, Indiana. Another professor attending had previously been an instructor at Rochester when I was a student.

In a workshop discussing grading of students, I stated my strong preference for purely objective grades without any personal evaluations. After the discussion, this pathologist said, "Arthur, I'm surprised at the stand you took on grading. Back at Rochester they always placed great emphasis on the personality of the student, how he behaved, etcetera." I said, "That is *precisely* what I don't want to do." He was puzzled. "Let's make it simple," I continued. "Some people were anti-Semitic at Rochester." The pathologist hesitated a moment, and then, as if to console me, said, "You know, they didn't like Italians either."

Later, at Stanford, I was visited by the president of the University of Rochester to inquire about my interest in becoming dean of the medical school. I told him I wasn't interested in being a dean. "Don't you, out of loyalty, have a sentimental attachment to Rochester?" he asked. When I told him of the discrimination that had deprived me of a research fellowship he said, "You know, I was at Stanford at that time, and the problems were the same here." It was universal.

I've wondered many times why very decent people at Rochester and elsewhere condoned discrimination. At Rochester these people included some important scientists. It could be Jews, Italians, or blacks. They went along with it. I guess they reasoned that, since there was little chance of these minority people becoming distinguished academicians, there was no sense in wasting precious fellowships on them. Let them just go and practice medicine among their own people.

Prejudice against women in science is the same. When women trained in precious scientific slots fail to find jobs compatible with marriage, they then abandon science. You then tend to discriminate against women rather than remove the barriers to their academic careers in science.

■   That's a circular kind of reasoning.

A vicious cycle of reasoning. Now we are trying to make up
for the earlier prejudices by showing preference, whenever
possible, for women and blacks.

■   We still haven't discussed what got you into research. What were the
influences that worked upon you in medical school?

I can cite both negative and positive ones. First, the negative. I had seen doctors in white coats going in and out of the
laboratories. These were internists doing research. I thought, I
could never spend all that time in the laboratory without
seeing patients. These role models didn't inspire me. I had no
interest in medicine as a business, nor could I see myself in a
strictly laboratory setting. I was further discouraged by an
early attempt at research. I asked a clinical endocrinologist
(Doran Stephens) for something to work on during the summer after my second year.

He gave me some boxes of slides to take home. They contained sections of thyroid glands from experimental animals,
used for assays of thyrotropic hormone. I was supposed to
measure the height of the acinar cells. In Brooklyn that hot
summer with my primitive microscope, I tried to make these
measurements. I simply could not make any reproducible
measurements and was totally frustrated. I decided, "I'm just
not cut out to do research."

■   Famous last words!

After trying for a week I gave it up as a bad job. On the
positive side I was a good student, acquisitive of information. I
collected no fauna or flora as a youngster, nor did anybody I
knew. I collected matchbook covers as a kid, and my father
would risk getting trampled to death in the subways trying to
pick up a matchbook cover that was not in my collection.

I don't recall asking any highly interesting or original questions of a scientific nature, but then something happened

that, as I look back on it, did represent an evidence of scientific initiative. A classmate noticed that my sclerae were yellow. He said, "You ought to have your icterus index measured." This was a colorimetric test in which the intensity of the color of serum was measured against a standard to indicate any degree of hyperbilirubinemia, or jaundice. Sure enough, mine was up, and although I felt well, they started investigating my gallbladder. I cooperated by developing some gastrointestinal symptoms, having earlier recovered from several fatal diseases I'd read about. There were even suggestions of removing my gallbladder.

Fortunately, this didn't progress but stimulated my interest. I later obtained some blood from the samples taken from the new medical school class and measured icteric indices. I found one guy who had a value even higher than mine and some others in the abnormal range.

A year or so later I was given a grant of one hundred dollars by the chairman of the Department of Medicine, Dr. William S. McCann, to buy bilirubin to do bilirubin tolerance tests on patients. I just selected some patients on the wards, gave them bilirubin, and collected blood samples over several hours to see how well they removed it.

■ It's a good thing the statute of limitations has run out.

I remember a kid who spiked a high fever and the resident came raging around asking, "What the hell is going on here?" Someone told him, "Kornberg has been here giving him bilirubin." I had some very anxious moments until that kid was okay. Anyway, my first paper, published in the *Journal of Clinical Investigation,* described this work. It was a prestigious journal even then, and the title of the paper was "Latent Liver Disease in Persons Recovered from Catarrhal Jaundice and in Otherwise Normal Medical Students as Revealed by the Bilirubin Excretion Test." I was one of the students, of course.

I still have mild fluctuating jaundice, as does one of my sons, and we obviously have Gilbert's syndrome [a mild congenital form of hyperbilirubinemia unrelated to liver disease]. In the paper to describe the patients I used the term "catarrhal jaundice," which was in vogue because we didn't know about viral hepatitis then.

There was an amusing incident related to this research on jaundice. When the army was inducting troops in the mobilizations of 1941 and 1942 they were injecting them with yellow fever vaccine and experiencing a tremendous incidence of serum hepatitis. Soldiers were coming down with severe cases, with some of them dying. The army didn't know what to do and was looking for help anywhere they could find it. A team came to Rochester to see the professor of pathology and dean, "The Great Whipple,"[b] but they also wanted to consult with Kornberg because of that paper I had just published. Whipple was nonplussed when they asked to see me too.

■   You have expressed an admiration for Dr. McCann, who was obviously of a different stripe from any of the other faculty you encountered as a student.

William S. McCann was chief of medicine while I was a student and intern at Rochester and one of the few people who gave me encouragement in research. I mentioned his getting me money for those bilirubin tolerance studies. As a department head, he was also free of prejudice in dealing with students and house officers. His was the only department that had a Jewish chief resident while I was there. He was also politically liberal, with moral strength and personal courage. In the years immediately preceding World War II, there was a very strong isolationist sentiment in this country, the America First movement. Whipple and many of the Rochester group were strong and vocal supporters of it. They opposed aid to Britain, for example, when England was alone in fighting the Nazis. To speak in support of American aid to Great Britain in that kind of environment, as McCann did, I thought was very admirable.

■ It was the war that ultimately led you to the NIH. How did that come about?

After the attack on Pearl Harbor in December 1941 everybody began to be mobilized for the armed forces. I would be finishing my internship in medicine in mid-1942 and considered where I should go. McCann wanted me to go into the navy with him, but I chose the Public Health Service. It wasn't that I was frightened of military duty. It was because my professor of bacteriology, George Packer Berry, indicated that the Public Health Service might provide more of an opportunity to learn something while in the service of the country.

There was one other member of my class who had research experience and seemed interested in a research career. Leon Heppel[b] had come to medical school after earning a Ph.D. in physiology. He had made a very important discovery. Using newly developed isotopic techniques, he had shown that, in the potassium-deprived laboratory animal, sodium would enter cells in its place. It was a major discovery. He supported his research while in medical school with a small grant from a local pharmaceutical company. Heppel and I joined the Public Health Service.

Heppel was immediately assigned to the NIH, which at the time was rather small, mainly an infectious disease laboratory, and only a small part of the Public Health Service. I was first assigned to Boston to examine recruits for the Coast Guard and then was assigned to sea duty. Heppel kept mentioning to the NIH director, Rolland Dyer, that he had a talented friend by the name of Kornberg who would be a great addition to the NIH staff.

At first I enjoyed my sea duty in the Gulf of Mexico and the Caribbean. The ship was based at St. Petersburg and made its way up and down the coast of Florida. It was the first vacation I had ever had. But then I began to get bored and started to collect blood from seamen to check bilirubin levels. During all this I was increasingly annoying to the captain. I knew nothing of naval etiquette and, unwittingly, assumed authority as the physician that belonged to the captain of the ship. I got off on the wrong foot with him when I refused to give this healthy, plethoric man the vitamin shots that the previous doctor did. My reasonable actions often irritated him no end. For example, on one occasion, when we had a seriously ill seaman aboard and were heading into port, I arranged to have an ambulance at the dock to take the sailor to the local hospital. When the captain saw the ambulance and asked, "What is that ambulance doing there?" someone told him that the doctor had ordered it. "The *doctor* had ordered it!" He was furious.

When my transfer orders to the NIH came, the captain was not unhappy about seeing me go.

At the NIH I was assigned to the Nutrition Section headed by W. Henry Sebrell. This was the laboratory that had been established by Joseph Goldberger,[b] one of my heroes of medicine and one of the great vitamin hunters. Sebrell had worked under Goldberger and had inherited his mantle and later became the director of the NIH.

By the time I arrived Sebrell was already distracted by administrative matters, and the lab was really being run by Floyd Daft, who became my immediate supervisor. I was put to work on rat nutrition. Heppel and I both looked upon our positions there as temporary—much like the other tours of duty in the military, with transfers every year or two.

Thomas Parran, the surgeon general then (when this post really carried authority), changed all that. He said the Health Services had traditionally wanted well-rounded officers, but what it needed were officers who were "less well rounded and sharper at the edges." As a result, Heppel and I stayed on at the NIH for more than the traditional tour of duty.

I fed rats with purified diets, looking for the exacerbation or induction of nutritional deficiencies. After about a year I felt that I could do this work full-time with a great deal of pleasure and gave up the idea that, inevitably, after the war I would go back to clinical practice. It is significant that I did not agonize over this decision. Heppel, for instance, years after we were at the NIH, would periodically brush up on his obstetrics and gynecology, etcetera, in anticipation of having to take state licensing examinations to return to the practice of medicine. Other friends of mine in similar positions also tried to keep their feet on both shores, straddling basic research and clinical medicine. This indecision dilutes your efforts. For me it seemed easy just to leave clinical medicine and focus on basic research.

Things went well at the NIH. I became resourceful in establishing a large rat colony and published many papers. After three years of this, I did something my friends at the NIH thought was mad. I quit the rat work and left to study biochemistry.

Sebrell was shrewd enough to see that this a was a good move. He knew that vitamin hunting was nearing its end. You could no longer "kick your feet in the dirt" like a gold prospector and come up with a big "nugget," a new vitamin. Almost all the vitamins were discovered by 1945. He thought he would let this ambitious young man "pick somebody's brains," as he said, and then come back and discover new enzymes.

■ This led to your year in New York with Severo Ochoa[b] in 1946 and then to a year with the Coris, Carl and Gerty, [b] in Washington University in St. Louis. What was this like?

I went to work with Ochoa, and it was a very fortunate choice, because he had no other postdoctoral people at the time. He had only one student. He was actually working in somebody else's laboratory space at New York University Medical School. Ochoa impressed me greatly, and we have been close friends ever since. Ochoa had the unusual capacity of being critical and yet seeing the bright side of things. He would ask if *this* could be interpreted in any other way or *that* could have come about through other circumstances. But he was always optimistic.

It was an exciting time even though there were some personal hardships involved. It was right after the war, and the housing situation in New York was impossible. I was still in uniform, so the Officers' Service Club was helpful, but my wife and I stayed in some of the worst hotels in New York. Every day or two, we would find ourselves moving out of one dive into another. But it was a great experience at NYU, and I could spend hours talking about it. My curve of learning was exponential. I could stay up until one in the morning reading papers in German, which was difficult for me, but then start off early the next day with tremendous drive. This new language and new culture was so invigorating. Instead of waiting four to six weeks for a rat to develop a nutritional deficiency, I was doing spectrophotometric assays that were complete in a minute. Setting up these experiments and seeing the needles move was very exciting.

I remember back at the NIH, when I was similarly enthusiastic about my nutritional experiments, there was a fellow researcher in nutrition, Milton Silverman, who asked me one day, "What are you so excited about?" I said, "This work is enormously interesting. Don't you get excited about your nutrition work?" Actually, his work on microbial nutrition was more important than mine on rats. "The only nutrition that excites me," he answered, "is the nutrition of Milton Silverman." Looking back, I did have an enormous enthusiasm, the quality I admired in Ochoa. You appreciate it when you see it, but you cannot give it to anyone.

I managed to extend my stay with Ochoa from three months to six months and then to a year. I don't know how I wangled it, but I got permission to go on to the Coris laboratory in St. Louis to learn more biochemistry. At that time, right after the war, it was a haven for ambitious, gifted people from all over the world to study with Carl and Gerty Cori. In the eight months I spent with them, my curve of learning continued to be steep. I had very little background in biochemistry. Mildren Cohn reminded me recently of that.

Just last week I gave a Mildred Cohn Lecture at the University of Pennsylvania honoring our most eminent female biochemist. She was with the Coris when I arrived there and years later told me how appalled she was at my ignorance. Following my stay with the Coris, I returned to the NIH. I had an interesting reception. I was not concerned with salary, housing, and other benefits, but I assumed that I would be given adequate laboratory space, even though I had not made specific inquiries before returning. Sebrell and Daft had decided to tease me a bit, so when I returned they led me to a little room off a kitchen where rat diets were prepared and told me that this was where I would be working. I took one look and told them, "I guess there is no place for me here. I will find somewhere else to work." I was ready to quit on the spot. They were embarassed by my response and immediately revealed the joke they were trying to play. I then set up the first Enzyme Section at the NIH.

This was a fortuitous time, not only for me, but for Heppel and another friend of mine, Bernard Horecker,[b] a biochemist who had done enzyme studies in graduate school and resumed them at the NIH before I left for New York. Palace revolutions were constantly going on at the NIH, and both Heppel and Horecker had just been displaced from their laboratories. I was able to get them laboratory space under my administrative direction in a newly designated Enzyme Section. Both have had very eminent careers.

Gerty Cori once came to visit in Washington, D.C., during this period. She was an extraordinary woman. She was suffering from aplastic anemia and had to be wheeled to the meetings of the National Science Board. She was fond of me and said sympathetically how sad it was that I had to work in a government laboratory rather than in an academic institution. I assured here that there was no reason to feel this way, because the atmosphere we had at the NIH was academic and supportive. Heppel, Horecker, Herbert Tabor, and I established, among other things, what has now become a worldwide practice. We had noon seminars during our lunch hour. We discussed scientific material rather than politics or other matters. We were educating ourselves in biochemistry every day by presenting papers at these sessions.

Things began rolling, and the pattern of my future work began to take shape. This was to make an extract of a cell and try to reconstruct the reactions responsible for some cellular event of great interest.

I was interested in how a coenzyme was synthesized. The coenzyme was then called DPN [diphosphopyridine nucleotide] and is now known as NAD [nicotinamide adenine dinucleotide]. Within a couple of years I had published several papers which attracted attention in the biochemical community, which at that time was very small. Although people generally associate me with later work on DNA, it was in 1952 that my popularity was near its peak. Applications for postdoctoral fellowship work with me around that year came from Paul Berg,[b] Gordon Tomkins, Bruce Ames, Ed Korn, and others.

By 1952 the Enzyme Section at the NIH had been in operation for five years, and I was becoming unhappy with government restraints and pressures toward more administrative roles at the NIH. Then I was offered the chairmanship of the Department of Microbiology at Washington University in St. Louis. This school had a great tradition going back to the nineteenth century and was one of the few medical schools with a major commitment to research before this became popular, with people like Joseph E_langer[b] in physiology, Evarts Graham[b] in surgery, the Coris in biochemistry, Oliver Lowry[b] in pharmacology, and Barry Wood[b] in medicine. To be invited to become their youngest departmental chairman was a great honor, and I went there in 1953.

The facilities in the laboratories were dismal—bare light bulbs, tiny sinks, broken-down benches. Nevertheless, I assembled a group of colleagues, most of whom have stayed together. These people, now in their late fifties, have been innovative and have become leaders in biochemistry.

■ It was at Washington University that you began your work on DNA. Perhaps this point is as good a time as any to bring this into our discussion. You started off as an M.D., went into enzymology and biochemistry, then headed into microbiology. You seem to have incorporated almost every aspect of molecular biology into your own experience.

People are confused about what "molecular biology" really is. I would like to read to you from something I have written about it.

What are the origins of genetic chemistry, more popularly referred to now as "genetic engineering"? The isolation, analysis, synthesis and rearrangement of DNA genes and chromosomes are generally regarded as the achievements and domain of molecular biology. Assuming this to be largely true, what is molecular biology and what are its origins? Narrowing our focus on the molecular biology of DNA, I would cite several diverse origins.

One origin is in medical science. Oswald Avery, in his lifelong and relentless search for control of pneumococcal pneumonia, became the first to show that DNA is the molecule in which genetic information is stored.

The second origin of molecular biology is in microbial genetics. Microbiologists, some of them renegade physicists, chose the biology of the small bacterial vi-

ruses, the bacteriophages, to illustrate the functions of
the major biomolecules: DNA, RNA and proteins.

The third origin of microbiology is in the refined
structural chemistry of these biomolecules. Analysis of
the x-ray diffraction pattern of proteins revealed their
three-dimensional structure. The DNA patterns gave
us the double helix and a major insight into its replication and function.

The fourth origin of molecular biology is in biochemistry. The enzymology, analysis and synthesis of
nucleic acids. The nucleases that cut and disassemble
DNA into its genes and constituent building blocks.
The polymerases that reassemble them; the ligases that
link DNA chains into genes and the genes into chromosomes. These are the reagents that have made genetic
engineering possible. In the cell these enzyme actions
replicate, repair and rearrange the genes and the
chromosomes.

Molecular biologists practice chemistry without
calling it such. They identify and isolate genes from
huge chromosomes, often only one part in billions, and
then amplify by even larger magnitudes by microbial
cloning procedures. They map human chromosomes,
analyze their composition, isolate their components,
redesign their genetic arrangement, and produce them
in bacterial factories on a massive industrial scale. Not
even the boldest among us dreamed of this chemistry
ten years ago. Yet with all its success, molecular biology is making halting progress in answering some of
the profound questions of cellular functions and development. What governs the rearrangements of genes to
produce antibodies? What determines that a primitive
cell will develop into brain or bone? What underlies
growth and senescence of cells? The current ap-
proaches of molecular biology falter when they ignore
the products of the DNA blueprints, the enzymes and
proteins that represent the machinery and brainwork of
the cell.

The tides of fashion in science erode one beach to
create another. In the rush and excitement surrounding

the new mastery over DNA, the training and practice of enzymology have been neglected. Most of our students are introduced to enzymes as commercial reagents and find them as faceless as buffers and salts. As long as this relative inattention to enzymology persists, the basic issues of cell growth and development, degenerative disease and aging, will not be resolved. Molecular biology has successfully broken into the bank of the cellular operations, but for lack of biochemical tools and training, it is still fumbling to unlock the major vaults.

■ This was the message that I received in a section you wrote for a festschrift honoring Ochoa on his seventieth birthday. You called it "For the Love of Enzymes," and the first sentence reads: "I have never known a dull enzyme." You must realize that most physicians are either scared to death or bored to death by enzymes, usually a combination of the two. But after reading that piece by you, I asked myself, "What have I been missing all my life?" I wanted to go back to my chemistry books and find out all I could concerning enzymes . . .

I'm glad it had that effect.

■ . . . so now all you have to do is go out and convince the rest of the 375,000 physicians in the United States.

Not only physicians, but molecular biologists, genetic engineers, and developmental and cell biologists, who are on the current frontiers of science and who are just as untutored and insensitive in this regard. If you look at an enzyme, you will find that it is as intricate as an ant or some marine creature. The excitement about it is that if you can understand its anatomy and its movements, you can then understand how it handles a molecule.

I am engaging in a campaign to resurrect an interest in enzymology. I have had several encounters recently in which former students of my department have told me, for example, "I had forgotten all about enzymology." In working on the development of a worm—the developmental genetics of *Drosophila* or rearranging the SV40 chromosome, the power and beauty of enzymology had somehow receded from their attention.

■ Let's pick up your chronological history again. You were at Washington University for six years, until 1959. What made you leave for Stanford?

We could talk for hours about that, but basically, there were some things that were attractive about Stanford and some that were less attractive in St. Louis.

At Washington University I was a junior member of the faculty, and although I was listened to politely, I really did not swing an awful lot of weight among all the "hoary greats." Furthermore, I was a biochemically oriented individual responsible for teaching microbiology. Instead of teaching students about the diagnostic tests for syphilis and corynebacteria, we were doing something revolutionary. We were teaching students the genetics and chemistry of microbiology. It was the wave of the future but not recognized by the students as such. They simply weren't receptive and called the course "Biochemistry II." Later on, some of these students would come back and tell me how fortunate they felt, having been in our classes at Washington University, but, in reality, I was a biochemist masquerading as a bacteriologist. When I switched officially to biochemistry at Stanford, it was sort of like "coming out of the closet."

There were many things that attracted me to California, even though many of my friends and senior advisors felt that, if I left St. Louis for anywhere, it should be a place like Harvard. But I had been introduced to California when I worked in H. A. Barker's lab in the summer of 1951 and again when I took C. B. van Niel's microbiology course in Pacific Grove in the summer of 1953. California is a lovely place. Academically and intellectually, Stanford impressed me as representative of the West in its receptivity to new ideas and ways of doing things. California can be wacky and weird, but you don't find an atmosphere in its institutions that you might at institutions hundreds of years old, where people are apt to tell you, "This is the way we've always done it" at Harvard or Washington University.

I was offered a bright new building and department at Stanford and asked to be one of the leading people in developing a new curriculum, a new school, and a new outlook, all in an attractive setting. So I came to my group and asked if this was what they would like to do. They were all enthusiastic and wanted to come with me to Stanford. So we all went together and have remained pretty much together since.

■ I take it, then, that your years at Stanford have been very satisfying.

People tell me that as a department chairman I ought to be terribly proud of what I have done. I simply did what I thought was sensible. I didn't regard myself as a "professional chairman." I used what common sense I had and did what I thought was decent and helpful. It was and is a democratic department. When the chairmanship was taken over by Paul Berg, then by Robert Lehman, and now by Dale Kaiser, I found that I was doing very much the same things as before in the department. Being chairman meant that one had additional responsibilities for extradepartmental functions that were burdensome and frustrating. Within the department it was like a family, and my relationships with my colleagues have always been warm, cordial, and rewarding.

■ Your feelings about trying to educate medical students have not, apparently, been as sanguine as your thoughts about your faculty. You sent me a copy of a letter you wrote in 1956 to Carl Moore, who was then dean at Washington University and heading a committee on the purpose of medical education. It obviously is important to you still, so I want to quote from it: "The most striking impression of the three years that I have been here is that we have a faculty with a rich and wonderful tradition of unswerving dedication to research while our medical students are about as congenitally free of an understanding of the scientific method as any non-scientific group in society."

My son, Roger, who is on the Stanford faculty, began to take an active interest in these matters, as I did twenty-seven years ago at Washington University. I dug this letter out of my files and showed it to him and Bob Lehman. They just shook their heads; they couldn't believe that in twenty-seven years nothing had changed.

■ It seems to me that if an individual just doesn't have that spark in him there is nothing you really can do about it. Look at your own history: there was nothing in your background to push you into research.

I agree. My family, my friends knew nothing about science. I came to it, as I told you, in a most circuitous and unlikely way. Students come for counseling as to whether they should go for the M.D. or Ph.D. degree. I used to waste an enormous amount of time, trying to provide this guidance. I finally took the advice Bob Lehman gave me. He said that if they have to ask for someone else's opinion about this choice, advise them to take the M.D.

■ Your sons, however, did have some direction. I read that your oldest, Roger, as a twelve-year-old was playing with biochemical experiments in your laboratory at Stanford.

My wife and I have been very fortunate with all three of our sons. Roger has a marvelous chemical background and is doing work that awes me. My second son, Tom, who is an associate professor of biochemistry, has gone more toward genetics, and he is doing very, very imaginative work studying the developmental genetics of *Drosophila*. My third son has a more artistic bent. He is an architect, specializing in laboratory design. In the past year he has become the most sought after man in his field because he has a sensitivity for what laboratories should be as attractive, living places in which to work.

■ There is one more subject I would like to cover, and that is the relationship between science and industry, more specifically, scientists and industry. This is certainly nothing new but seems especially critical now. I would like to mention to you just three news items of the recent past and get your response.

1. Genentech was established in 1976. In 1980 the *Wall Street Journal*

estimated that Herbert Boyer's[b] stock shares were worth forty million dollars at that time.

2. Walter Gilbert,[b] like yourself a Nobel laureate, during an interview unabashedly makes the remark that he considers himself both a businessman and a scientist.

3. All kinds of pharmaceutical houses and technological firms are making special deals with institutions like the Massachusetts Institute of Technology, Harvard, and even Stanford.

What effect will all this have on the progress of science?

You realize that I am myself involved. Yet, I have never been interested in the entrepreneurial aspects of science. Not only did I not seek our consultantships, I avoided them. But universities are entrepreneurial and need money. Stanford has always encouraged professors to use one day a week for this kind of extracurricular activity. Silicon Valley, near Stanford, and the home of much of the computer industry and related technology, is the product of this enlightened policy. Even the NIH, years ago, urged that its investigators be granted patents so that basic research would be applied and investigators and the institutions would be rewarded for their efforts.

I am aware, as you implied, of resentment of some scientists who have gotten disproportionately wealthy from work that others have done. On the other hand, why should business tycoons get such rewards for even less good reasons? These entrepreneurial scientists are certainly more deserving than some business people who have gained wealth through intricate financial maneuvers.

There is a danger, however, to entrepreneurial activity for a research scientist. If a professor is consumed with promoting his business and exploits the work his students are doing to obtain patents for financial gain, it is bound to warp relationships. If his thoughts while shaving in the morning are about improving a patent position or besting his business competition rather than about some fundamental question, it is unfortunate.

The solution to these problems will be as diverse as the people and the institutions involved. If we were in China or the Soviet Union, it would be arranged by the government. But in our capitalistic society it has to be different. After all, for a basic discovery to become a valuable new drug, who but the pharmaceutical industry will invest fifty million dollars for the research to develop it? A tremendous amount of time and money are needed, and we must rely on industry to do it.

■ What about constraints on the free flow of ideas, which is essential for effective communication among scientists? Is this not impeded by such agreements between scientists and industry?

Not really. I am doing something along these lines that I find encouraging. Paul Berg, Charles Yanofsky, and I helped Alex Zaffaroni start a small biotechnology venture called DNAX. It is an industrial operation supported by Schering-Plough Corp. Students, postdoctoral fellows, and professors move freely in it. The scientists' identity, freedom, and openness are as great as in a university. This has come about through the influence of Zaffaroni, formerly president of Syntex Research and now head of Alza, a company he founded fifteen years ago.

I have been a scientific advisor at Alza since its inception. Zaffaroni is an intimate friend. He is humane, intelligent, a shrewd businessman—but mostly humane. He has proven that secrecy makes even less sense in industry than it does in academia. Nobody seems to believe it, but he has practiced it and proved it. We are trying to deliver that message at DNAX and at Schering-Plough. You may feel cheated on rare occasions, but in the long run you gain by being open and able to sop up the basic information that you need, almost all of which is being supplied by academia. In this posture industry is not seen just as a sponge or, if so, at least a sponge that can also be squeezed.

■ Looking back on it all now, would you have done anything differently?

I could have been a better physical chemist. I could have acquired a broader view of biology as well as of chemistry. But I do look back on my clinical training with some pleasure. It was entertaining and enriching in giving me another view of people and society and another approach to learning about biology. I found medical school absorbing. I enjoyed anatomy; I enjoyed medicine. I was a good physician and had fine rapport with patients. I enjoyed the challenge of a neurological diagnosis. But when I later realized that I didn't understand structural chemistry and lacked a firm foundation in genetics, I was disappointed in my command of these languages that I needed in my work. But I have not regretted what I have done. People generally don't.

■ DNA has filled much of your life.

We discovered DNA polymerase, the enzyme that lengthens chains. I have stuck to DNA replication or it has stuck to me for thirty years. I have done other things, but they don't match my enthusiasm and accomplishments with DNA replication. We probably still only know ten percent of what we should about it. But there is a question I often think about, and most everybody in biology does too: How a cycle of replication starts? What sets if off? And what stops it?

We evolve from simple cells, and we must pick those experimental opportunities that are relatively uncomplicated by the size of a molecule or the intrusion of adventitious activities. We wasted years picking the wrong model or the wrong place to look. Finally we have learned how to dissect out the part of the *E. coli* chromosome which we regard as the "switch" where the major commitment is made as to whether a cell is going to make DNA or not. That work is going quite well, and some people have commented that it is the best work we have yet done.

■ That must be nice to hear at this late date. How old are you now?

I am sixty-five.

EPILOGUE

After over five years of researching, conducting, and preparing these interviews for publication, I could not help but be tempted to draw some general conclusions about these remarkable personalities. What is it about their backgrounds and the way they conducted their lives that possibly reveals to us something about ourselves and about those who are just beginning their lives in medicine?

Certainly, with only sixteen subjects, all chosen with some degree of personal prejudice, no claim to any statistical significance could possibly be entertained. Furthermore, no specific plan was initially made to examine systematically the social, economic, and psychological aspects of their lives. Yet, in retrospect, some features were so striking that they cried out for exposition.

Because only two women are included among the group, I can judge their achievements only in the same light as that for other American women entering medicine in the first half of this century. All of them had to be extraordinarily intelligent, determined, self-sacrificing—and lucky.

As for the men, if one were to assemble all the ingredients for success, based on this limited sample the first requisite would seem to have been a father who, in their youth, was either dead, distant, or indecisive in guiding them into maturity. Bailey, Pickering, Johnson, and Good were all deprived of this role model in their childhoods. Because of socioeconomic conditions beyond their control, the fathers of Wintrobe and Kornberg had little influence on the career decisions of their sons. One suspects that George Dock, although a towering medical figure of his time, was not overly solicitous of his son, William, who seemed much more impressed by other figures, male and female, both within and outside of the family circle. Only André Cournand, in the course of our talk, mentioned a paternal influence that could be construed as profound, with the case seeming much less so for Drs. Wangensteen and Kolff.

As striking as the absence of fathers was the dominating presence of mothers. Without the encouragement of enlightened, strong-willed matriarchs, it is doubtful that many of these men would have persevered as they did.

Poverty also seemed to be a necessary spur for many of these men. It runs like a leitmotif throughout their stories. Interestingly, though, economic deprivation did not serve as an incentive to become wealthy, but rather as a rigorous exercise in preparation for the other vicissitudes they were to encounter in pursuit of their goals. Racial, religious, and sexual discrimination within the world of medicine are aspects of which younger physicians might not be fully aware in an era during which much is being done to eliminate them. Yet these were hard facts of life in the recent past, as the interviews reflect.

What of the tradition of medical families? There are, without question, distinguished families of doctors spanning successive generations: the Mayos, the "surgeons-Warren," and others where the torch has been passed from father to son to grandson. In terms of achieving greatness, however, these are probably exceptions to the rule. Only Dock and Kolff had physicians as fathers (Lena Edwards's father was a dentist), and only Dock's father was preeminent in his field. It is comforting to be reassured that in a democratic society outstanding physicians and scientists can spring from any walk of life.

The types of training these physicians received for the roles they wished to play in medicine indicated similarities as well as contrasts. Whether their international recognition stemmed from one major discovery (e.g., Murphy and pernicious anemia, Bailey and mitral commissurotomy, Kolff and the artificial kidney) or, as was more often the case, from an accumulated lifetime of teaching and research, almost all these individuals experienced at one point in their lives an intense exposure to a scientific discipline. This most often took the form of the effort to complete requirements for the doctor of philosophy degree (Wangensteen, Wintrobe, Johnson, Good, Kolff, Weinstein). For those such as Francis Moore and Arthur Kornberg who never formally took this route, there was a sense of dissatisfaction in the incompleteness of their training for the work that lay ahead, although they compensated for this admirably. This tells us something about the equipment future medical scientists may need if they are to make really important contributions to our body of knowledge. It suggests that the "holistic" approach to medicine, now somewhat in vogue, may have little to do with scientific excellence.

Good physicians have always felt insecure about the extent of their knowledge and understanding. They often refer to themselves as "lifelong scholars"—a cliché but nonetheless true. Keeping up is a problem. Dr. James B. Herrick, whose name appears several times in the book, exemplified this. At the age of forty-three, in the midst of a busy consultative practice, he began to take courses in chemistry at the University of Chicago. He then temporarily deserted his practice to run off to Germany to study with a leading chemist because he felt that it was in this discipline that the future of medicine lay.

Even the great William Osler was not immune to fears of being engulfed by the onrushing tide of "modern" medical advances. In his memoirs, Herrick recalled a meeting of the American Medical Association at Saratoga Springs, New York, in 1902. He and Osler were seated next to one another at a scientific session while a speaker began by drawing a benzene ring on the blackboard and then proceeded to add, subtract, and rearrange various radicals around it. Osler, according to Herrick, "turned to me and said seriously, wistfully and pathetically, 'Herrick, I wish I were nineteen and had it all to do over again.' "

Can the complete physician and complete scientist coexist within the same body? About this question there seems to be a dichotomy of opinion, with the opposing views best articulated by Francis Moore and Arthur Kornberg. The former defends the role of the clinical investigator as the "bridge tender" spanning the gulf between clinical medicine and basic research. Kornberg opts for hopping ashore on one bank or the other if one is to accomplish what he sets out to do. They are probably both right, although in somewhat different contexts.

As stated before, the participants were selected, in the main, for their overall contributions in order to provide, as a group, a panorama of the American medical scene over the past fifty years. In a few cases, however, the introduction of a new idea or treatment was the highlight, and in these instances it is instructive to review the attitudes with which these tasks were undertaken. Murphy, Bailey, and Kolff are the most exemplary in this regard.

A certain amount of ruthlessness, I suspect, is mandatory when anything new is proffered to the inevitably skeptical and conservative medical community. One wonders if the mild-mannered, self-effacing Murphy could have succeeded without the collaboration of George Minot, whose character, one gathers, was imbued much more with a will of steel. Or was this a hidden element of Murphy's personality, not readily detected? Many influential surgeons of the day viewed Charles Bailey's intense, almost monomaniacal effort to promote mitral commissurotomy with much distaste because of what they considered his disregard of medical ethics. Even today a bitter residue of that feeling persists in certain quarters. When Willem Kolff speaks about his own past and recent efforts in the field of artificial organs and the opposition he has had to overcome, there is detectable in his demeanor what can only be described as a kind of ferocity in his resentment of this interference.

Samuel Taylor Morrison, in reference to another discoverer, has written, "Columbus was a man with a mission and such men are apt to be unreasonable and even disagreeable to those who cannot see their mission." Perhaps explorers on uncharted medical seas must be gifted with the same intolerance of those less visionary than they if they are to reach their destination.

There was an element of sadness in bringing this collection of interviews to an end. Born into and living in an antiheroic age, I stubbornly cling to the belief that there are real heroes to whom we can turn for learning and inspiration. During the writing of this book some of these have died and will never see the result of this effort. There are others whom I would have wished to include but who, for various reasons, do not appear. One misses the joyful anticipation of that next trip, that next interview, and all the benefits that it might bestow. Yet the line must eventually be drawn, and it is hoped that with those completed the overview of American medicine that had been planned has been achieved.

My being a physician-researcher-educator was my passport to my meeting with those I had come to admire so deeply and sharing vicariously in their exciting adventures and triumphs. In the end, that has been the greatest personal reward of *Conversations in Medicine.*

BIOGRAPHICAL NOTES

For those who are discussed to any extent within the preceding chapters a notation is made to refer to the index for the appropriate pages.

Abel, John Jacob (1857–1938)
Professor of pharmacology at Johns Hopkins University (1893) and director of the Laboratory for Endocrine Research (1932) at the same institution. Besides invention of the first artificial kidney, he isolated a form of adrenaline (epinephrine) and crystallized insulin (see index).

Albright, Fuller (1900–1969)
Brilliant endocrinologist at the Massachusetts General Hospital who contributed greatly to the understanding of hormone function and abnormalities in man, especially involving the parathyroid gland (see index).

Aschoff, Karl Albert Ludwig (1866–1942)
German pathologist who described the reticuloendothelial system as well as the inflammatory nodules seen in heart tissue following rheumatic fever (Aschoff's bodies).

Aub, Joseph C. (1890–1973)
Product of Harvard Medical School and the Massachusetts General Hospital where, among other major contributions, he did his most famous work on lead poisoning.

Austrian, Robert (1916–)
Hopkins-trained physician who worked at Downstate Medical Center in Brooklyn, 1952–62, best known for his long-term studies there of pneumococcal infections that led to the recognition of persistent

high mortality despite antibiotics. His work on pneumococcal capsular polysaccharides has contributed to the development of the polyvalent vaccine in use for highly susceptible subjects. Currently John Herr Musser Professor of Research Medicine, University of Pennsylvania School of Medicine.

Banting, Sir Frederick G. (1891–1941)
Canadian physician who, with Charles H. Best, working at the University of Toronto, was the first to devise a method for obtaining from the pancreas of dogs the active principle that controls blood sugar (insulin). This discovery in 1921 led to the modern treatment of diabetes mellitus and the saving of innumerable lives of sufferers from this disease. He was corecipient of the Nobel Prize in medicine and physiology in 1923 for this work.

Barcroft, Joseph (1872–1947)
Cambridge scientist who made a lifelong study of the "respiratory function of the blood." He measured oxygen-dissociation curves and showed the influence of various salts and acids upon them; he discovered different kinds of hemoglobin; and he contributed to studies of high-altitude effects upon cardiopulmonary function.

Barnard, Christiaan (1922–   )
South African surgeon who, after completing doctoral (Ph.D.) studies at the University of Minnesota (1956–58), returned to Cape Town and Groote Schuur Hospital where he headed a team of surgeons who performed the first human heart transplant (in Louis Washkansky). Although this first patient soon died from noncardiac complications, this attempt led the way for further operations of this type in man both in Cape Town and elsewhere.

Bauer, Walter (1898–1964)
Internist-rheumatologist and, for much of his career, professor of medicine at Harvard and chief of medicine at Massachusetts General Hospital.

Bean, William B. (1909–   )
Gifted clinician, medical researcher, and historian who has spent the bulk of his medical career at the medical schools of the University of Cincinnati and the University of Iowa.

Beeson, Paul B. (1908–   )
One of the most distinguished living American internists, who has worked under Soma Weiss and Charles Janeway at the Peter Bent

Brigham Hospital, Oswald Avery at the Rockefeller Institute, and Eugene Stead at Duke. Besides having held the Nuffield Chair at Oxford, he has headed the Department of Medicine at both Emory University and Yale University. His research interests have been in fever and infectious disease. He has coedited the *Cecil-Loeb Textbook of Medicine* and is currently at the Veterans Administration Hospital, Seattle, Washington.

Berg, Paul (1926–   )
Biochemist and longtime associate of Arthur Kornberg at Washington University, St. Louis, and Stanford, where he is currently professor of biochemistry. He received a Nobel Prize in chemistry in 1980 for "his fundamental studies of the biochemistry of nucleic acids, with particular regard to recombinant DNA."

Bernard, Claude (1813–78)
Major French figure in the development of nineteenth-century biological and physiological thought. In addition to developing the technique of cardiac catheterization, he pioneered in studies on gastric juice, pancreatic function, the autonomic nervous system, and neuromuscular transmission, to list only some of his contributions. Perhaps he is best remembered for his concept of the internal environment ("milieu interieur"), which held that the body fluids of higher animals provide a medium that makes possible the conditions for existence of the cells they surround and nourish (see index).

Best, Charles H. (1899–1978)
Canadian physiologist, most noted for his work when still an undergraduate student at the University of Toronto with Frederick Banting in the discovery of insulin. In 1923 he was excluded from the Nobel Prize that was awarded to Banting and to the head of the laboratory where the work was performed, J. J. R. Macleod. Outraged at this injustice, Banting gave half of his prize money to Best, who had a distinguished career thereafter, heading the Physiology Department at the University of Toronto (1929–65)

Billings, Frank (1854–1932)
Leader in Chicago medical circles who also performed research, developing the doctrine of focal infection.

Billroth, Theodor (1829–94)
Surgeon, teacher, and scientist who worked mainly at the surgical clinic of the University of Vienna. He was one of the first to introduce antisepsis on the Continent, the first to resect the esophagus

and to perform total laryngectomy. The types of gastric resection he developed still bear his name today (i.e., Billroth-1 and Billroth-2) (see index).

Blalock, Alfred (1899–1964)
Johns Hopkins vascular surgeon who, among other accomplishments, with Helen Taussig's urging (see listing below), devised an operation diverting unoxygenated systemic blood back into the lung circulation to improve survival and allow later total correction of congenital heart defects in "blue babies" (Blalock-Taussig operation) (see index).

Bland, Edward F. (1901–   )
Prominent Boston cardiologist, especially known for his work in rheumatic fever.

Bloomfield, Arthur L. (1888–1962)
Distinguished physician and teacher at Johns Hopkins (1912–26) and later Stanford, where he headed the Department of Medicine (1926–54).

Blumgart, Herrman L. (1895–1977)
Outstanding physician-cardiologist at Harvard and at Boston's Beth Israel Hospital where he headed research and clinical programs from 1928 until retirement in 1962.

Boyd, William (1885–1979)
Scottish-born pathologist who spent most of his professional life in Canada at the University of Manitoba and the University of Toronto. A great teacher and author of an extremely popular textbook of pathology.

Boyer, Herbert W. (1936–   )
Professor, Division of Genetics, Department of Biochemistry and Biophysics, University of California at San Francisco.

Boylston, Zabdiel (1679–1766)
Massachusetts surgeon responsible for the introduction of smallpox inoculation in the United States (see index).

Brock, Sir Russell (1903–   )
Guy Hospital surgeon who performed the first pulmonary valvotomy for obstruction to outflow tract of the right ventricle (pulmonic stenosis) as well as pioneering surgery for mitral stenosis in England (see index).

Bunker, John P. (1920–)
Anesthesiologist, Stanford University Medical Center (see index).

Cannon, Walter B. (1871–1945)
Harvard physiologist (1898–1942) who was the first to use X rays in physiological studies (gastrointestinal tract), among many other achievements involving the nervous system. His autobiography, *The Way of An Investigator* (1945), remains an enlightening and uplifting guide for those trying to tread a similar path in science.

Carlson, Anton J. ("Ajax") (1875–1956)
Swedish-born physiologist who headed the Department of Physiology at the University of Chicago from 1914 to 1940. He was active in many academic areas, and was the president of the American Physiological Society (1923–25) and the American Association of University Professors (1937).

Carrel, Alexis (1873–1944)
French-born experimental surgeon who emigrated to the United States in 1904 and developed many of the cardiovascular techniques that were later incorporated into clinical surgery involving the heart and blood vessels as well as transplantation. Much of this work was done at the Rockefeller Institute. He was the first American citizen to be awarded the Nobel Prize in physiology and medicine (1912).

Cartwright, George E. (1917–1980)
Distinguished hematologist and successor to Dr. Wintrobe as chairman, Department of Medicine, at the University of Utah from 1967 until his death.

Castle, William B. (1897–)
Boston hematologist and discoverer of the "instrinsic factor" leading to the elucidation of the cause of pernicious anemia (see index).

Chesney, Alan Mason (1888–1964)
Early thyroid researcher who later became faculty member, then dean at Johns Hopkins Medical School. In the latter post he served twenty-four years of a four-decade span at his alma mater (see index).

Christian, Henry A. (1876–1951)
Pathologist and internist at Harvard who authored many papers as well as textbooks of medicine but is probably remembered best as chief of medicine at Boston's Peter Bent Brigham Hospital over a great many years (1910–39), during which time many future leaders of American medicine trained under him (see index).

Churchill, Edward D. (1895–1972)
Surgical researcher and teacher who served as chief of surgery at Massachusetts General Hospital for many years beginning in 1933, interrupted only by distinguished World War II service. His major contributions included surgery for hyperparathyroidism, constrictive pericarditis, and bronchiectasis. Many future outstanding surgeons trained under him.

Cobb, William Montague (1904–   )
Physical anthropologist, anatomist, and physician who taught at Howard University's medical school from 1928 until 1973, mainly in the Anatomy Department, which he headed between 1947 and 1969.

Coller, Fred A. (1887–1964)
Head of Department of Surgery at the University of Michigan Medical School, Ann Arbor, from 1930 to 1957. Author of many investigations, including those involving thyroid disease, water balance and electrolytes, and cancer.

Cooper, Irving S. (1922–   )
Neurosurgeon who has specialized in the surgical destruction of certain parts of the brain in order to relieve the symptoms of Parkinson's disease.

Cooper, Theodore (1928–   )
Surgeon-physiologist-pharmacologist who served as assistant secretary, Department of Health, Education, and Welfare (1975–77), and who shouldered much of the responsibility for use of "flu" vaccine during the 1976 outbreak. Currently executive vice-president, Upjohn Company, after serving as dean at Cornell University School of Medicine.

Cope, Oliver (1902–   )
Harvard-trained surgeon active mostly at the Massachusetts General Hospital from the time of his internship (1928) until 1969. He was the first to concentrate on the function and surgical treatment of parathyroid disease as well as making critical studies in fluid and electrolyte balance (see index).

Cori, Carl F. (1896–   ), and **Cori, Gerty T.** (1896–1957)
Classmates in medical school at the University of Prague, the Coris married in 1920 and became scientific collaborators as well. Between 1931 and 1957 both were at the Washington University, St. Louis, heading the Biochemistry Department to which Arthur

Kornberg, among others, came for training. They received a Nobel Prize (1947) for their work on how glycogen is catalytically converted.

Crile, George W. (1864–1943)
Innovative Cleveland surgeon who distinguished himself in thoracic surgery, the use of nerve-block anesthesia, and the development of blood transfusions. Founder of the Cleveland Clinic Foundation.

Cushing, Harvey (1869–1939)
Father of neurosurgery who trained under the legendary Halsted at Johns Hopkins but was also influenced by Osler, whose biography he wrote and for which he received a Pulitzer Prize (see index).

Cutler, Elliott Carr (1888–1947)
Moseley Professor of Surgery at Harvard, where he succeeded Harvey Cushing, and chief surgeon at Peter Bent Brigham Hospital in Boston (see index).

Dennis, Clarence (1909–   )
Protégé of Dr. Wangensteen at Minnesota; he later became chief of surgery at State University of New York Downstate Medical Center in Brooklyn (1952–72). Now at SUNY–Stony Brook (see index).

DeWall, Richard A. (1926–   )
Thoracic surgeon who trained under Dr. Owen Wangensteen and developed the bubble oxygenator, which allowed for bypass during open-heart operations (with Walton Lillehei). Chairman, Department of Surgery, Chicago Medical School (1962–66). Currently at the Cox Heart Institute, Ohio.

Dixon, John (1923–   )
Utah surgeon who, after graduating from medical school at the University of Utah (1947), later returned to serve as professor of surgery and dean.

Dragstedt, Lester R. (1893–1975)
Starting as a physiologist-pharmacologist and protégé of Anton J. Carlson (see index) at the University of Chicago, Dragstedt, at the age of thirty-two, started a second career, becoming a surgeon. Working at the University of Chicago where he finally became chairman of surgery (1947–59), he concentrated on the physiology of the stomach, especially peptic ulcer, for which he introduced vagotomy (division of the vagus nerve) to reduce acid secretion.

Edelman, Isidore S. (1920–   )
Chairman, Department of Biochemistry, Columbia University College of Physicians and Surgeons. He has conducted outstanding research in body water and electrolyte metabolism as well as in sodium and potassium transport and endocrinology.

Edsall, David L. (1869–1945)
Noted medical educator and researcher, first at the University of Pennsylvania, then at Harvard, specializing in public health and industrial medicine problems. He influenced greatly the growth and development of research at the Massachusetts General Hospital (see index).

Effler, Donald B. (1915–   )
Colorful and enterprising thoracic and cardiovascular surgeon who was at the Cleveland Clinic during the development of open-heart surgery and especially coronary bypass surgery, at which that institution was an early leader. Currently chief cardiac surgeon at St. Joseph's Hospital in Syracuse, New York, and clinical professor of surgery at State University of New York Medical Center in Syracuse.

Ehrlich, Paul (1854–1915)
One of the giants of nineteenth-century medicine who, at Robert Koch's Institute in Berlin, made important contributions to hematology, immunology, and chemotherapy. His discovery of the arsenical, Salvarsan, represented the first effective treatment for syphilis (see index).

Einthoven, Willem (1860–1927)
Dutch scientist and physician who invented the string galvanometer electrocardiograph, which is still used today. He received the Nobel Prize in medicine for this (1924).

Eliot, Charles W. (1834–1926)
President of Harvard responsible for reformation and raising of its standards during his forty-year tenure beginning in 1869.

Erlanger, Joseph (1874–1965)
Johns Hopkins M.D. who spent most of his professional life at Washington University, St. Louis, as professor and head of the Physiology Department, becoming emeritus in 1944. He received a Nobel Prize in medicine (1944) with Herbert Spencer Gasser for "discoveries regarding the highly differentiated functions of nerve fibers."

Fitz, Reginald (1885–1953)
Son of the famous pathological anatomist, Reginald H. Fitz (1843–1913), he, himself, became a distinguished physician, with most of his professional career at Peter Bent Brigham Hospital in Boston. His broad interests in medicine were matched by those in medical history.

Gibbon, John H., Jr. (1903–73)
Philadelphia surgeon who, beginning in 1935, pioneered the development of the heart-lung machine and thus paved the way for the introduction of open-heart surgery.

Gilbert, Walter (1932–   )
Harvard molecular biologist who in 1980 shared a Nobel Prize with Frederick Sanger for developing methodology for the sequencing of DNA.

Gilman, Alfred (1908–   )
Pharmacologist formerly at Yale and coeditor of *The Pharmacological Basis of Therapeutics* (6th Ed., 1980), with Dr. Louis S. Goodman. Professor emeritus of pharmacology, Albert Einstein College of Medicine, Yeshiva University.

Gilman, Daniel Coit (1831–1908)
First president of Johns Hopkins University, which opened in 1876, and primarily responsible for the organization and selection of faculty for the medical school which opened in 1893.

Goldberger, Joseph (1874–1929)
Called the "Forgotten Hero of Common Health" by William Bean (he is not even mentioned in the *Encyclopaedia Britannica*), Goldberger served for over thirty years in the U.S. Public Health Service and made many outstanding contributions to the field of nutrition and epidemiology. He is primarily remembered for the demonstration that pellagra is a disease due, not to an infectious agent, but rather, to a dietary deficiency, later found to be nicotinic acid.

Gorer, Peter
In 1937 identified the major histocompatibility complex in mice, the genetic site containing information regarding tissue typing and a forerunner of a similar locus in man.

Graham, Evarts A. (1883–1957)
Professor of surgery at Washington University School of Medicine,

St. Louis. For thirty-two years, until 1951, chief surgeon at Barnes Hospital, St. Louis. He was the first to use radiopaque media for visualization of the gallbladder and its ducts (cholecystography), as well as the first to remove a cancer of the lung by pneumonectomy.

Gregg, Alan (1890–1957)
Influential figure in medical research and education through his positions at the Rockefeller Foundation in the Divisions of Medical Education and Medical Science (1922–31), and thereafter as vice-president of the foundation. His service in the field of public health, medical education, and research spanned over forty years (see index).

Gross, Robert E. (1905–   )
Surgeon at Children's Hospital in Boston who in 1938 performed one of the earliest operations for cure of a congenital cardiac defect by ligating a patent ductus arteriosus (an abnormal postnatal persistence of a connection between the pulmonary artery and aorta).

Halsted, William S. (1852–1922)
One of the original quadrumvirate selected to head the clinical departments at Johns Hopkins Medical School. A vascular surgeon who also excelled in many other areas of this discipline and who was responsible for the training of many others (see index).

Hamman, Louis (1877–1944)
Johns Hopkins physician-educator remembered most, now, for the inflammatory fibrosing lung disorder he described (Hamman-Rich syndrome).

Harken, Dwight E. (1910–   )
Thoracic surgeon at Harvard and Peter Bent Brigham Hospital in Boston. In addition to his contemporary work at the time Charles Bailey introduced mitral commissurotomy, he inserted the first intracardiac ball-in-cage heart valve and made other contributions to the field of cardiac surgery, e.g., counterpulsation and anticoagulation (see index).

Harrison, Tinsley R. (1900–1979)
Alabama physician-cardiologist who, among other posts, developed three new departments of medicine (University of North Carolina, Bowman Gray, and University of Alabama). Major contributions included his monograph *Failure of the Circulation* (1938) and his textbook of medicine.

Harvey, Réjane M. (1917–   )
Professor of Medicine, Columbia University College of Physicians and Surgeons, and director, Pulmonary Division, Department of Medicine at Presbyterian Hospital since 1973.

Harvey, William (1578–1657)
Physician during the time of James I and Charles I who, through publication of his findings in *De Motu Cordis*, described for the first time the true circulation of the blood through the heart and its vessels.

Hecht, Hans H. (1913–71)
Swiss-born cardiologist and member of the nucleus of outstanding internists assembled by Dr. Maxwell Wintrobe in building his department at the University of Utah. He left there after a number of years to become departmental chairman in medicine at the University of Chicago.

Heppel, Leon A. (1912–   )
Biochemist and physician who was a classmate of (M.D., 1941), and worked with, Dr. Arthur Kornberg at the NIH (1942–53) and later at the National Institute of Arthritis and Metabolism (1958–67). He is currently in the Department of Biochemistry at Cornell University in Ithaca, New York.

Herrick, James B. (1861–1954)
Distinguished Chicago physician whose investigations covered a number of medical areas. He is most remembered for his publication in 1912 of the report, "Clinical Features of Sudden Obstruction of the Coronary Arteries," in which he pointed out that patients could survive from this disease, which had previously been thought to be uniformly immediately fatal (see index).

Horecker, Bernard L. (1914–   )
Biochemist whose work has involved isolation and characterization of respiratory enzymes, hemoglobin study, and enzymology. He was at the NIH between 1941 and 1953, collaborating for much of this time with Arthur Kornberg. He is now at the Roche Institute for Molecular Biology.

Howell, William Henry (1860–1945)
Early major figure of American physiology who was first to head this department at the Johns Hopkins Medical School (1892). At Hopkins

he studied mainly the effects of inorganic salts on the heartbeat, action of the vagus nerve, and coagulation of the blood. He isolated thrombin in 1910 and worked on heparin.

Huggins, Charles B. (1901–)
American surgeon and researcher best known for his finding that the injection of female hormones could control cancers of the male prostate gland. This introduced the whole field of endocrine inhibition of tumor growth to the cancer field.

Hunter, John (1728–93)
English surgeon, anatomist, and physiologist with wide-ranging interests in many branches of natural history. At his death, in addition to a number of medical works, he left his personal museum containing over 10,000 items, which were finally donated by the government to the Royal College of Surgeons.

Ingelfinger, Franz (1910–79)
Leading Boston gastroenterologist and editor of the *New England Journal of Medicine* (1967–77).

Ivy, Andrew C. (1893–1978)
Prominent physiologist at Northwestern University where he headed the Physiology Department (1925–46) and worked mainly in gastrointestinal physiology. His final years were clouded by the Krebiozen controversy in which he and coworkers claimed that this substance could limit or even cure some cancers. This was never proved and led to indictment for fraud by the Food and Drug Administration in 1965. He was found not guilty. Ivy's reputation was nonetheless severely damaged by this, although he continued to work on anticancer substances thereafter.

Jasper, Herbert Henry (1906–)
American-born neurophysiologist who has held important teaching positions in both the United States and Canada. Now emeritus professor of neurophysiology at the University of Montreal.

Jenner, Edward (1749–1823)
English physician best remembered for the introduction of vaccination for the prevention of smallpox. As such, he must be considered the founder of modern immunology (see index).

Jones, Chester M. (1891–1972)
Founder and for thirty-six years Chief of the Gastroenterology Section of Massachusetts General Hospital until the time of his retirement (1957). A great teacher, he was also noted for his research, which included studies concerning metabolism of bile pigments and digestive tract pain.

Jones, T. Duckett (1899–1954)
A graduate of the medical school of the University of Virginia, his home state, he later migrated to Boston, working at Harvard, Massachusetts General Hospital and especially the House of the Good Samaritan, where he directed the research department from 1929 to 1947. His major contributions included devising of the Jones criteria for the diagnosis of rheumatic fever (1944), his primary interest, thus creating some order out of the preexisting diagnostic chaos that had previously led to many errors.

Joseph, Sir Keith
In England, secretary of state for social service, 1970–74, and secretary of state for education and science since 1981.

Joslin, Eliot P. (1869–1962)
World-famous researcher in diabetes mellitus whose Boston clinic was the focus of many advances in the study and treatment of the disease. Dietary control for prevention of diabetic complications (infection, heart disease, etc.) was the hallmark of the clinic, at which bronze and gold medals were conferred upon those patients surviving for extended periods of time.

Kantrowitz, Adrian (1918–   )
Innovative surgeon with early interest in heart transplantation and the intraaortic balloon assist device. Currently professor of surgery at Wayne State University in Michigan (see index).

Keefer, Chester Scott (1897–1972)
Prominent medical figure who, following training at Johns Hopkins, Billings Hospital (Chicago), and Peiping Union Medical College, came to Boston in 1930 for ten-year stint at the Thorndike Memorial Laboratory of Boston City Hospital. He moved to Boston University where he became chief of medicine (1940–59) and later dean (1955–72).

Koch, Robert (1843–1910)
Following immediately in the footsteps of Louis Pasteur, Koch was

one of the founders of the science of microbiology. As a provincial German physician, he built his own laboratory where he first demonstrated the life cycle of the anthrax organism. Called to Berlin, he later isolated the bacterium causing tuberculosis, the "white plague" of Europe at the time, among other important discoveries at the institute named for him. Koch's postulates in infectious diseases: to establish that a specific microorganism is the cause of a disease it must be present in all cases of the disease, cause the disease when injected into other animals, and be obtainable from the latter, once affected, in such a way that it can again be propagated in pure culture (see index).

Korotkoff, N. C. (1874–1920)
Russian vascular surgeon who discovered the auscultatory method of measuring arterial blood pressure (1905). The sounds by which we measure systolic and diastolic blood pressure today still bear his name.

Krogh, August (1874–1949)
Danish physiologist whose fundamental studies on the circulatory system and on respiratory control were major contributions to the understanding of this function in lower animals and man.

Kronecker, Hugo (1839–1914)
German-born physiologist who spent a large part of his career at Bern, Switzerland, where he headed Department of Physiology. His research involved heart muscle, mechanisms of swallowing, and mountain sickness.

Kuttner, Ann G. (1895–1968)
Johns Hopkins graduate who served on the faculty of the New York University College of Medicine.

Lahey, Frank H. (1880–1953)
Founder and director of the Lahey Clinic in Boston where he also made a great many contributions to clinical surgery, especially in regard to the thyroid.

LeCount, Edwin R. (1868–1935)
Pathologist at Rush Medical College for several decades following graduation there in 1892; took further training at Hopkins, the Pasteur Institute in Paris, and Berlin.

Levine, Samuel A. (1891–1966)
Professor of medicine at Harvard and cardiologist at Peter Bent Brigham Hospital. Author of the books, *Clinical Heart Disease* (5th ed., 1958) and *Coronary Thrombosis* (1929). An esteemed teacher of his specialty for many years in Boston as well as on the national scene.

Lewis, F. John (1916–   )
Minnesota surgeon who performed the first successful open-heart surgery. This was done using hypothermia to close an atrial septal defect.

Lewis, Sir Thomas (1881–1945)
Welsh-born clinician and cardiovascular physiologist who was one of the earliest physicians in Great Britain to recognize the potential of the electrocardiograph. His books, *Clinical Disorders of the Heart Beat* (1912) and *Diseases of the Heart* (1933), became immediate classics. From the University College Hospital, London, his professional home from 1902 until his death, his continuous output of research and clinical teaching strongly influenced subsequent generations of cardiologists in Great Britain and elsewhere (see index).

Lillehei, C. Walton (1918–   )
Minnesota surgeon who has made many important contributions to open-heart surgery, especially in the areas of congenital defects and valvular heart disease.

Locke, Edwin A. (1874–1971)
Influential Boston physician who in 1924 organized the first group practice in that city. His major interest was in chest disease, especially tuberculosis. He was active both at the Boston Sanatorium as physician in chief and at Boston City Hospital, where he was also physician in chief of the Fourth Medical Service.

Long, Perrin H. (1899–1965)
Best known for his work on the introduction of sulfonamides in the treatment of infections. After twenty-two years at Johns Hopkins, he became chairman of the Department of Medicine at the State University of New York, Downstate Medical Center in Brooklyn. He held his post ten years (1951–61) until illness forced his resignation.

Longcope, Warfield Theobald (1877–1953)
He received his M.D. from Johns Hopkins in 1901 and, for the major portion of his career (1922–46), was professor of medicine at his alma mater, where he exerted a major influence on its faculty and students.

Lowry, Oliver H. (1910–)
Distinguished Professor Emeritus, Department of Pharmacology, Washington University School of Medicine in St. Louis. He is known as much for his devising of medical instrumentation and methods for measuring minute quantities of enzymes and substrates as for his research involving these aspects of pharmacology.

Luisada, Aldo A. (1901–)
Italian-born Chicago cardiologist who has made the investigation of the physical diagnostic aspects of normal and diseased hearts his primary activity.

MacCallum, William C. (1874–1944)
Successor to William H. Welch, the first chairman of the Department of Pathology at Johns Hopkins, and a distinguished pathologist and educator in his own right.

Matas, Rudolph (1860–1938)
New Orleans surgeon who made many important contributions, including the use of spinal anesthesia, a device for assisting respiration intraoperatively, and improvement of techniques for surgery involving arterial aneurysms.

Mayo, William James (1861–1939), and **Mayo, Charles Horatio** (1865–1939)
Sons of William W. Mayo (1819–1911), and founders of the Mayo Clinic in Rochester, Minnesota. The elder Mayo was retired when the clinic opened, and it was his sons who developed the institution at St. Mary's Hospital. The clinic opened in 1889 and the Clinic building was added in 1914. (see index).

McMichael, Sir John (1904–)
One of the earliest cardiologists in Great Britain to use cardiac catheterization for the study of human heart disease, he served as director, Department of Medicine, at the Postgraduate Medical School (Hammersmith) between 1946 and 1966 (see index).

McQuarrie, Irvine (1892–1961)
Outstanding figure in pediatrics who headed the Department of Pediatrics at the University of Minnesota School of Medicine from 1930 to 1956.

Means, James Howard (1885–1967)
A protégé of David Edsall at the Massachusetts General Hospital

who was sent to study with leaders in medical science such as August Krogh in Copenhagen and Joseph Barcroft in England. Returning to Massachusetts General Hospital in 1913, he was given laboratory space in which he began studies on metabolism and thyroid disease, for which he became famous. He succeeded Edsall as chief of Medical Service of Massachusetts General Hospital and inspired other researchers at the famous Ward 4, about which he later wrote a history (see index) .

Meigs, Joseph Vincent (1892–1963)
Gynecological surgeon, primarily at the Massachusetts General Hospital, who made important contributions to the understanding and management of endometriosis (the presence of uterine lining tissue, endometrium, in abnormal pelvic locations) and infertility. He is best remembered now for the Meigs syndrome: the presence of abdominal cavity fluid (ascites) and chest fluid (pleural effusion) sometimes associated with fibroma of the ovary.

Meyer, Adolph (1866–1950)
Swiss-born psychiatrist who emigrated to the United States in 1892 and was also an eminent neurobiologist and pathologist. He became head of psychiatry at Johns Hopkins in 1910, and between 1900 and 1946 was considered one of the most influential psychiatrists of the time.

Minot, George R. (1885–1950)
Recipient, with George Whipple and William P. Murphy, of the Nobel Prize for physiology and medicine in 1934 for the introduction of successful liver treatment of pernicious anemia. This and other work was performed during his tenure at the Massachusetts General Hospital, Huntington Memorial Hospital, Peter Bent Brigham Hospital, and Thorndike Memorial Laboratory (Boston City Hospital), where he served as director from 1928 until his death (see index).

Morton, William T. G. (1819–68)
Massachusetts dentist who discovered the use of ether as a general anesthetic and, in a dramatic gesture at the Massachusetts General Hospital (1846), demonstrated in the surgical amphitheater (now called the "ether dome") the use of general anesthesia in a patient with a vascular tumor in the neck, which was removed by Dr. John Collins Warren, surgeon.

Nickerson, Mark (1919–)
Canadian pharmacologist-physician formerly associated with Louis Goodman, and currently professor of pharmacology and therapeutics at McGill University in Montreal, Quebec.

Nier, Alfred O. (1911–)
Professor of physics, University of Minnesota, and known for his work in mass spectometry and aeronomy.

Nutting, Mary Adelaide (1858–1948)
With Lavina Dock, one of the pioneers in the development of American nursing. Canadian-born, she did not enter nursing training until age thirty when she attended the newly opened Johns Hopkins School of Nursing, where she met Dock who was an instructor there. After Dock and the superintendent of the school, Isabel Hampton, left, Nutting stayed on to guide it for eleven years, until 1906. From 1907 to 1925 she headed nursing training at Teachers College, Columbia University, in New York City and was active in many nursing activities even after retirement. Coauthored with Lavina Dock an exhaustive in-depth four-volume *History of Nursing*, which was first published in 1907.

Ochoa, Severo (1905–)
Spanish-born physician who, following graduation from the University of Madrid, studied muscle biochemistry and physiology in Otto Meyerhof's laboratory in Heidelberg. His next stop was Oxford, working on thiamine with R. A. Peters; he then went to Washington University, St. Louis, working with Carl and Gerty Cori for a year. In 1941 he went to New York University where he spent a number of years doing work that led to the discovery of RNA (ribonucleic acid) polymerase and to his sharing of a Nobel Prize in 1959 with Arthur Kornberg.

Ochsner, Alton (1896–1979)
Prominent surgeon who, in 1942, founded the New Orleans clinic that bears his name. Among many contributions to medicine and surgery, his work linking cigarette smoking to cancer and other maladies was probably the most important.

Oliver, Jean Redman (1889–1976)
Professor of pathology, State University of New York, Downstate (formerly Long Island College Hospital), he was most noted for his work on kidney structure through microdissections.

Osler, Sir William (1849–1919)
Most distinguished of all American physicians, although Canadian-born and destined in later years to become Regius Professor of Medicine at Oxford. Greatly admired for his bedside teaching, textbook of medicine, and general philosophy, he was one of four clinical figures who established Johns Hopkins Hospital as a great medical institution (see index).

Page, Irvine H. (1901–   )
Hypertension researcher whose investigations led to the discovery of the vasopressor substance, angiotensin. Much of his work was done at the Cleveland Clinic (see index).

Park, Edwards A. (1877–1969)
Key member of the first American full-time Department of Pediatrics at Johns Hopkins where he later became chairman. In addition to distinguished work in bone disease, especially rickets, he was instrumental in developing careers of many outstanding pediatricians, Helen Taussig among them.

Pauling, Linus C. (1901–   )
Nobel laureate chemist (1954, for work on nature of the chemical bond), whose work on the molecular flaw in sickle-cell anemia provided one of the earliest major thrusts in the development of molecular biology. Also very active politically, he received the Nobel Peace Prize in 1962 (see index).

Peabody, Francis Weld (1881–1927)
Harvard and Peter Bent Brigham physician, who also served the important role as early director of the Thorndike Memorial Laboratory at the Boston City Hospital.

Rammelcamp, Charles H., Jr. (1911–81)
Infectious disease expert who, after a brief Boston training period, spent the bulk of his career at Western Reserve University and the Cleveland Metropolitan General Hospital (1946–79). Starting with World War II service, he devoted himself to the study of streptococcal infections and the sequelae of rheumatic fever and glomerulonephritis, among other contributions to the field.

Richards, Dickinson Woodruff (1895–1973)
Physiologist-physician at Columbia University's College of Physicians and Surgeons and Presbyterian Hospital in New York, and

lifelong collaborator with André Cournand, with whom he shared the Nobel Prize in medicine in 1956 (see index).

Roentgen, Wilhelm Conrad (1845–1923)
German physicist and discoverer of X rays, for which he received the first Nobel Prize in physics (1901).

Sabin, Florence Rena (1871–1953)
One of the earliest women graduates of Johns Hopkins and later the first woman professor there, where her work on neurological and vascular anatomy built her reputation. In 1925 she opened a laboratory devoted to the cellular aspects of the immune response at the Rockefeller Institute in New York.

Sauerbruch, Ernst Ferdinand (1875–1951)
Brilliant German surgeon who first made his mark while at Breslau where he developed a negative pressure cabinet that would permit operations on the opened chest without collapse of the lungs occurring (1904). He moved on to Zurich and later to the Charité Hospital in Berlin, where he dominated German surgery for years until the unhappy end to his career when he was overtaken by senility, which he did not recognize, with disastrous results to his patients, necessitating legal action to prevent his continued practice of surgery.

Sherrington, Sir Charles (1857–1952)
Professor of pathology at the University of London, then professor of physiology at the University of Liverpool (1895–1913) and Oxford (1913–35), who investigated almost every aspect of mammalian nervous function over a period of fifty years of experimentation. He was awarded a Nobel Prize in physiology and medicine for his work in 1932.

Shumway, Norman E. (1923–   )
Head of cardiac transplantation team at Stanford University where approximately a third of the entire world's heart transplantations have been performed (see index).

Smith, Homer W. (1895–1962)
Professor of physiology and biophysics at New York University School of Medicine. He was at the core of much research done there during his tenure and as much a philosopher as investigator of kidney function. (*From Fish to Philosopher: The Story of Our Internal Environment*, (1953) (see index).

Snapper, Isidore (1889–1973)
An acknowledged giant in medicine, the Dutch-born Snapper became professor of medicine at the University of Amsterdam at the age of thirty. With the impending invasion of the Netherlands just prior to World War II (1938), he left for Peiping Medical College in China. Captured by the Japanese, he was exchanged for a Japanese general during the war and joined his family in the United States, where he held teaching posts at Mt. Sinai in New York, Cook County Hospital in Chicago, and later at Beth-El Hospital (now Brookdale Medical Center) in Brooklyn. He made both clinical and laboratory contributions in many areas of internal medicine. Part of his manifold gifts may be savored through reading his *Multiple Myeloma* (1953) and *Bedside Medicine* (1960), both of which have appeared in several editions.

Starling, Ernest H. (1866–1927)
Physiologist at the University of London among whose many contributions was an explanation of the basis of fluid exchanges between tissues (the Starling hypothesis) and the development of a heart-lung preparation in dogs that enabled him and other investigators to determine the various factors governing the metabolism and performance of the heart (Starling's "law of the heart") (see index).

Starr, Isaac (1895–)
Philadelphia-based physician and cardiovascular physiologist who has spent almost all his professional life at the University of Pennsylvania. Most noted for his invention in the 1930s of the ballistocardiograph, an apparatus that recorded, noninvasively, the movements of the body that resulted from the beating of the heart (see index).

Sweet, Richard (1901–62)
Prominent Boston surgeon associated with the Massachusetts General Hospital and New England Deaconess Hospital.

Szent-Györgyi, Albert (1893–)
Colorful Hungarian-born biochemist who is most noted for the discovery of vitamin C as the antiscurvy factor as well as of the muscle components necessary for contraction. Awarded Nobel Prize in 1937. Still active in cancer research at the Institute for Muscle Research, Woods Hole, Massachusetts.

Taussig, Helen B. (1898–)
Probably the outstanding woman physician worldwide of this cen-

tury. As a pediatrician at Johns Hopkins, she specialized in cardiology and convinced the surgeon Alfred Blalock to carry out the surgery she devised for alleviating the lack of blood oxygenation resulting from abnormal communications in congenital heart disease. (These patients were commonly referred to as "blue babies.") This connection of systemic artery to pulmonary artery to reroute unoxygenated blood back through the lungs was called the Blalock-Taussig operation and was responsible for keeping thousands of these children alive until open-heart surgery development allowed for full correction of the defects (see index).

Thayer, William S. (1864–1932)
Harvard-educated assistant to Osler at Johns Hopkins, where he remained on staff until the end of his life. He was known for his monographs on malaria and infective endocarditis.

Thomas, Lewis (1913–)
Greatly influential and diversified physician who has held professorships in pediatrics, pathology, and medicine at various institutions. He headed Memorial–Sloan-Kettering Institute for Cancer Research in the 1970s and is author of popular books in medicine and biology, *Lives of a Cell* (1974), *The Medusa and the Snail* (1979), and *The Youngest Science: Notes of a Medicine Watcher* (1982).

Thorn, George W. (1906–)
Harvard endocrinologist who made fundamental contributions to the understanding of adrenal disease. Through his influential administrative positions in Boston at the Peter Bent Brigham Hospital and Harvard he was able to initiate and obtain support for many other worthwhile research projects, one being the construction of the Kolff-Brigham artificial kidney, which became the first widely used model in the United States.

Tidy, Sir Henry (1877–1966)
Consultant physician, St. Thomas's Hospital, London.

Trotter, Sir Wilfred (1872–1939)
English surgeon and sociologist. His surgical career was spent at the University of London, and he was also honorary surgeon to King George V (1928–32). He authored *Instincts of the Herd in War and Peace* (1916), which was at one time widely studied by those interested in prevention of war (see index).

Visscher, Maurice B. (1901–83)
Minnesota-born Dean of American Physiologists, who was one of the last fellows to work with Ernest Starling in England. He also spent time with A. J. Carlson at the University of Chicago before returning to the place of his undergraduate studies, the University of Minnesota, where he was to head the Physiology Department for forty-one years (1936–68) (see index).

Warner, Homer R. (1922–   )
Innovative physician, physiologist, and bioengineering expert who, early on, introduced computer science to medicine, especially with respect to the cardiovascular system. His work has been performed almost exclusively at the Latter-Day Saints Hospital and at the University of Utah in Salt Lake City.

Warren, John Collins (1778–1856)
One of a long line of a family of prominent Boston surgeons dating from the Revolutionary War period. He succeeded his father, John Warren, a founder of Harvard Medical School, as professor of surgery and anatomy and performed the first surgical operation under ether anesthesia (see index).

Waterhouse, Benjamin (1754–1846)
Medical successor to Zabdiel Boylston (see index) in introducing immunization against smallpox to the United States. After visiting Jenner in England, he returned to Boston and vaccinated his own four children and three servants before exposing them, without harm, to smallpox (1801).

Weiss, Soma (1899–1942)
Hungarian-born physician-cardiologist who emigrated to the United States in his youth, joining the Harvard medical faculty in 1925. A brilliant career that led to his appointment as Hersey Professor there was ended by his untimely death at forty-three from a brain tumor, which he, himself, had diagnosed.

Wenckebach, Karel F. (1864–1941)
Dutch-born cardiologist whose major pioneering work in the field was done during his tenure as professor at Groningen and Vienna (see index).

Whipple, George Hoyt (1878–1976)
University of Rochester pathologist who shared the Nobel Prize in

medicine (1934) with Minot and Murphy for demonstrating the effects of diet on anemia (see index).

White, Paul Dudley (1886–1973)
One of the world's best known and beloved cardiologists, Dr. White was based at the Massachusetts General Hospital for virtually the whole of his professional life. His activities as author of an important monograph on heart disease; as a founder of the American Heart Association; and as investigator of, among other subjects, the epidemiology of coronary heart disease, made him well known to the medical world. His public recognition derived from his treatment of President Eisenhower during the latter's myocardial infarction in 1955.

Williams, Robert H. (1909–80)
Hopkins, Harvard, and Vanderbilt-trained endocrinologist whose textbook on the subject became the leader in the field in the United States. Professor and chairman, Department of Medicine, and head of Endocrinology at the University of Washington in Seattle from 1948 until 1963. He was still active at the University of Washington in endocrinology until his death.

Wilson, Frank N. (1890–1952)
Early researcher in various aspects of electrocardiography who applied and extended much of the earlier work of Einthoven (see index).

Wood, Paul H. (1907–62)
Brilliant cardiologist at Postgraduate Medical School at Hammersmith who was responsible for numerous important clinical studies and a textbook, *Diseases of the Heart and Circulation* (1950), that has become recognized as a classic. A great researcher, clinician, and teacher, he was also known for his occasional vitriol.

Wood, W. Barry, Jr. (1910–71)
Hopkins-trained physician-bacteriologist who was chairman, Department of Medicine, at Washington University, St. Louis (1942–55), before returning to Hopkins, where he headed the Microbiology Department from 1959 until his death. His important contributions covered the problems of pneumonia, antibiotics, chemotherapy, phagocytosis, and fever.

Yunis, Edmond (1929–)
Pathologist who collaborated with Dr. Robert Good during the Min-

neapolis years. He is now chief of immunogenetics at the Sidney Farber Cancer Institute and professor of pathology at Harvard in Boston.

Zollinger, Robert M. (1903–)

Professor and chairman emeritus, Department of Surgery, College of Medicine, Ohio State University in Columbus. Although a respected teacher of many generations of surgeons, he is probably best known as one of the two who described the Zollinger-Ellison syndrome (recurrent peptic ulcer disease associated with pancreatic tumors).

ACKNOWLEDGMENTS

Although this book is entitled *Conversations*, a great deal of background material was required in order to place the sixteen contributors in clear and proper historical perspective. Much of this information was derived from the writings of the physicians, themselves, and from my personal files covering the period.

There were other sources within hardcover, however, that were invaluable and to which the reader might wish to refer. The two-volume *Advances in American Medicine: Essays at the Bicentennial,* published by the Josiah Macy, Jr., Foundation and the National Library of Medicine, and John Duffy's *The Healers: The Rise of the Medical Establishment* were of great assistance. In the field of surgery the Wangensteens' *The Rise of Surgery: From Empiric Craft to Scientific Discipline* and the gemlike book on cardiac surgery, *The Scalpel and the Heart,* by Robert G. Richardson are highly recommended. For information on American blacks, Herbert M. Morais's *The History of the Negro in Medicine* was very helpful. A good idea of the changing role of women in medicine may be gleaned from *Women in White* by Geoffrey Marks and William K. Beatty.

For the typing of the major portion of the manuscript I am indebted to the speed and good humor of Mrs. Marilynn Pittman. Mrs. Esther R. Meiboom, librarian at the University of Medicine and Dentistry of New Jersey Library in Newark, was of invaluable assistance in tracking down names, dates, and biographical data.

Many individuals were most generous of their time and effort in assisting in the completion and correction of the manuscript. With the death of Dr. Wangensteen occurring before he was able to review his chapter, Sarah D. Wangensteen and Dr. Clarence Dennis were kind enough to go over this material and provide suggestions for improvement. A similar role was assumed by Lady Carola Pickering following the death of her husband. Of course, without the cooperation of the contributors in conducting the interviews and in subsequent editing of the manuscript there would have been no book, and for their acquiescence I am eternally grateful.

Several colleagues at the New Jersey Medical School were most helpful in reviewing the background material contained in the introductory pages of each chapter as it pertained to their areas of expertise. These included Drs. Norman Lasker, Mary Ann Michelis, Arnold D. Rubin, Benjamin F. Rush, Jr., and Richard P. Wedeen.

Finally, I wish to thank my wife and children for their forbearance during the many long hours when I was incommunicado and Colin Jones, Director of New York University Press, for his unflagging enthusiasm and support for this project.

Allen B. Weisse, M.D.

NAME INDEX

Initial entries in boldface indicate listings in *Biographical Notes* section.

SUBJECT INDEX